BREATHING
FREE

BREATHING FREE

**The Revolutionary 5-Day Program to Heal
Asthma, Emphysema, Bronchitis,
and Other Respiratory Ailments**

TERESA HALE

FOREWORD BY LEO GALLAND, M.D.

Harmony Books
New York

616.2
H164

This book is intended as a guide to people who want to improve and maintain their health. If you are concerned in any way about your health, you should seek medical advice.

Published by Harmony Books, 201 East 50th Street, New York, New York 10022. Member of the Crown Publishing Group.

Originally published in Great Britain by Hodder and Stoughton in 1999.

Random House, Inc. New York, Toronto, London, Sydney, Auckland www.randomhouse.com

HARMONY BOOKS is a registered trademark and Harmony Books colophon is a trademark of Random House, Inc.

Printed in the United States of America

Library of Congress Cataloging-in-Publication Data
Hale, Teresa.
Breathing free : the revolutionary 5 day program to heal asthma, emphysema, bronchitis, and other respiratory ailments / Teresa Hale.
p.   cm.
Includes bibliographical references and index.
1. Respiratory organs—Diseases—Treatment. 2. Breathing exercises. I. Title.
RC731.H34   1999   99-30267
616.2'0046—dc21   CIP

ISBN 0-609-60424-4

10   9   8   7   6   5   4   3   2   1

First American Edition

*To my mother Vee Hale,
my late father William Hale,
and my grandfather Alfred Steel,
who suffered from asthma
and could never breathe freely.*

Contents

CONTENTS

CONTENTS

CONTENTS

Foreword

LEO GALLAND, M.D.,
Director, Foundation for Integrated Medicine

Techniques of breathing are of great importance in many traditional healing systems, especially those of India and China, where healers believed that how you breathe influences your health. Modern Western doctors, in contrast, emphasize the effect of health on breath. If you breathe abnormally, it is because you have a disease. In the December 1998 issue of *The New Republic,* the editor of the prestigious *New England Journal of Medicine* launched a caustic attack on alternative medicine by stating that your health determines how you breathe, but how you breathe has no effect on your state of health. Despite his protestations, there is considerable sicentific evidence that how you breathe impacts on your health. Not only does health affect breath, breath affects health as well.

The main reason for breathing, of course, is to replenish your body's supply of oxygen. If your lungs are healthy, obtaining oxygen from the air is rarely a problem. The complex effects of breathing on health have less to do with oxygen than with *carbon dioxide.* We're taught that carbon dioxide is a waste product, the final result of the burning of fuel in the body, a gas that we expel each time we breathe out. However, carbon dioxide is much more. It is a chemical that regulates the acid-alkaline balance of your blood and of your cells. An excess of carbon dioxide in your blood causes an excess of acidity. A deficiency of carbon dioxide produces a state of excessive alkalinity. Because the main route for eliminating carbon dioxide from your body is the lungs, how you breathe affects the carbon dioxide level in your blood. Severe lung disease produces an excess of carbon dioxide by interfering with its elimination. Far more common are deficiencies of carbon dioxide that result from overbreathing, a condition called "hyperventilation." Hyperventilation may result from anxiety or more commonly from acquired habits of breathing that may be shaped by chronic stress.

The effects of hyperventilation on the body are well-known. The increase in alkalinity of the blood causes both calcium and magnesium in the circulation to become attached to the blood's major protein, albumen. This protein-binding lowers the level of free calcium and magnesium, creating a virtual deficiency of these important minerals. The major consequence is muscle spasm that affects both the voluntary muscles that permit you to move and the involuntary muscles that line the arteries, the intestines and the bronchial tubes. Spasm of the voluntary muscles may produce pain and stiffness. Spasm of the involuntary muscles may cause narrowing of the blood vessels and the bronchial tubes and cramping of the intestines. Narrowing of the blood vessels interferes with blood flow to many parts of your body. It may produce cold hands and feet, chest pains and palpitations, dizziness and difficulty with concentration. Spasm of the bronchial tubes may cause shortness of breath.

These effects of carbon dioxide deficiency are aggravated by another effect of carbon dioxide: its influence on the way in which oxygen is carried by the blood. Oxygen is transported from the lungs to the cells of your body in the red blood cells, where it is bound to hemoglobin, a protein that gives blood its red color. When the blood is excessively acid, hemoglobin gives up its oxygen more readily, making it more accessible to your body's cells. When the blood is excessively alkaline (when there is a deficiency of carbon dioxide, that is), hemoglobin is *less able* to release oxygen to your cells. The result is a relative deficiency of oxygen.

Carbon dioxide deficiency, therefore, can wreak havoc with the normal functioning of your body by preventing calcium, magnesium and oxygen from reaching the cells. These facts are undisputed. There is no controversy about them. Controversy surrounds the questions, How common is this condition? How often does it produce ill health? What role does it play in diseases like asthma, migraine headaches and panic disorder?

In the United States most doctors have believed that hyperventilation only occurs as an acute, dramatic illness that is the result of anxiety and that produces dizziness, breathlessness, numbness and tingling of the mouth and the hands, creating more anxiety. In Europe, on the other hand, researchers have described a state known as *chronic hyperventilation,* in which a person's habitual pattern of breathing causes a chronic deficiency of carbon dioxide and chronic, fluctuating symptoms that may involve any or all of the body's muscles. Chronic hyperventilation may cause dizziness, lightheadedness, fatigue, muscle tension, muscle cramps, intestinal or bladder spasms, palpitations, chest pains, and headache. Strangely enough, chronic hyperventilation also creates a shortness of breath, which leads to more hyperventilation, producing a vicious cycle. The shortness of breath resulting from hyperventilation may have three causes: (1) a decrease in blood flow to certain parts of the brain resulting from spasm of blood vessels in the brain; (2) spasm of the bronchial muscles which narrows the air passages to the lungs; and (3) decreased release of oxygen to the cells of the body, even though the oxygen level in the blood appears normal. There have been different approaches to solving the problems caused by chronic hyperventilation: training in a variety of breathing techniques, breathing into a paper bag so that the carbon dioxide you expel with each breath is breathed back in, vigorous exercise to increase the production of acid in the body, magnesium and/or calcium pills, relaxation and stress management training, and even sedative drugs.

Teresa Hale brings to our attention a revolutionary, modern technique of breath control, developed by the Russian physician Konstantin Buteyko. Buteyko was researching the breathing problems of people with asthma, a disorder that has increased dramatically in the past fifty years. He discovered that people with asthma frequently hyperventilate. This observation was not a surprise. Every emergency room doctor knows that many patients with asthma become more and more short of breath the harder they breathe. For these patients breathing more slowly and less deeply is essential for asthma control. Butekyo, however, reached a profound conclusion from this obervation. He surmised that hyperventilation was the *primary* cause of asthma, that the lungs of asthmatics responded to chronic overbreathing with spasm and swelling of the bronchial tubes. His theory extended the impact of hyperventilation beyond its known ability to cause muscle spasm. He believed that asthma was the body's attempt to compensate for the loss of carbon dioxide by making breathing more difficult. He developed a therapy based upon progressive training in breathing less while doing more. This book describes his theory in detail and provides the reader with comprehensive instructions for learning and utilizing Buteyko's technique. Even if the theory is wrong, the technique itself is valuable and has been shown in controlled clinical research conducted in Europe and Australia to improve the symptoms of people with asthma, to increase their capacity for exercise and to decrease their need for medication.

One important component of the Breath Connection program is that the dramatic improvement made to your respiration will enable you to avoid drugs that artificially dilate the bronchial tubes (bronchodilators). In my recent book, *Power Healing* (Random House, 1988), I warned of the dangers of bronchodilator drugs, which are usually taken as inhaled sprays. When these drugs were first used in the 1940s, the death rate from asthma immediately increased. Research during the 1980s revealed that continuous use of bronchodilators was associated with deteriorating lung function and an increased death rate. Respiratory therapists, who are routinely exposed to bronchodilator mists in the course of their work, develop asthma at a rate four times greater than would be expected *after entering their profession*. The adverse outcome of continuous bronchodilation indicates that bronchial spasm is indeed part of a protective response that bronchodilation prevents. Conventional treatment strategies for asthma are a disaster and the Buteyko program is part of the solution.

For those people who suffer from the other effects of chronic hyperventilation, whether asthma is part of the problem or not, the Buteyko program provides a structured and effective method of breath control, which may be of great benefit, especially when incorporated into a comprehensive approach to health restoration that include sound nutrition, regular physical exercise, effective stress management and the cultivation of a healthy physical and social environment. *Breathing Free* presents a welcome addition to the arsenal of holistic and complementary therapies available in the United States today.

Acknowledgments

Professor Konstantin Buteyko, whose discovery linking our breathing patterns to so many diseases became the inspiration behind this book.

My literary agent, Al Lowman, an asthma/emphysema sufferer whose life was transformed by the Breath Connection Program. It was his vision, dogged persistence, and encouragement that resulted in this book being written.

Chip Gibson, the president and publisher of Crown, whose insight and courage was a vital ingredient in the publication of this book.

The patience and commitment of Doug Pepper, my editor at Crown, was greatly appreciated.

My eternal gratitude to Susan Hill, whose inspired editorial skills enabled the content of this book to be expressed so clearly.

Ralph Morris, Danielle Braender, Bianca Foot, and all the administration team at the Hale Clinic, whose hard work provided me with the time in which I could write *Breathing Free*.

Rodney Paul, who portrayed the Breath Connection exercises so well in diagrammatic form.

Finally, my deepest thanks to Sue Carter, who was able to type the manuscript from my illegible writing, which even I can't read.

Introduction

Asthma kills thousands of people every year. Millions of others are severely debilitated by related respiratory illnesses every day of their lives. And asthma is on the increase—it is now the only disease in the Western world that is increasing in epidemic proportions. Perhaps most frightening, modern medicine practices have done nothing to reduce the number of asthma-related deaths, and we are no closer to a cure than we were forty years ago. Over that time, the number of cases, and the number of deaths, has continued to rise. Doctors have little idea of how to prevent this disease, and its cause has remained one of medicine's modern mysteries.

But there is hope. This book introduces a program that will dramatically reduce the symptoms of all asthmatics and anyone suffering from bronchial disorders within as little as five days. By following the program, you can improve your health without the need for drugs or any of the traditional methods used to treat respiratory conditions. Most important, you will make fundamental changes to the way your body works, and, over time, all kinds of niggling health problems will be addressed.

This program involves learning to breathe. Across time, we have been led to believe that deep breathing is good for

1

us because it increases our oxygen intake. In fact, the reverse is true. The more we breathe, the less oxygen actually reaches the cells of our bodies.

Breath Is Life

Gentle, regular breathing is a reassuring sign of peace and healthy rest. Most of us consider the calm rise and fall of the chest, the soft, steady rhythms of breathing itself, to be evidence of good health. Indeed, the physical act of breathing indicates that we are alive. It's not surprising, therefore, that people find it difficult to understand the concept that breathing shouldn't be an obvious function. When we breathe correctly, our chests do not expand and sink. Healthy breathing is quiet and shallow, and our chests barely move.

We breathe from the moment we are born. When an obstetrician gently slaps a new-born baby's bottom, that baby is encouraged to take his or her first deep lungful of air. The baby's noisy cry of protest as he or she releases that breath is evidence that he or she is alive and well, and there are few parents who don't breathe a deep sigh of relief themselves. But how ironic it is that a baby's first breath should be deep—causing the baby to inhale much more oxygen than his or her tiny body needs and encouraging a damaging pattern of breathing that will be with the child for the rest of his or her life.

This may sound like an unusual concept. If breathing is an involuntary process, how can taking a natural, deep breath be wrong? The answer is quite simple. Breathing is not just involuntary. There are many factors that can cause us to breathe more or less, including stress, panic, emotion and—most important—habit. We can also adjust our rate of breathing, as we do when we hold our breath under water or blow out bursts of air when we exercise.

Most of us breathe incorrectly out of habit, and there are many reasons why this occurs. We are literally trained to overbreathe and have been led to believe that deep breathing is healthy. In times of stress, deliberation, or emotion, we are encouraged to take a deep breath. We have been taught that with every breathing motion we inhale healthy oxygen and exhale a toxic gas called carbon dioxide. Big, deep breaths of fresh air provide us with masses of essential oxygen; exhaling releases the poison. Oxygen is the gas of life, while carbon dioxide is the waste gas.

Therein lies the confusion.

The Carbon Dioxide Myth

Carbon dioxide is not a waste gas. It is one of the most important chemical regulators of the human body, and it is essential for the activity of our hearts, our blood vessels, and our respiratory systems. Carbon dioxide enables oxygen to do its work and, in reality, we need far more carbon dioxide than we do oxygen.

When we overbreathe—that is, breathe more than the physiological norm—we are actually getting less oxygen, not more. This happens because our bodies need to maintain a certain level of carbon dioxide in our blood in order for the red blood cells to release the oxygen we need. When we overbreathe, the balance between carbon dioxide and oxygen in the bloodstream is upset. We may be taking in more oxygen, but we are also breathing out more carbon dioxide, and without the carbon dioxide, our bodies cannot use the oxygen we inhale. We need certain levels of carbon dioxide in our bodies for them to function correctly. When those levels are too low, the chemical bond between oxygen and hemoglobin (which carries oxygen through our blood) increases. In real terms, that means that hemoglobin will not let go of the oxygen it is carrying, which makes it difficult for the cells of our brains, hearts, kidneys, and other organs to get the oxygen they need. As a result, the deeper we breathe, the less oxygen our bodies get.

We now know that all asthmatics overbreathe, and that this rate of overbreathing occurs during asthma attacks. If you stop overbreathing, your asthma will go away. The cause of asthma is hyperventilation, and the way to prevent it is to retrain your breathing.

This book seeks to educate all of us about the way we breathe. It is aimed particularly at asthmatics, parents and carers of asthmatics, and those who suffer from other respiratory conditions. But the fact is that we will all benefit from breathing correctly. We will show that scores of other debilitating conditions, from heart disease to emotional stress, can be relieved and in many cases helped by adopting our new approach to breathing and breath control.

I'm Out of Breath. Out of Breath . . .

It's a common playground cry, as familiar as "It's not fair." But while one child may be panting after competing in and completing a school sports day race or rushing for a catch during a game of football, another child may wheeze and squeeze out the words in desperate pain. For an increasing number of parents, this cry strikes a chord of fear in their hearts. At least one in 10 children in the United Kingdom suffers from asthma, and every week 40 people die from an asthma attack.

It is a tragedy that so many children suffer from asthma and it can be terrible for their parents to watch helplessly as they endure spasms and attacks that could be life-threatening. Asthma reduces quality of life, and whole families can be affected by the needs of one member. Some parents may even feel illogically responsible for the constraints that asthma can place on the lives of their whole family. And despite the fact that asthma is commonly regarded as a childhood affliction, many adults have also been sentenced to a life of fear, one in which a potential attack looms with every deep breath or act of physical exertion.

But it doesn't have to be this way. *I'm out of breath* need never again mean something akin to being out of luck, out of time, or out of funds. Our program is designed to change breathing patterns so that there will never be a need to take great gulps of air after exercise. By retraining breathing and learning correct breath control, gasping for breath becomes unnecessary—for adults, children, asthmatics, and even sports professionals.

Even those of us who find the mildest of exercises—such as walking or carrying home a heavy load from the shops—strenuous will experience an amazing respite from wheezing and heavy breathing. When you have learned to breathe properly and are able to abandon drugs that may have hindered rather than helped you in the past, you will feel better than you could ever have imagined. Your asthmatic child will sleep in peace and grow ever stronger as he or she learns to follow the simple steps that we suggest here.

Healthy breathing should be a birthright, and for many people it is. But for those thousands of people who die each year through asthma and related conditions, breathing became impossible. For the hundreds of thousands of others who have had the quality of their lives destroyed by asthma, breathing is a challenge they face day after day. Most of us don't even think about breathing; asthmatics are forced to think about it constantly.

It's important to remind ourselves that asthma is a killer disease. It is sometimes underestimated or even dismissed because its victims can seem so well most of the time, with no visible bandages, crutches, rashes, temperature, or pain. Yet in the grip of an attack, an asthmatic can feel and indeed be close to death. Such attacks are all the more frightening for the speed at which they occur and their unpredictability.

More and more of us are suffering. Despite, and possibly because of, advances in drug-related treatment, the numbers of sufferers are continuing to soar. Coupled with an outdated and dangerous form of breathing that has become the norm in most Western countries, this epidemic is likely to reach even more frightening proportions.

But we are entering a new age in health care. The god of modern medicine has been proved fallible, and we are, increasingly, looking for alternatives to conventional medical treatment. We are beginning to rely less on a medical system that is overdependent upon drugs and beginning to take some responsibility for our own health. Happily, that means that we are beginning to listen more closely to the messages preserved by older cultures, cultures in which treatment is aimed at uncovering the cause of a condition and actually curing it rather than relying on a barrage of drugs that mask the symptoms and do little at all to effect a cure.

A Drug-Free Life

We do not advocate that all asthmatics should abandon all their drugs and medicines immediately, but we will show here that they can dramatically reduce dosages within five short days. Carefully prescribed steroids may continue to play an essential role in the day-to-day lives of some asthmatics and dosage should only be reduced upon the advice of a general practitioner or a Breath Connection counselor. But for those sufferers who experience milder symptoms, our program will dramatically reduce the need for drugs. And that's not all. Whether you suffer from asthma or a respiratory condition, you will experience better, more peaceful sleep, weight control, emotional balance, professional efficiency, and a sense of well-being that imparts confidence and a renewed zest for life. The threat of other conditions ranging from heart disease to muscular disorders will also be minimized. Even more importantly, you will be given a priceless sense of freedom to live life to the fullest and to reach your individual potential.

Perhaps this sounds too miraculous, too good to be true. Give us five days and we will prove it to you.

Maybe you simply experience occasional panic attacks. If so, you know how debilitating—even terrifying—they can be. Imagine being asthmatic and experiencing the daily dread of something 50 times worse. Imagine attacks that can strike you in professional situations, in public places, or, more frighteningly, at home alone. Panic attacks are close relations of asthma attacks: Both are caused by hyperventilation.

What Is Hyperventilation?

In this book we use the term *hyperventilation* to describe any condition that is caused by overbreathing. *Hyper* means "too much," and *ventilation* refers to lung ventilation, or breathing.

As we discussed earlier, overbreathing, or hyperventilation, starves the body and brain of something it actually needs more than oxygen: carbon dioxide, or CO_2. Carbon dioxide is now known to be essential to every aspect of our good health. Outdated ideas about CO_2's poisonous qualities took root a century ago, around the time when the trees in London's parks were described as the city's lungs. But how would those splendid trees have grown so tall and stood so long without the correct interaction of the carbon dioxide that their trunks and leaves absorbed and the oxygen that was subsequently emitted?

It's time to review old theories and assumptions. Carbon dioxide is now known to be our friend. By breathing more shallowly, lightly, and carefully, we will not lose so much of this essential gas when we exhale. With higher levels of carbon dioxide in our blood, the oxygen will be released more quickly and more steadily from our red blood cells. Whether you suffer from asthma, bronchitis, emphysema, or any other respiratory disorder, you will benefit from correct breathing and your general health will improve dramatically.

Retraining

You may wonder how something as automatic as breathing can be retrained. Isn't the process completely natural? We promise you that the relearning is fast and easy. The deep breathing that many of us were brought up to regard as healthy isn't natural at all. In many parts of the world, people are not taught to breathe deeply, and in those regions the incidence of bronchial disorders is significantly lower than it is here in the West.

Perhaps you are also wondering why reeducating breathing patterns requires a whole book or even attendance at a group session. For most readers, a study of these pages will be sufficient; for others, the benefits of group learning will be more helpful. In either case, it is a matter of positive application, an understanding of the basically sound and scientific principles upon which the Breath Connection program is based, and a little education. A small amount of effort and application will be handsomely rewarded.

Conventional medicine has never really addressed the causes or effects of hyperventilation. Putting it simply, when we hyperventilate, we take in too much air, and we breathe out too much precious carbon dioxide. This means that the body is unable to absorb the small but essential amount of oxygen it needs for all of its interrelated systems to function properly. The Russian professor Konstantin Buteyko discovered that hyperventilation not only causes asthma and other respiratory illnesses, but it lies at the root of nearly 200 other disorders.

We do advise certain dietary changes, and to begin with you will need to concentrate on your breathing exercises for 30 or 40 minutes each day. We also gently recommend that you appraise your general lifestyle, which is ultimately crucial to your overall health and well-being. So, it may take some time and effort over these next days or weeks, but look upon this as the best investment you can possibly make. You'll be investing in yourself—your health and your future. Take a little care, time, and trouble to follow our guidelines and the results and benefits can be immeasurable.

A Revolutionary Approach

The inspiration behind this book and the Breath Connection program of which it forms a part is a distinguished Russian scientist and doctor, Professor Konstantin Buteyko, whose research and work with asthmatics and others with bronchial disorders has only recently been available outside the former Soviet Union. We'll talk more about Professor Buteyko and his pioneering work later in this book and we urge you to study the background of this revolutionary program. Professor Buteyko's discovery is a fascinating one and it is gathering increasing support among both the conventional and complementary health professions.

Here at the Hale Clinic, we have always searched for different approaches—both old and new—to treating the widest range of illnesses and I believe our record speaks for itself. Tried and trusted assumptions about health are never dismissed and we are aware that there is a wealth of advice, gathered across the centuries, that is as applicable today as it was thousands of years ago. We always seek to find complementary solutions to disorders and work in a holistic way with all our patients. Very occasionally, something wonderful and new comes along, such as Professor Buteyko's method—a revolutionary approach to a health problem that challenges one of our most basic instincts: breathing. The Breath Connection program sets out to question the established thinking and to change the way in which we have been taught or trained to breathe. It is an exciting discovery, and the results are unquestionable.

On a personal level, I see the Breath Connection program as one of the most important medical discoveries of the century—and one that will come of age in the next. Although it is our belief that no one system of medicine has all the answers to all the disorders that can strike, we know that Breath Connection has already saved many lives, has transformed the lives of thousands more, and has the potential to help millions.

Just as air cannot be bottled, Breath Connection research cannot be patented. But this is fine with us—we welcome and encourage further research that could do so much for the general health and well-being of millions of people—not just asthmatics. It will be a great day when carefully monitored and assessed collaboration exists—ideally worldwide. For obvious reasons, we cannot expect much encouragement from international pharmaceutical companies who stand to lose from such research, but doubtless they will adapt and we will find our funding elsewhere. Charities could help and so could governments and academic research foundations. Already our work has solicited the supportive interest of some such bodies. It won't happen overnight, but it *will* happen.

Perhaps we are most eager to establish a partnership with the conventional medical establishment. It will be another great day when we work in greater formalized harmony toward the aims of Breath Connection—aims that are, surely, shared by everyone.

Coexistence: Conventional and *Complementary Medicine*

First of all, let me introduce myself. I am Teresa Hale, founder of the Hale Clinic. The clinic was opened in 1988 by the Prince of Wales, whose interest in complementary medicine is well known. My aim was to offer treatments that could integrate conventional and alternative medicine. The strengths of both systems would be called upon to treat patients in a unique setting. Since its inception, the Hale Clinic has explored ideas and treatments from around the globe, and we remain firm in our belief that the most successful kind of health care is one that calls upon the doctrines and methods of a variety of disciplines. No single discipline holds the answer for every patient, and we are able to come up with an individually tailored treatment plan for all types of patients, based on the very best of leading therapeutic systems around the world. As a result, the clinic has become a sort of United Nations for complementary medicine and the fact that we continue to grow suggests that we have simply addressed a need that was waiting to be met. The clinic is based in central London, but we hold courses all over the United Kingdom. We are strong believers in the power of self-help, so no readers should feel disadvantaged if they are not within easy reach of us. We see health as a personal journey for the individual, and it is important to find the right path for each of our patients. With over 100 practitioners offering a broad range of conventional and holistic treatments, we are well placed to meet specific needs.

A few years ago, I was intrigued by the enthusiasm of a fellow professional who had heard about Professor Konstantin Buteyko's extraordinary work with asthmatic patients in the former Soviet Union. There wasn't much to read at that stage, but I was impressed by his results and managed to speak to some people who had taken part in his courses. Their responses ranged from being hugely enthusiastic to positively evangelical. From them and from his preliminary research I learned about his Breath Control methods and resolved to delve further, holding a course at the Hale Clinic based on his work. I was startled by the improvements observed in both the attitude and the health of asthmatics.

It wasn't just the fact that bronchial problems had been dramatically diminished, or even the fact that all of the patients who visited the clinic had either abandoned previous medication entirely or had greatly reduced their need for it. What also caught my attention were the other, unexpected benefits to the treatment. Peoples' appetites had become balanced and stabilized so that even the very overweight were shedding pounds while dangerously underweight patients had recovered an interest in the right kinds of food and were building up strength. Balanced breathing had led to balanced eating. There also seemed to be an awakening of confidence and a general increase in energy as well as relief from distressing sleep patterns and the daytime fears and discomfort that most asthmatics endure.

I was amused to learn that English patients who received treatment with Professor Buteyko's method in Russia had enjoyed little of the cozy bedside manner that we prize so much in Britain. The system had been explained to them, they were told to follow the guidelines and expected to get on with it. Oddly, this brusque attitude rather impressed the English patients who reasoned, correctly, that no clinic attempting to peddle a dubious treatment would treat the patients with so little pampering. I became more and more intrigued, making it my business to learn as much as possible about Buteyko's methods.

I learned that although his findings are now treated with the greatest respect in Russia, this wasn't always the case. For years, his work had been undervalued, and certainly, before the rapprochement between East and West, there was little interest in his work from doctors outside the Soviet Union. Unwittingly, my interest in his work has helped to bring a revolutionary and truly lifesaving technique to the West.

I, too, was full of enthusiasm when I found myself talking about the method to an American journalist, after speaking to a group of businesswomen at a dinner in London. She showed more than a polite interest and suggested that I meet her agent, Al Lowman, when I was next in New York. Al, she said, had such severe asthma that his doctor had recommended a lung operation that would cost in the region of $90,000. When I met him soon afterward, I did not promise that the clinic could cure his asthma but I was pretty sure that we could enable him to reduce his medication, to suffer far fewer attacks, and to walk upstairs or along a corridor without gasping for breath every few steps.

Although by nature skeptical, Al was impressed by my absolute confidence and general approach. Soon afterward, he braved a flight to London—during which he endured a near-fatal asthma attack—to visit us at the clinic and to learn about the incredibly simple shallow-breathing techniques that have spared the lives of thousands of asthmatics and others suffering from related illnesses. Al was adamant that I should write this book. It would have been impossible for him to return to The Hale Clinic for follow-up treatments, and he was well aware that few of the 6,000 Americans who die from asthma every year could do so either. He was right. This book is of real value both to those who suffer as severely as Al does and to the scores of thousands more who have milder but nonetheless distressing symptoms.

I decided to stress how a revised diet and exercise regime can help many people and to point out the importance of educating people to understand the nature of the asthma and its severity. By coincidence, as I was in the early stages of planning this book, there was an outstanding BBC1 TV documentary, produced by Norman Stone, about the effectiveness of Professor Buteyko's techniques. It raised questions about why the established medical profession seemed to be dismissive. This cutting-edge program closely reflected my own interest in the area. A phenomenal 7 million people watched the show and the BBC was inundated with requests for further information about Professor Buteyko's method.

I was more determined than ever to spread the word about the Buteyko principles. It also inspired me to do all I could to ensure that Breath Connection classes and workshops were accessible to people in every major city in the United Kingdom. This book will be the perfect complement to those classes, and if you are, for whatever reason, unable to attend the classes, it will provide the basic grounding you need to understand the principles behind this unique treatment. This book sets out to relieve you, or anyone you care for, from the shackles of asthma and other bronchial or respiratory illnesses for life.

Like me, Norman Stone was alarmed to discover that a killer disease such as asthma had no cure. Conventional medicine addresses the symptoms and eases the suffering, but it does nothing to treat or uncover the root cause. In the program, he featured three seriously ill asthmatics who followed a five-day course. After that short period, all were well on their way to leading normal lives again. People whose lives were seriously restricted were enjoying sport; an anorexic demanded food. Norman Stone also drew attention to the fact that no medical research establishments in Britain were set up to investigate this horrifying disease. This is, perhaps, a sad reflection of our approach to the condition. Despite the fact that it kills thousands each year, asthma is still not receiving the attention that it deserves.

Indeed, despite his landmark successes, Professor Buteyko's ideas were largely ignored if not actually impeded in Russia for nearly 40 years. Better late than never, however, for the millions worldwide who endure this underestimated and almost invisible disorder.

It is extraordinary to think that work begun by a young Russian doctor would result in over 45 years of practical and scientific research into the major causes of over 200 medical conditions currently considered to be incurable by conventional medicine. The simplicity of Buteyko's theories— namely, that asthma is caused by hyperventilation—should not lead anyone to underestimate the depth, extent, and complexity of the scientific research that led to this momentous discovery. His studies are a cause for celebration for anyone who stands to benefit from them.

In the past, Professor Buteyko expressed his hope that freer societies would provide people with the right to choose their medical treatment without constraint. The society in which he lived and practiced did not allow patients the luxury of choice, and his 40-year battle during the pioneering stages of his work led him to the conclusion that people must be able, and encouraged, to choose the treatment system that is right for them and their individual conditions. Most importantly, treatment should be readily available to all who need it. Let us hope that in Britain, the United States, and other Western countries, this vision will become a reality. Bodies such as the National Health Service in the United Kingdom need to recognize the importance of the Breath

Connection program and to make its benefits freely available to every one of the huge population of asthma sufferers.

Our Promises

We promise to utilize everything that modern science, communication, and technology can offer, as well as our own tried and tested methods, to help improve every aspect of the quality of your life. We promise to respect you as an individual and to offer support at every level. These are not shallow or hollow promises. Even if you follow the program for only five days, there has to be effort and commitment on your part—particularly if you decide to keep going for weeks, or even months. It is never easy to break a habit or to learn a new skill, and it's only human to consider lapsing from time to time. We believe that the results that can be achieved by practicing the program for just a short time each day, over five days, will encourage you to keep going. Soon, the Breath Connection program will become second nature, and you will continue to reap the benefits.

In the meantime, here is an introduction for everyone who wants to breathe more easily and to be freed and released from the unnecessary constraints of any one of a host of health conditions. Whether you suffer from antisocial snoring or life-threatening asthma, this book addresses no more than the breath of life—*and no less.*

1

Into the Next Century

Breathing is our first affirmation when we enter the world. Our last breath signals our departure. Death is an experience beyond human understanding, and our ways of approaching it range between calm and panic. Personal spiritual beliefs may well play a major part in the way we see death, but they are far beyond the remit of this book. What we are concerned about is life, and our certain belief that your earthly life can be enhanced long into the next century by the ideas we embrace.

For those of you who are depressed or discouraged by your asthma, or another health condition, it is worth remembering that huge advances have been made in medicine in the twentieth century. So far, we have focused on the fact that asthma is underestimated and that we are no nearer to a cure than we were decades ago. But in all fields, not just medicine, the daily quality of our lives has improved dramatically, and there is no reason to suppose that this exponential improvement in our general comfort and well-being will not continue in this lifetime. Think about the advances and improvements in the quality of our lives and leisure time or the disappearance of such diseases as polio and small pox, which were regarded as common only a few decades ago. Our age has seen the emergence of some new, or newly identified, illnesses, such as AIDS and CJD (Creutzfeldt-Jakob disease), but on the basis of past successes, aren't we right to believe that these can be managed and conquered just as the killer diseases were in the past?

Many of us have grown up in the age of huge scientific advance and may simply take these wonders in our stride. We live in an amazing time, and now, more than ever, we can use the significant scientific discoveries and the wealth of information from around the world for our own personal benefit. We are relearning about our bodies and their miraculous ability to respond to treatment of all kinds.

We should welcome our new century with confidence. We have the benefit of a rich past to call upon, and we can open our eyes to the new discoveries of the future.

Even the most fundamental aspects of our lives are now being given attention. It is, perhaps, surprising that breath and breathing—the most basic and necessary element of our daily lives—have received so little attention. Considering the number of extensive studies undertaken on nutrition and exercise, breathing has been the subject of very little medical research. Firm in the belief that all treatment should be holistic, we at the Hale Clinic believe that research into all of the body's functions and systems is equally important and necessarily interlinked.

Asthma has, until recently, remained a mystery. More cases were reported in the former West Germany, where access to sophisticated medicines and treatment were readily available, than in the less technically advanced and highly polluted East. In Britain, asthma is as common in the cleanest parts of the countryside as it is in London. While pollution may exacerbate the condition in asthmatics, we now know that it is not the cause. This is where the Breath

Connection program has a great deal to offer. After decades of research, Professor Buteyko has finally uncovered the cause of asthma. We still have a great deal to learn about this life-threatening condition, but the Breath Connection program has made extraordinary strides in both the understanding and educational training for asthma. We can offer much more than relief for your respiratory problems. Using a unique preventative health program, we now have the means by which to give our children the basis of sound health for life. And all of us can experience better health as a result of the training offered through the program.

This Is What We Promise

The Breath Connection program requires no medication, no special equipment or technology, and simply aims to reeducate people about how to breathe in a balanced, healthier way. Apart from helping you to overcome a debilitating illness and to enhance your health generally, we hope that this book will encourage further research into the importance and value of carbon dioxide. In Appendix B, we discuss a host of other illnesses that have responded to the Breath Connection program. We hope this book will draw attention to these ailments and inspire more studies and research. All doctors, nurses, physiotherapists, and other hospital professionals need to learn the Breath Connection methods as part of their training. They can be utilized alongside the best of the current conventional and complementary techniques and offer the first real hope of a breakthrough in the treatment of asthma, and a host of other conditions, to date.

An asthmatic who has contracted pneumonia could, for example, be treated with antibiotics in the first instance, and then taught Breath Connection so that his or her immune system is strengthened and the risk of recurring illness lessened. Heart surgery could, for many patients, be avoided if a hospital specialist had worked with a Breath Connection practitioner. I also hope to see many practitioners in the complementary fields—such as acupuncturists, homeopaths, and chiropractors—utilizing the tool to help their patients. As a remedy for common, but nonetheless distressing, conditions such as colds, flu, sinusitis, and sore throats, Breath Connection has a wide range of uses, the first and foremost being an ability to encourage the immune system in a way that antibiotics will never do. The British government has acknowledged the futility of prescribing antibiotics for viral conditions that simply do not respond to them and has urged doctors to be more wary in prescribing them, to prevent a surge of superbugs that are resistant to antibiotics. By using the Breath Connection program, the need for antibiotics is diminished, and because it works to boost immunity, the overall health of the population will improve.

In the business community, I see Breath Connection being used to enhance concentration and performance. Businesspeople in all walks of life would experience greater energy and could function well with less sleep, something that may become an increasing necessity in our competitive world. Good health is essential if we are to cope with stress in the workplace, and Breath Connection offers fast stress relief, quite apart from its other benefits. The additional effects of this would be a reduction in absenteeism, as well as increased alertness and productivity. In the future, employees may be entitled to sue their employers for conditions caused by stress in the workplace, so it makes sense that employers should endeavor to prevent stress before it becomes a serious problem. By supplying basic facilities, such as a quiet room and regular breaks for staff to perform Breath Connection exercises at work, employers would reap the benefits of a healthier, more productive workforce.

Schools also need to consider the implications of the Breath Connection program. It is, in particular, helpful for hyperactive children, as well as those with attention deficit disorders, allergies, and a range of respiratory conditions. Children will have a better ability to focus on the job at hand and will learn more quickly and efficiently. If the exercises are learned at an early age, children will undoubtedly achieve better results at school, as well as experience a dramatic decline in illnesses. If mothers practice breath control while pregnant, more oxygen will reach their babies' bodies and brains, giving them a good start in life.

Adopting the Breath Connection program on a broad scale across nations would have ramifications for everyone. Governments would save vast amounts of money on unnecessary treatments. Premiums for private medical insurance should, logically, be reduced for the same reasons. In the 1998 QED program documenting Professor Buteyko's work, Dr. Gerald Spence said that the annual cost of drugs per annum, for each asthmatic patient, fell by two-thirds once Professor Buteyko's method had been employed. Breath Connection could save Britain's strained National Health Service about £330 million every year. In the United States, where medical care is often dictated by the level of health insurance and health maintenance policies, this is even more significant.

And costs will be reduced for a whole host of other ailments as well. For example, we now know that impotence is largely caused by vascular problems, and Breath Connection is a far cheaper alternative to Viagra. Better circulation, as a result of the program, ensures that blood reaches the penis and both achieves and sustains an erection.

International sportsmen and -women, such as the 1994 Australian football team, have found that Breath Connection enhanced their stamina and performance. The techniques can reduce symptoms of high physical stress, such as headaches, blocked noses and fevers, psychological pressures, and the problems experienced while training and competing in unfamiliar climatic conditions. Performance at the highest level can be enhanced by the athlete's increased ability to cope with pressures of every kind. Even at local park kick-around level, Breath Connection can help to improve performance and increase enjoyment.

Even more crucial for the Western world is the fact that Breath Connection enables people to reach their natural weight. Reconditioned breathing speeds up the metabolism and balances the hormonal system. Carbon dioxide influences the function and performance of the pancreas, which controls our blood sugar, our metabolism, and, through that, our weight. In a relatively short time, the overweight can shed pounds and experience a reduced appetite, while the underweight will begin to eat healthily again. We are not in the beauty business, but there is no question that overweight and underweight can lead to health problems. We want to see a normalization of our patients' weight, and we have observed startling changes in eating habits and weight as a result of the Breath Connection program.

The Will to Be Well

As you can see, Breath Connection offers a simple program to rebalance the whole body and to improve the quality of every area of your lives. The success of the program depends on you, and your willingness to set aside a little time for just a few days. If your problems are more severe, you may need to invest a little more time, but we can promise that you will begin to see encouraging results in as little as five days. You must also resolve to make a few dietary and lifestyle changes if you want the program to fulfill its promise of changing your life for the better—forever.

Each of us has to decide how much we want to make changes—how much regeneration we want to see, and how willing we are to accept degeneration in our bodies. It goes without saying that the majority of us do want to reach our own full potential, but there are some of us—with our own complex psychological reasons, which we will discuss later— who cling to the familiarity and comfort of illness. Nothing worth achieving comes easily, and to achieve the best, you have to be prepared to give your best. Always remember that you are investing in yourself and your future health. While the majority of us may not be ill in the accepted medical sense, chances are that we are not functioning at our full potential. It is often the case that we don't realize that we did feel unwell until we experience the full benefits of optimum health and well-being. Whether or not you have a recognized illness to confront, you can be helped by the Breath Connection program.

I have a term for certain people who seem to be functioning well, with little effort: *the vertically ill*. These people may be standing up straight and coping on a day-to-day level, but beneath the surface, their body systems are working double shifts to keep them that way. The body does not have unlimited resources, and when it is forced to work hard to maintain an equilibrium, there will, eventually, come a time when it is unable to continue. All of us can benefit from Breath Connection, whatever our age or level of health and fitness. In fact, people who do not suffer from an obvious illness will find the program remarkably easy to adopt, and it takes no time at all to get into the habit of practicing the Breath Connection exercises almost anywhere. With the exercises under your belt, and a few dietary and lifestyle changes, you will feel stronger and more energized in every possible way. By achieving your own individual potential, all aspects of your life will be changed: You will sleep better, work more efficiently, look great, and enjoy life more fully. You don't need to spend money on special equipment, gyms, or extra treatments—the improvements will be evident through breathing alone.

A simple Control Pause will tell you if you stand to benefit from Breath Connection. If you can't hold your breath out comfortably for 45 seconds, there is a strong chance that you will experience illness later in life. Don't put something as vital as your health on hold. That back burner may be slow, but it allows things to simmer. . . .

If you do suffer from a life-threatening illness, such as emphysema, you need to ask yourself if you want to be dependent upon drugs for the rest of your life, without any guarantee that they will improve its quality. Or would you prefer to control the illness our way, alleviating its symptoms and allowing you to start participating in your life again. It's up to you. At the very least, you stand to gain a vastly improved stake in the control of your life. In a later chapter, we will show that you don't have to continue down the drugs route and that making changes really is possible.

If you can find the time to spend half an hour leafing through a magazine or polishing the kitchen floor, you can find the time for Breath Connection. Think about your retirement and any money you may be paying into a pension fund. How wasteful it will prove to be if you aren't well enough to enjoy the last third of your life. Think about your children. You want to be healthy enough to watch them grow up, and, even more importantly, you want to watch them do well in life. By investing the time and energy now, your whole family can benefit in the years to come. It's all time that can be clawed back in other forms. For example, the Breath Connection program encourages deeper, more restful sleep, and you'll find that you need far less of it. You can use part of the time you have gained to practice a program that will affect your whole life.

Many of the treatments we now practice, such as herbalism, ayurveda, and acupuncture, are, in fact, based on age-old wisdom. They are now becoming accepted in the conventional medical system and have encouraged a new holistic view of treatment. It is rare when something recent and modern, not involving drugs, comes along. Professor Buteyko's findings are just that—a real breakthrough in the history of medicine based on modern research and a recent discovery. It is my dearest wish that the Buteyko principles will become accepted in the same way that ancient wisdom has experienced a renaissance. We are all working toward the same goal, that of relieving unnecessary pain and suffering, and we need to have the vision to embrace discoveries, both new and old, with equal fervor.

There is a great deal of evidence that the act of helping oneself can encourage positive health, and Professor Buteyko's methods are based on self-help. We live in an age when health is becoming a priority, and more and more of us are taking steps to ensure that we are getting the best, and doing the best we can, for optimum health and well-being. Public demand encourages change. Supermarkets now stock a wide range of organic foods because the public insisted they wanted them. Herbs and homeopathic remedies are available at most pharmacies, when only five years ago they were considered by many to be distinctly alternative. If the same interest and enthusiasm is shown for the Breath Connection program, the demand will encourage the changes we want to see in our health services, and the way we address health in general.

Explain what you want to your doctor. With luck he or she will be sympathetic and helpful. The results speak for themselves, and no doctor can fail to be interested in something that provides genuine relief from ill health of any description. We can only hope that conventional medicine will see the light and begin to offer this treatment alongside, or in place of, drugs. In the meantime, take heart from the guidance we offer here and show, by shining example, that you, as the owner of your body, know best.

The Expansion of Health

We often see the phrase *optimal health* in books and articles. It sounds like a vague term, even if it is a laudable aim. The importance of ginger tea, or broccoli, food combining, special exercises, and even cider vinegar have all been attributed with the power to provide optimal health. So many regimes promise instant perfection, and most of us are, of course, healthily skeptical. There is no such thing as perfection, but what you are aiming for is what is the best for you. *Optimum* or *optimal health* means achieving the best health you possibly can, for you as an individual. We don't promise perfection. We offer a result in five days which acts as a foundation to good health, a springboard from which you can only get better.

The teachers of ancient systems such as acupuncture and

the Indian system of life, ayurveda, considered good health to be an equilibrium within the body. Massages, needles, and herbs were employed to balance energy through meridians or channels that run through our bodies. Yoga, T'ai chi, and Qi Gong programs were adopted to encourage equilibrium, and those same disciplines are used today with equally good results. Breath Connection follows these same principles. We believe that good health can be achieved and maintained through correct breathing. When the body has a correct balance of oxygen and carbon dioxide, the right environment is created for the expansion of our health. You will see how balanced breathing not only prevents disease, but expands our capacity for good health.

In the West, the average life span is 78 years. This may sound like a long time until we consider the longevity of people living in remote enclaves of the Himalayas or the Andes. In these regions, some people are known to live for 120 or even 150 years without enduring ill health or degenerative disease as they grow older. So, the possibility of expanding not only health but life span clearly exists. The long life that is common to these regions is full and pain-free. At Breath Connection, we believe we know how to establish similar patterns that will work here in the West.

We have spent a great deal of time, energy, and financial resources effectively fire fighting. We have lost the knack of preventing the fire in the first place. It can never be repeated too often that prevention is better than cure. Health expansion begins with monitoring your daily progress by checking your pulse and measuring your breathing rate with a daily series of Control Pauses (see page 48). Early improvements in the way you look, feel, and sleep will encourage you to continue with the program until every vital system in your body is primed to last long beyond that 78-year mark.

Reading and understanding the principles that underpin this book are excellent ways to begin your journey on the road to a long, fulfilling life. You will experience improved mental and physical function for as long as you live. As we have stressed earlier, you can achieve a great deal by yourself. With the help of a Breath Connection course or workshop, you can go even further. Classes are now held in cities across the United Kingdom and the United States, and many people find it easier to retrain their breathing under the supervision of one of our counselors. If you think you need extra coaching, try the classes. Or, put your time and energy into learning the methods described in this book for a lifetime of better health. You may wish to extend your life well into your second century, enjoying children, grandchildren, and even great-grandchildren, and for this you may need some extra help. It's a little like playing tennis or any other sport. If you want to enjoy your game, you can do so by practicing on your own and following simple guidelines. However, if you want to get to Wimbledon, or even aspire to being a local champion, you need a first-rate coach and you need to begin work as soon as possible. Whatever your goals, we think you will be startled and delighted by the results you will achieve with Breath Connection. Anyone can embark on this journey of life expansion, and you can improve the quality and depth of your life as well as living much, much longer.

This journey is for everyone, from pregnant mothers wishing to give the best possible start to their unborn babies, to the elderly; from children of all ages to people in their middle ages. Whether you are well or have a history of frailty, you will experience positive change with this program.

Regeneration

As soon as you begin the Breath Connection program, your digestive system starts to function more efficiently. Sluggish metabolisms are given a kick-start, and food is more swiftly converted to energy. Nutrients are more easily absorbed by the body, and toxins are more easily excreted. Food cravings will reduce as the pancreas functions correctly, and the pH balance of your body will be corrected, leading to improved resistance to food allergies and a stronger immune system.

The body's elimination system will also start to function better. This is not merely bowel function, but the pores and sweat glands that are crucial for the excretion of toxins. We need to absorb and extract goodness from food while losing, as quickly as possible, any toxic residues. Much of our food is sprayed with pesticides and fertilizers, and then processed. Our bodies need to take what nutrition our food has to offer, and then excrete the harmful additives and chemicals before damage can take place.

We also need to start thinking about hygiene. Naturally, you wash daily and launder your clothes regularly. Your house may be immaculate, especially your kitchen. You need to apply the same care to your body that you do to your home. If you don't flush out toxic waste from your body, it would be just as damaging, or offensive, as not flushing your toilet for several days, or allowing old food to molder in a filthy refrigerator. Give your liver, kidneys, and bowels a helping hand by breathing correctly so that they function well.

To ensure that your heart is strong enough to take you through a long life, you need to look after your cardiovascular system. With Breath Connection, circulation will improve, and the danger of high blood pressure, palpitations, and any form of collapse will be reduced. Respect the complex network of your hormonal system. It's not just the thyroid gland that ensures the healthy working of your endocrine system. The pineal gland, the pituitary, and the thymus are all connected and important. They in turn affect the pancreas, itself an important endocrine gland, which affects other parts of the body. Breath Connection is holistic, which means that it is aimed at treating all of you, not just one single part.

The nervous system also needs to be well-tuned to cope with the inevitable pressures of life. Good health and strength can make any pressure easier to bear, but when all systems are working at their peak level, problems are more quickly and efficiently dealt with. We can't promise you a life without anxiety or stress, but we can promise you a better way of dealing with the challenges. Once you are eating properly, breathing correctly, and sleeping well, you are far better placed to cope. Extra blood reaching the brain through correct breathing will make it easier to concentrate upon and solve intellectual dilemmas and to deal with emotional ones as well. The calm and peaceful sleep that you will experience increases this effect.

Perhaps you don't want to live until you are 120; perhaps your aim is to experience good health and well-being in the here and now. The process can begin at any age. We want to help you to empower yourself.

It begins with a simple, single breath.

2

Overbreathing

*And what it is to cease breathing but to free the breath
from its restless tides, that it may rise and expand and seek
God unencumbered?*

Kahlil Gibran, *The Prophet*

What does the word *hyperventilation* mean to you? For some, it may mean rapid, shallow gasps and for others fast, deep gulps. Almost everyone will conjure up a picture of someone panting, red-faced and distressed, possibly after overstrenuous exercise or during an asthma attack. Medical dictionaries usually define it as "abnormally rapid deep breathing."

By Professor Buteyko's definition, *hyperventilation* is what happens when someone habitually breathes more than four to six liters of air into their lungs every minute. This quantity of air is the correct amount for all adults and children—but obviously varies between three and six liters depending on whether you are a child or a large man—and leads to very quiet, gentle, and almost undetectable breathing, rather like that of a sleeping baby. Nine out of 10 of us, however, overbreathe. We have become so accustomed to breathing deeply that we regularly lose vital carbon dioxide when we exhale.

Try the Control Pause test on page 48. This simple test is designed to assess your risk of suffering from hyperventilation-related diseases.

Studies have shown that asthmatics inhale anything between four and eight times the amount of air they need for optimum health, often breathing through the mouth, rather than the nose. This type of overbreathing, or hyperventilation, puts tremendous strain on our body systems, such as the digestive, hormonal, circulation, cardiovascular, and elimination systems. This dysfunctional breathing can be corrected by the Breath Connection program.

Deep Breathing Test

This quick test will help to show you how harmful deep breathing can be. Do not try it if you are a severe asthmatic or epileptic.

Breathe rapidly through your mouth, as if you have been taking part in a fast run. Try to maintain this for several minutes. Have a pencil and paper on hand and make a note of how quickly you experience any of the following symptoms:

- Dizziness
- Chest pains
- Palpitations
- Blocked nose
- Coughing
- Feeling faint
- Headache

These effects will have occurred because your physiological systems have been starved of carbon dioxide.

Now begin to breathe slowly and shallowly through your nose. We call this type of breathing *balanced breathing*, in which the equilibrium between levels of oxygen and carbon dioxide in the respiratory system is maintained. See how quickly the symptoms of overbreathing are reversed.

We should stress that our definitions of deep and shallow breathing relate to the amount of air that is inhaled and we're often asked to explain why in many yogic exercises people are, conversely, encouraged to take deep breaths. It's not actually so very different. When practicing yoga, you are encouraged to breathe very slowly, and through the nose. You do not hyperventilate because the amount of air you take in is restricted. Other techniques, such as rebirthing,

Yogic breathing

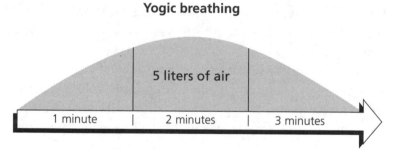

5 liters of air breathed over 3 minutes.

Asthmatic breathing

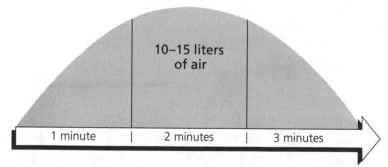

10–15 liters of air breathed over 3 minutes.

encourage shallow, rapid breathing, called *panting*. We do not feel that this is a healthy way to breathe.

Why Orthodox Modern Medicine Can't Cure Asthma and Emphysema

Every idea in this book is underpinned by the strongest belief in a holistic approach to health. All of our advice must be considered alongside diet, sleeping, and exercise habits—your lifestyle in general. These are all important aspects of your health, and addressing only one tiny part will not have the same effect as broadscale measures that take into consideration all of the factors that make you and your lifestyle individual. In later chapters, we address other essential aspects of our holistic approach. Here, however, we offer some very specific information and answers to what has been one of the most crucial health challenges of our age.

Asthma and emphysema are defense mechanisms against hyperventilation, created by the body to counter a loss of carbon dioxide. This mechanism induces spasms of the bronchotubes, creating inflammation and excess mucus or a reduced lung capacity. Any attempt to treat asthma or emphysema without dealing with hyperventilation as the underlying cause is doomed to fail. Dealing with hyperventilation, or overbreathing, is the central tenet of the Breath Connection program.

Many therapies and some drugs, including the use of nebulizers, can provide some temporary relief, but artificially suppressing what is actually the body's natural defense mechanism will further increase hyperventilation and cause the body to implement some other line of defense. By suppressing your asthma, you could develop emphysema, pulmonary fibrosis, heart disease, diabetes, epilepsy, or cancer in its place because your body still has to find some means of preventing you from hyperventilating and expelling too much carbon dioxide. Further, the more often you resort to using a bronchodilator or taking steroids, the more you will come to depend on them. Asthma is not cured by modern medical treatments, its symptoms are merely suppressed. The cause still remains and if we continually ignore our body's message that something is wrong, the condition will become much, much worse.

Many asthmatics start with the occasional puff on an inhaler for quick relief, but soon depend on a battery of nebulizers and steroids. Some may need hospital treatment. The reason for this dependency and the overall degeneration of the condition is solely because doctors have been treating symptoms rather than the disease itself.

The conventional treatment for asthma and emphysema is drugs or physiotherapy—both of which actually cause hyperventilation. This is akin to treating an alcoholic with vodka or a diabetic with sugar. This practice is not to be confused with the considered homeopathic principle of treating like with like.

The Respiratory System

The Lungs
The right lung has three lobes and the left two, each comprising numerous lobules bound by connective tissue. Within each of them is a group of air chambers bearing small pouches called *alveoli*.

During inhalation, air passes through the windpipe into the main airways attached to each lung. The oxygen in the air dissolves into the alveoli and is diffused through these cells and through capillary walls into blood plasma. From the plasma, the oxygen molecules combine with hemoglobin in the red blood cells to form oxyhemoglobin. This process allows the blood to carry approximately 70 times more oxygen than it would normally. Once this blood reaches the body cells where oxygen in required, its oxygen load is released. The trigger for this release is carbon dioxide which, converted to carbonic acid, allows it to be freed. When there is insufficient CO_2 due to overbreathing, the amount of oxygen available to the brain, heart, kidneys, and every other organ in the body is restricted. As a result, essential functions are impaired. Oxygen starvation excites the breathing center of the brain and thus the desire to hyperventilate increases.

Oxygen and carbon dioxide are, thus, partners and not enemies within our system. Carbon dioxide also regulates the body's acid/alkaline balance (also called pH), which is essential for a healthy immune system.

Asthma attack

| Normal breathing | Asthmatic's breathing |

Bronchotubes open
Normal level of CO_2 and O_2

Broncho restriction
Less than normal level of
CO_2 and O_2

The illustration on page 37 is a simplified representation of what happens to the bronchotubes during an asthma attack. The fairly straight line (*top left*) represents shallow breathing, or normal breathing. Both oxygen and carbon dioxide can move through the clear bronchotubes. To the right you can see the jerky depths and peaks of asthmatic breathing and the bronchial restriction caused by inhaling and exhaling too deeply. The asthmatic is losing too much CO_2 so the bronchotubes have narrowed as the body fights to retain the carbon dioxide which is essential for so many of its functions.

The Causes of Overbreathing and Hyperventilation

Even before we are born we may be affected by the deep-breathing exercises that our pregnant mothers followed so trustingly. Then we were probably encouraged to announce our safe arrival with an outraged scream followed by a deep breath. Later, at school and beyond, we were encouraged to take deep breaths if we felt faint, giddy, or exhausted after strenuous exercise.

Apart from being taught to deep breathe, we have also created a scenario where our oxygen needs are higher, which encourages us instinctively to overbreathe, or to breathe more deeply in a misguided attempt to satisfy our oxygen needs.

Take, for example, our eating habits. A high-protein diet—until quite recently regarded as healthy and desirable—places severe strain on many of our bodies' systems and creates a pattern of overbreathing. The amount of oxygen energy needed to digest a protein meal, whether it is made up of vegetable or animal proteins, is similar to the amount needed for a brisk walk. More information about diet and nutrition follows in a later section of this book where we describe the foods that will help you not to overbreathe.

Sleeping correctly is enormously important, and very little advice has been given about the correct way to sleep. Many of us have a tendency to sleep on our backs, which causes breathing to deepen. Sleeping with our mouths open compounds the problem. Most epileptic fits, strokes, and paralysis happen at the end of a long sleeping period when the sleeper is about to waken. It is no coincidence that these occur after a long period of deep breathing.

Meditation and controlled relaxation encourage shallow breathing. Stress and emotional pressure tends to make breathing heavier. Try to avoid stressful situations and emotional confrontations late at night, which can cause breathing to deepen. Restful, peaceful sleep relies on calm, shallow breathing. Overheated, polluted, and confined spaces at night should also be avoided. Arrange your pillows to the left side to help prop you into a correct position (see pages 52–53). Your breathing will be shallower throughout the night as a result. Even Professor Buteyko has no scientific explanation for this phenomenon, but he has observed, in thousands of cases, that it works.

One technique we recommend is to tape your mouth up at night, thus ensuring that you breathe through your nose. This can be particularly effective for children (see Chapter 10) and is not as drastic as it may sound. There is a special tape that is light and painless to remove and apply. We suggest you use this tape until you have learned to breathe through your nose.

If we ensure that we get plenty of carbon dioxide at night, hyperventilation, anxiety, insomnia, and, quite possibly, irritability, stress, and panic attacks will decrease.

The Link Between Carbon Dioxide Starvation and Disease

By now we know about the importance of the natural collaboration between oxygen and carbon dioxide and how their partnership helps our bodies to function at full strength every day. And we know that hyperventilation deprives us of the benefits of that partnership. What follows is a short list of some of the many roles carbon dioxide plays in helping us to maintain a healthy, balanced body:

- Oxygenation of vital tissues and organs.
- Maintenance of the acid-alkali (pH) balance necessary for a strong, healthy immune system, without which we are prone to allergies and recurrent infection.
- Smooth muscle dilation, which helps to prevent the sort of spasms which lead to migraine as well as asthma attacks. Such spasms also narrow the arterial vessels, causing varicose veins and hemorrhoids. A spasm is the body's way of preventing the loss of too much CO_2 and is yet another example of the body's defense mechanism against over-breathing.
- Regulation of nervous system activity which prevents the body from going into an unnecessary "fight or flight" mode that can exacerbate stress levels.
- Regulation of a healthy cardiovascular system without which we can suffer from abnormal blood pressure, hypertension, angina, chest pains, and strokes.
- Maintenance of a healthy digestive system, particularly the level of gastric juices needed for efficient breakdown of ingested foods.
- The natural elimination of toxic substances.

As you can see, the Breath Connection program is not only for asthmatics or people suffering from respiratory problems. Dealing with the devil of hyperventilation provides massive benefits for everyone. Oxygen is not the only gas of life. We need carbon dioxide, too. We need to change a previously unchallenged way of thinking and accept that the demon is not a toxic gas, but a way of breathing.

At The Hale Clinic, we are convinced that, despite extraordinary success with our program for those with asthma and other related disorders, the crucially important role of carbon dioxide in holistic health has only just begun to be explored.

These are the facts about hyperventilation, which could remain an invisible killer well into the twenty-first century:

• Up to 90 percent of people in the developed world suffer from illnesses caused by hyperventilation.

• The root cause of so many of these illnesses—ranging from asthma to chronic fatigue—is not yet recognized by orthodox medicine as being hyperventilation. Conventional medicine can greatly alleviate symptoms of these and other illnesses, but it has been unable to reach any firm conclusions about the causes.

• Doctors don't study hyperventilation at medical school and are, therefore, unaware of its very real dangers.

• Most doctors are unable to recognize, diagnose, or treat hyperventilation except in its most acute form.

• Even those few doctors who treat hyperventilation do not do so very effectively.

• Modern medicine uses drugs and deep-breathing exercises to treat hyperventilation, treatments which may relieve symptoms in the short term, but which aggravate the condition in the long term.

• Modern medical theory has not established, nor attempted to establish, the link between hyperventilation and respiratory diseases. Asthma and other respiratory diseases are blamed on a host of unrelated causes and triggers, including the environment, stress, smoking, cats, dogs, cut grass, red wine, butter, salt, sugar, cholesterol, calories, *Candida,* the weather, flu, colds, and dust mites. Some of these may indeed be triggers for some people, but they are not the cause of asthma or any other respiratory disease. Blaming these triggers for asthma is akin to blaming rats for the Black Death plague of the fourteenth century. Certainly the rats transported the bacilli that spread the plague but they didn't create the plague or the disease itself.

• The common ignorance of the physiology of breathing has lead to a situation where the killer phrase *take a deep breath* has become the most popular—and dangerous—advice offered in stress management. This advice is offered to combat panic attacks, anxiety, asthma, and emphysema within fitness classes, schools, hospitals, and sporting establishments.

• More and more people, including—tragically—children, breathe through their mouths. Yet doctors and teachers rarely offer advice against this fast track to hyperventilation. A general national awareness of the importance of breathing through our noses would make a massive difference to public health. Most asthmatics and emphysemics have been advised to deep breathe, little realizing this will deprive them of oxygen rather than supply it.

• Pregnant mothers are taught to deep breathe during labor. If a woman hyperventilates during pregnancy there is a danger that her child will be affected by her hyperventilation habits while it is in the womb and certainly when it is born.

• Various deep-breathing techniques and exercises, including lessons in breathing from the diaphragm, rebirthing, some Yoga exercises, blowing balloons, blowing out candles, peak flow meters, coughing techniques, voice therapy, and many others encourage us to breathe more deeply. Some of these examples may seem to be innocuous occurrences in our daily life, but they set us on a dangerous course.

• Doctors, in the main, are not yet aware that breathing, like other physiological functions, has a normal functioning state, so they rarely check or treat it. They should examine this aspect of their patients every bit as carefully as they check pulse or blood pressure, temperature, or cholesterol level.

Every one of these points suggests that our knowledge of breathing, respiration, and its link to illness remains dangerously insufficient. It's clear that unless something dramatic is done to change the way we think, and the way we breathe, hyperventilation will remain a killer for the next generations. And, the many diseases and health conditions caused or exacerbated by hyperventilation will continue to plague the population.

But it's not all gloom and doom. For those of us who have already experienced or witnessed the extraordinary effects of Breath Connection, there is help at hand. We may be a small minority of the population at present, but word is spreading, and this program is set to change the way we view illness forever.

There are, already, hundreds of people whose lives have been radically and triumphantly changed by the growing new awareness of the dangers of hyperventilation. This is John's story:

JOHN

People tend to associate ME (myalgic encephalomyelitis) or chronic fatigue syndrome with women, but men can be vulnerable, too. John, a university student, enjoyed various sports in his leisure time and was reasonably fit. He drank socially and didn't smoke, but he had a tendency to regular colds and flu, and he took medicines for this, occasionally using a nasal spray at night.

After one particularly nasty bout of flu, he remained weak, giddy, and generally unwell for weeks. His doctor prescribed antibiotics and vitamin supplements but after further weeks of illness, further drugs, and further assurances from his GP that all would be well soon, he despaired. After months of the same debilitating symptoms, he was finally diagnosed as suffering from ME. By that time he was sleeping for up to 14 hours a day, had dropped out of his course, lost contact with most of his friends, and spent most of his few waking hours in bed. He had no strength to leave his bedroom, let alone even consider resuming his old lifestyle. John also found it difficult to read or concentrate and became both so angry with his doctor and depressed at life in general that he seriously considered suicide.

He soon began to have difficulty breathing—and it was this final symptom that saved him. John's mother saw an advertisement for a Breath Connection workshop and somehow John found the energy and motivation to attend. The first time he attended his Control Pause (CP) was a frightening 8 seconds. He was weak and pale after six months indoors, and his symptoms were as crippling as ever. Yet, after the second day, he began sleeping for only eight or nine hours a night and his muscular pains lessened. After a week, with his CP improving all the time, he began to go out walking and shopping. Less than two months later, John had resumed his studies and three months later was back playing basketball, his CP a very sound 45.

We'll be giving you lots of inspiring examples like John's story throughout our book, and they may just be the impetus you need to make changes that will affect the rest of your life.

Points to Remember

• Most people are inhaling more air than their bodies need. This has an adverse affect on the delicate balance between carbon dioxide and oxygen levels, triggering the compensatory defense mechanisms which we call *disease*. More than 200 disorders can be reversed or eased with correct breathing (the most common of which are listed in Appendix B).

• Your body needs a precise level of carbon dioxide for oxygen to reach its vital tissues and organs.

• Carbon dioxide was once considered to be a waste gas and a poison to the body. Professor Buteyko's discoveries herald a new appreciation of the important, indeed vital, role that it plays in health. The key to optimum well-being is the natural balance between oxygen and carbon dioxide.

• Much of the advice offered by medical experts, physiotherapists, sports trainers, and even some complementary therapists to breathe deeply has been based on scientific misunderstandings that have only been challenged relatively recently. Don't imagine the old rules are all still valid.

• Our CP (Control Pause) test can indicate if you are hyperventilating, whether or not you know it.

• The Breath Connection program exercises have been responsible for a 90 percent improvement in the condition of people with asthma and have contributed toward further dramatic improvement in the condition of people suffering from other illnesses.

3

Breath Connection Basics

Before we go on to discuss the exercises for individual health conditions, it is important that the basic Breath Connection techniques are clearly understood. The exercises that form the basis of the program are easy to understand and to implement, and within five days you will see outstanding benefits. The exercises can be adapted according to your individual needs, and with the help of a Breath Connection counselor, you can come up with the ideal formula for you. If you plan to practice the exercises from home, there are a few safety notes to consider. We'll discuss these alongside the basic exercises that form the treatment.

The most important part of the program is the Control Pause. It is both a test, a monitor, and a tool for controlling your breathing. Here's how it's done.

The Control Pause

Four to six liters of air per minute are all you need to supply your blood with oxygen. More than that, particularly if you are breathing deeply or erratically, can destabilize the central nervous, cardiovascular, immune, hormonal, excretory, and digestive systems. It can also lead to general fatigue and sleeping problems. It is very easy to breath more air per minute without seeming to be overbreathing, and most of us do it. As a result we are all, unknowingly, damaging our health on a regular basis.

To discover if you are unconsciously hyperventilating, try the Control Pause (CP) test. This simple exercise is central to the Breath Connection program.

1. Sit comfortably in an upright chair close to a clock with a second hand, or hold a stopwatch.
2. Relax and breathe in and out gently, mouth closed.
3. Pinch your nose with your fingers, after the exhalation.
4. Keeping your mouth closed, count how many seconds you can comfortably last before you need to inhale again.
5. Don't push yourself too hard. The accuracy of the test depends on you stopping before you reach the threshold of discomfort.
6. Remember: you are not holding your breath in, you are emptying your lungs and then counting.
7. When you breathe in again, try not to take in large gulps of air, control your breathing, keep your mouth closed.
8. Do *not* push your Control Pause above 60. This can only be done under the guidance of a Breath Connection Practitioner. These breathing exercises, like medication, must be administered correctly.

• A control pause of 50 to 60 seconds or more suggests that you are in excellent health. Holding for 25 seconds means that your health requires attention.
• If you can only manage 10 seconds or less, a serious

hyperventilation problem exists. This might already have manifested itself as asthma or some other illness.

• Anyone with a control pause of less than 30 seconds needs to follow the exercises outlined in this book. The exercises are necessary for your general health and well-being and will help to prevent the creation of a fertile environment for more than 200 different health disorders (see page 253 for a list of the most common ones).

Take 60 as the ideal Control Pause. Now divide that number by your own CP. The answer tells you how many people you are breathing for—or, more importantly, how severely you are threatening your health. If your CP is 20, divide that number into 60. The answer is 3, which means that you are, effectively, breathing 3 times as often as you should be, or breathing for 3 people.

If you have ever suffered from any sort of respiratory disorder, you may feel daunted at the prospect of modifying the way you breathe—tampering with something that seems absolutely natural. We promise you that it isn't difficult and it certainly isn't dangerous. In many societies, past and present, breathing is naturally shallow normally, that is, shallow in terms of how much air is taken in. People in such societies have never been taught to breathe deeply, and so did not develop bad breathing habits such as breathing through the mouth. Everyone breathes in a much healthier way. We should not assume that our norm is what is right for us, particularly in light of the fact that we are, in the West, decidedly less healthy than our Eastern neighbors.

Try to see correct breathing as a form of nutrition. Just imagine how much harm you would be doing to yourself if you were eating for two, three, four, or more people.

You must always interrupt your CP test if you feel at all uncomfortable. Shallow breathe for a few minutes and start again without pushing yourself. Never forget that our exercises are as powerful and effective as some conventional medicines, so please follow the instructions carefully and never push yourself to get a higher Control Pause.

Shallow Breathing

Shallow breathing is the opposite of deep breathing. It involves taking in small quantities of air. The best way to achieve shallow breathing is to be aware of your breathing and to consciously regulate the flow in and out of the nose. Nasal breathing is the key to correct breathing. When we breathe through our mouths, we take in too much oxygen and breathe out too much carbon dioxide, which upsets the balance of these essential gases in our bodies.

It has been established that people with breathing disorders, such as asthma, often have nasal problems, too, such as sinusitis, rhinitis, or polyps. Most nasal problems—such as asthma—are one of the body's defense mechanisms against overbreathing. Breath Connection can teach you to get rid of nasal problems, and you will also learn how to get rid of asthma, which is another facet of the same problem.

After two or three days of practicing Breath Connection, your nasal passages will open up—and stay open—if you continue to breathe correctly.

Unblocking Your Nose

It may seem impossible to consider shallow breathing, or breathing through your nose, if you have chronically blocked nasal passages. We have a quick-fix method for unblocking your nose, which will provide relief for a few minutes, or even hours. Once you have practiced Breath Connection for a couple of days, your nose will stay clear, and this exercise will be unnecessary. This is what you do:

- Breathe in and out normally.
- Pinch your nose with two fingers after the exhalation.
- When you can no longer comfortably hold your breath out, let go of your nose, but keep your mouth closed and carry on breathing through your nose, which will now be open.

Try to move around while pinching your nose—the added movement will increase the carbon dioxide levels in your blood even further, and we know that carbon dioxide is a natural bronchodilator.

Taping

It can be difficult to remember to breathe through your nose, which is why we recommend taping. It's not as draconian as it sounds! We recommend a special type of tape, 3M micropore mouth tape, which is available from pharmacists and hardware shops. This tape can be applied and removed easily and painlessly, and because it has tiny pores, or holes, you will not feel completely suffocated. We suggest that you tape your mouth with a small piece of tape, placed vertically over the lips, while you learn the techniques and throughout the program. Obviously, this may not be appropriate if you are in an office or out and about throughout the day, but it should certainly be undertaken while you are at home, whenever you are alone, and definitely while sleeping. Children in particular need to be reminded to breathe through their noses, and this is an easy way to set a good habit in place. If your child or children are resistant, perhaps all members of the family can take part, so he or she will feel more involved. Taping is not essential, but it definitely improves your progress.

Sleeping Techniques

Asthma becomes worse at night and in the early hours of the morning because the horizontal position of your body during sleep increases hyperventilation. Professor Buteyko believes that this is because the natural position of our bodies is upright. Lying flat on our backs is not the optimum position for our breathing to function normally.

When we sleep, our breathing starts out being low and shallow. However, as we slip into deeper sleep, our breathing becomes deeper and deeper. When we are lying down, our breathing increases, so that our levels of carbon dioxide go down. So, how should we sleep?

The more upright you are, the better. Sitting up is the ideal position, but we accept that it isn't very comfortable— or practical. However, if your asthma symptoms are very bad, you might want to consider it. The next best option is to position yourself on a high pile of pillows, which should rest under your head and shoulders.

Always sleep on your left side, with your legs pulled up to your chest. This fetal position has been proved to be the most effective position for sleeping, although the reason is unclear. If you find it uncomfortable, switch to your right-hand side, which is, ultimately, much better than sleeping on your back. Lying on your back and breathing through your mouth is the worst possible way you can sleep. According to Professor Buteyko, children should sleep on their tummies.

Professor Buteyko recommends sleeping on a hard bed, such as a futon, or one with a thin mattress, and suggests that we should aim to reduce our time sleeping by as much as possible. The less you can sleep, the better. Here are some other tips for getting a good night's sleep:

- Don't go to bed until you are so tired that you cannot do anything else but sleep.
- Don't go to bed just because it is bedtime. Wait until you are genuinely tired before retiring for the night.
- Don't go to bed during the day. If you have had a sleepless night, take a 20- to 30-minute nap, sitting in a chair.
- Make sure your mouth is closed while you sleep and tape your lips to ensure that it stays this way. Breathing through your nose at night can reduce phlegm, prevent snoring, and provide a much more refreshing sleep. Most importantly, however, it can prevent asthma attacks.

Professor Buteyko noted that Native American women used their fingers to ensure that the mouths of their children were closed when they slept, until the children developed the habit of breathing through their noses. Doctors of the time noted that these children were often healthier than their Colonial contemporaries.

Taking Your Pulse

Before and after Breath Connection exercises you will take your pulse. Your pulse is a sure measure of the state of your health, and it's important that you learn how to measure it. Sit quietly for a few seconds before following these steps.

A pulse means that blood is circulating in the body. Check for a pulse:

- On the thumb side of the wrist, about 1.5 cm above the wrist crease and about 1.5 cm in from the side of the wrist.
- At the carotid artery in the neck, which runs up either side of the back of the Adam's apple. You'll find the

Taking your pulse

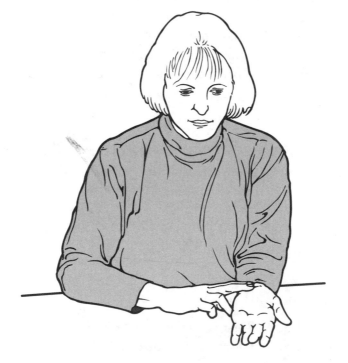

pulse in the hollow between the Adam's apple and the neck muscle.

1. Check for a pulse by pressing two fingers on either of the pulse points (not both). Never use your thumb to take a pulse since it has a pulse of its own.
2. If you do not feel something immediately, press a little deeper and move your fingers around gently to find the pulse point.

In general, 70 beats per minute indicates that your health is good. Up to 80 it is probably fair, but 100 is too high. There are very few people whose health is fine, even if they have a high pulse rate and body temperature, but don't take the risk that you may be one of them. When you normalize your breathing, your whole system becomes more efficient and less stressed—and so normalizes the heartbeat. Checking your pulse rate before and after doing the Control Pause exercises will demonstrate how breathing correctly has a direct bearing on circulation. As your CP goes up, your pulse rate will come down. You will be checking your pulse regularly to ensure that this happens. It is a very good way to gauge the effect of the exercises.

The Exercises

The Breath Connection program is made up of a series of exercises in which you learn to control your breathing. The exercises are suggested according to the severity of your symptoms, the condition from which you might be suffering, and what you hope to achieve from the program. In general, the exercises involve the Control Pause, which is used both to monitor your condition and to help control your breathing, shallow breathing techniques, and, at various stages, taking your pulse.

The program also involves learning to breathe through your nose and making adjustments to your day-to-day breathing techniques in order to learn normal breathing. In Breath Connection, you are taught to breathe less air, which is considered to be normal breathing. Abnormal breathing is the cause of many diseases; normal breathing, the Breath Connection way, will both improve your health and well-being. You'll start to see changes after only a few days. Now, let's begin.

4

Breath Connection for Adults with Asthma

Every asthmatic is an individual and no one series of steps will work for everyone. In this chapter, we look at the special needs of adult asthmatics and emphysemics, whether your levels of distress are high or relatively low. Later on, we look at the different problems that children and their caregivers face and the separate needs of those whose lives are blighted by related disorders.

Here, we address the appalling symptoms experienced during an asthma attack. Sufferers will be more than familiar with that terrifyingly severe shortness of breath, the pain, the panic, and the fear that you are going to die. An asthma attack can also be frightening to witness, but unless you are a sufferer there can be little understanding of the severity of the problem, and the overwhelming dread and fear that it produces.

When a person is breathing normally, the bronchotubes are open and there is no asthma. If we begin to overbreathe/hyperventilate and start exhaling too much carbon dioxide, the bronchotubes narrow in order to prevent the body from losing so much carbon dioxide. In an asthma attack, a bronchospasm occurs, and the hyperventilation can become even more pronounced. After using a reliever, the bronchotubes

A vicious cycle in asthma

1

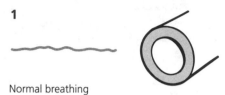

Normal breathing
Bronchotubes are open—no asthma

2

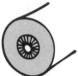

Asthmatic's breathing
Bronchotubes are narrowed (hyperventilation)

3

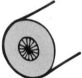

During asthma attack
Bronchospasm—hyperventilation is even greater

4

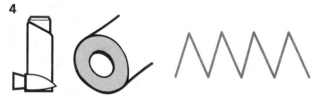

After use of reliever
Bronchotubes are open but hyperventilation is even worse

5

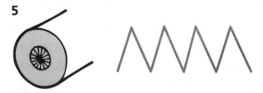

New bronchospasm and the need to use reliever again

are opened, the asthma symptoms are relieved, but the underlying problem of hyperventilation is even worse. A new bronchospasm forms and the asthmatic needs to use the reliever again. The vicious cycle is complete.

But, this cycle can be broken, and in a few short days you can experience huge relief. In this chapter, we provide invaluable advice on self-care for adult asthmatics. If you don't suffer from a respiratory illness, turn to Chapter 9, where we provide tips on Breath Connection for general health.

We begin with a word about the drugs and medication that you may well have relied upon for some time. Understanding them and correct usage is essential to your recovery.

Drugs and Medication

Some drugs, judiciously used, are helpful. Taken in partnership with the Breath Connection program, some medication can ease your symptoms as you travel the road to recovery. But remember: Any drug has the strength and power to damage as well as heal. Now is the time to assess your actual needs and decide whether a prescription that may have been appropriate for you years ago is relevant to your present condition. Every illness progresses, and there is every likelihood that the drugs you are taking now are unnecessary or even inappropriate. Perhaps you do need to continue with the same type of medication, but you should certainly query whether the dosage is right for your present needs. Consider whether these drugs have actually made you feel better over the years, or have they merely staved off attacks?

When you break a leg or arm you need to be protected by a plaster cast for a short period. You don't need that shield for the rest of your life. Try to think of prescribed asthma drugs in the same way.

Read this section on medication for asthma, emphysema, and other respiratory conditions with care. Be optimistic and try not to depend on crutches that you may no longer need. Pick up a crutch, by all means, when you are very weary, but learn not to depend on it as an everyday prop. You will see how a dependency can actually encourage the development, rather than elimination, of other disorders.

We know that some drugs and medicines, correctly administered, can be vital. But the sad fact is that sometimes drugs can actually aggravate asthma. We see conventional asthma medication as a very useful stop-gap, on which you can rely in times of need, while you learn the basics of the Breath Connection program and come to appreciate its fuller and longer-term benefits. Little by little, as your symptoms of asthma decrease, you can reduce your drug intake. It goes without saying that no medication should be discontinued or reduced without consulting your doctor, but we are confident that the Breath Connection program will make such a dramatic change that even your doctor will have to agree that drugs may no longer be necessary.

Many doctors may not have been aware of the Breath Connection program, and it is up to us to ensure that they are educated about this revolutionary system. While you are learning the techniques, your doctor can alter your drug intake as he or she sees fit. In partnership with Breath Connection techniques, some carefully prescribed drugs can be very helpful. Explain to your doctor what you are doing, and let him or her witness the results. You will find that your need for medication is reduced or even entirely nonexistent once you have started the program. Your body will be more balanced and in control, and the need for external treatment may well be completely unnecessary.

Understanding Your Drugs

All drugs have side effects. If you take an aspirin for your headache, the chances are that one or more of your other senses will be dulled. It's easy to ignore niggling side effects when you have been taking an asthma-related medicine for years. Indeed, the medicine may well have become a placebo. You may need to use a little amateur psychology to analyze this: Do you take those medicines because you know they will help you or because you subconsciously believe that they are a kind of insurance against an attack?

In the future, think more carefully about why and when you take that medication. Remember that taking drugs automatically could lead to further problems with hyperventilation and, in turn, lead to a stay in the hospital where further drugs will probably be administered. This is the cycle that we aim to break.

Most drugs are prescribed at the same dosage each day, occasionally at specified times. We do not agree with this method of treatment. We believe that as a patient's health or symptoms improve, the drug intake should be reduced. At the very least it should be varied, depending upon how you feel from day to day. A single prescribed level should be maintained only if you cannot see any change in your condition over a long period of time. Even then, don't let that situation carry on indefinitely. If you are chronically ill, and your medication has not made any improvement, chances are that the drug is not doing anything at all. Remember that all pharmaceutical drugs, including adrenaline, are prescribed to ease symptoms. They are not created to address the causes of illness, only its physical manifestations. The causes of many chronic illnesses remain unknown, despite the fact that the majority of them are treated regularly with prescription drugs.

Adrenaline, in particular, is used regularly for the treatment of asthma. Adrenaline derives from the adrenal cortex, a gland that produces natural corticosteroids. Asthmatics cannot produce enough of this natural steroid and often rely on synthetic substitutes. Experiments in Australia show that patients who follow Breath Connection are able to reduce their intake of artificial steroids by half. This clearly indicates that our bodies can learn to produce sufficient levels of this natural steroid on their own. Professor Buteyko maintains that the need for synthetic steroids is a direct result of hyperventilation, and the fact that the body produces its own, once it is back in balance, supports this view.

Shocking as it might seem, steady use of bronchodilators could worsen your asthma in the long run and could even be fatal. Recent asthma epidemics in the relatively clean environments of Australia and New Zealand have been attributed to the overuse of nebulizers.

KEY TERMS

• *Bronchodilators* are drugs prescribed to widen the bronchioles and improve breathing. There are three main groups of bronchodilators: sympathomimetics, anticholinergics, and xanthine drugs, which are related to caffeine. Corticosteroids are also used to reduce inflammation and suppress allergic reactions.

• *Bronchodilators* can either be taken when they are needed in order to relieve an attack of breathlessness that is in progress, or on a regular basis to prevent such attacks from occurring.

- Sympathomimetic drugs are mainly used for the rapid relief of breathlessness; anticholinergic drugs and xanthine drugs are used in the long term.

- Bronchodilator drugs act by relaxing the muscles surrounding the bronchioles.

- Sympathomimetic and anticholinergic drugs achieve this by interfering with the nerve signals passed to the muscles through the autonomic nervous system. Xanthine drugs are believed to relax the muscle in the bronchioles by their direct effect on the muscle fibers, although their precise action is unknown.

- Bronchodilator drugs usually improve breathing within a few minutes of administration.

- Corticosteroids usually start to increase the sufferer's capacity for exercise within a few days.

- All of these drugs have side effects: Sympathomimetic drugs stimulate a branch of the autonomic nervous system that controls heart rate and they may sometimes cause palpitations and trembling; anticholinergic drugs cause a dry mouth, blurred vision, and difficulty in passing urine; xanthine drugs may cause headaches and nausea. Corticosteroids may cause water retention, swelling, and an increase in blood pressure. They reduce the effect of insulin and may cause problems in diabetics, even producing the disease in susceptible individuals. They suppress the immune system, increasing the susceptibility to infection, and suppress symptoms of infectious disease. With long-term use, they can cause muscle wasting, peptic ulcers, osteoporosis, easy bruising, and a fat pad on the back.

• Inhalers or "puffers" release a small dose of a bronchodilator drug when pressed.

• Insufflation cartridges deliver larger amounts of the drug than inhalers and are easier to use because the drug is taken in as you breathe normally.

• Nebulizers pump compressed air through a solution of drug to produce a fine mist which is inhaled through a face mask. They deliver large doses of the drug to the lungs, rapidly relieving breathing difficulty.

• Ventilators are machines used to stimulate breathing in hospital.

COMMON DRUGS

Sympathomimetics
Bambuterol
Eformoterol
Ephedrine
Epinephrine
Fenoterol
Isoprenaline
Pirbuterol
Reproterol
Rimiterol
Salbutamol
Salmeterol
Terbutaline
Tulobuterol

Anticholinergics
Atropine
Ipratropium bromide
Oxitropium

Xanthines
  Theophylline/aminophylline

Corticosteroids
  Beclomethasone
  Budesonide
  Fluticasone
  Prednisolone

Other Drugs
  Antihistamines
  Ketotifen
  Nedocromil
  Sodium cromoglycate

There are some startling statistics, which bear out our worries:

• In 1930, when adrenaline first appeared, there was an increase in asthma-related deaths.
• Mortality was further increased following the widespread prescription and use of Isoprenaline, a bronchodilator, in 1960.
• Sudden respiratory arrests were reported among young asthmatics who had taken Salmetorol (Serevent) and in 1996 a group of Canadian scientists found that even as few as two puffs a day from a bronchodilator—about 200 milligrams—not only worsened the condition of asthma patients but contributed to a higher incidence of cataracts and glaucoma problems in asthmatics.

- According to a 1989 study, asthma mortality increased to epidemic proportions in New Zealand and was linked to inhaled Fenoterol.
- A 1990 study claimed that inhaled steroids were contributing to many psychiatric and endocrine disorders.

We offer these facts not to alarm you, but to point out the very real dangers of some drugs. It may help you to decide that the Breath Connection program, which uses only natural means by which to treat asthma and related conditions, is a healthier and safer alternative to long-term drug use. One of the aims of our treatment is to help you to reduce any existing drug dependency, and in consultation with your doctor you could soon be able to set aside your bronchodilator and steroid intake.

In our overstretched health service, GPs (general practitioners) are usually very busy. If your doctor does not have the time to discuss things as fully as you would like, we offer the following facts for you to consider for yourself. With this knowledge, you can consult your doctor about making possible changes.

Bronchodilators

These contain natural substances as well as manufactured drugs and have an honorable history going back to a Chinese doctor, Ma Huang, who devised one using the herb *Ephedra,* more than 4,000 years ago. Hippocrates, the father of modern medicine, was the first physician to identify asthma in the West. He called it *asthma,* which in translation means "hard to breathe." The first modern-day bronchodilators, which included ephedrine and adrenaline, were devised about 70 years ago. Before that, whisky, caffeine, tobacco, and chloroform had all been used to treat paroxysms of the bronchial tubes. Let us hope that the Breath Connection will in time be seen as another—but better—example of science's fragmented leaps and bounds.

Steroids

The steroids used for asthma and similar conditions are called *corticosteroids* and should not be confused with anabolic steroids, which are sometimes illegally taken by athletes to improve performance. When a medical pioneer was awarded the Nobel Prize for medicine for his discovery of steroid-related drugs and their anti-inflammatory effects, there was a rush to embrace them. People who had suffered for years from arthritis, skin disorders, chronic pain, and indeed asthma did not stop to query their possible side effects and the long-term damage they can produce. Diabetes sufferers gained relief and there was an almost universal, if hasty, welcome for the drugs and their spin-offs, many of which were lifesaving. Then came the backlash. Artificial steroids given to asthmatics and others produced some horrific side effects, including puffy faces, excess weight, excess facial hair for women, ulcers, osteoporosis, and serious problems for diabetics, including blindness, deafness, and memory loss. The regular prescription of most forms of steroid was halted for some time, while the medical profession reconsidered their uses. Over this period, nasal sprays and some skin creams were still widely available.

The overuse of artificial steroids suppresses the body's ability to produce natural steroids. Some people, particularly asthmatics, develop such a severe steroid dependency that they need to resort to drugs as their needs exceed their body's ability to produce the natural versions. The increased dosages and increasing use of these drugs will, over time, harm sufferers far more than they will help them. Some doctors have been unable to see the difference between the natural and unnatural steroids and have unwittingly colluded in the dangerous dependency of their patients. When the glands cease to produce natural steroids, due to artificial interference, the adrenal cortex is affected.

Other doctors, who may have been warned of the dangers of overprescribing steroids, actually underprescribe, which also puts their patients in danger. Steroids can be an effective, short-term treatment for a variety of illnesses, but their use must be assessed on a regular basis and regulated constantly.

Furthermore, few doctors actually understand how steroids work. Typically, oral steroids are prescribed for use in the morning, on the basis that they will tune in to the rhythms of the body. However, most asthmatic patients are at most risk early in the day, and since these types of steroids normally kick in after about six hours, they are virtually useless. Steroids are meant to be used on a preventative basis and not used to relieve an attack. It would be far better if they were taken at night so that problems early the next day can be avoided.

And why do doctors so often reduce the dosage of steroids by one tablet every three days, as if this treatment were set in stone? Why not every day, every two days, or every seven days? Surely these adjustments should be made after observing a patient's individual needs, which can change daily. The diagram below may help to explain things.

Steroid medication

a) Graphically, the steroid policy for a typical patient looks like this:

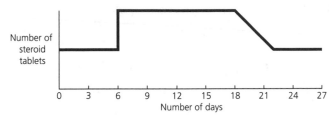

A doctor will increase the dose to 6–8 tablets in a day. The patient is then maintained on this high dosage for 10–12 days, after which it is gradually reduced by 1 tablet every 3 days, bringing it down to nothing. Professor Buteyko believes steroid intake should be adjusted for the particular condition of the patient in a more flexible way. In a typical case, with this sudden increase and decrease in dosage, the patient's health will improve and deteriorate just as quickly.

b) Often asthmatic patients have to go to the hospital where they can be given 200–1,000 mg of steroids. Graphically, this looks like this:

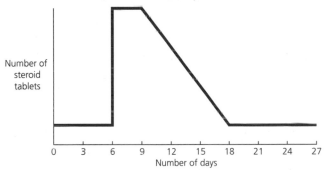

The patient is given a very high dose suddenly. When he or she leaves the hospital, the dose is reduced to nothing, endangering the patient's condition.

A Steroid Case

Let's take the case of an imaginary patient who visits his doctor and is prescribed oral steroids. Until now, the patient has been taking four puffs from an inhaler on most days. This amounts to a total daily dosage of one milligram of steroids (even more if the steroid prescribed was Beclomethasone).

He is now advised to take six to eight tablets, amounting to 30 or 40 milligrams daily, and typically advised to decrease this intake by one tablet every three days. This would likely produce the following scenario:

• The patient has now been prescribed 30 or 40 times more steroids than he has been used to (and even more if the choice of drug was Beclomethasone).

• The patient reduces this dosage by one tablet, or five milligrams, every three days. Therefore, he will take eight tablets on days one to three, seven on days four to six, and six tablets on days seven to nine, and so on over 21 days until he is taking no tablets at all.

Over three weeks, the patient has taken 128 tablets of oral steroids, each containing five milligrams. This means that he has ingested a total of 640 milligrams, a huge amount compared to the 21 milligrams he would have been taking over the previous three weeks.

In the first three days, the patient's body must adapt to an increase of 117 milligrams of steroids. This is cause for concern and raises the following questions: On what basis did the doctor prescribe the original four puffs a day? Why does this prescription tend to be offered fairly universally? If you suffer from diabetes your doctor will measure your blood sugar level and prescribe correct dosages of insulin accordingly. Patients' needs should be met on an individual basis. This practice has rarely, if ever, been considered for asthmatics.

Why was the new dosage of steroids increased 40-fold to cope with the problem? If a diabetic's blood sugar level suddenly jumped, his doctor would be unlikely to increase his insulin intake so dramatically.

It is easy to overdose on steroids, and their side effects are evident on even lower dosages, taken over a longer period of time. Administered correctly, there is no doubt that steroids can save lives. However, Professor Buteyko believes that the frequent and improper use of steroids is the cause of great discomfort and has even contributed to death. Not surprisingly, many people are becoming worried about taking them at all. His policy on steroids is very clear:

• Correctly prescribed steroids are a very effective means of preventing asthma attacks, subsequent deterioration, and even death from asthma.

• Ignorance in understanding their importance, reluctance, or refusal to take steroids can be fatal, as can medical negligence in failing to prescribe the right dosage.

• The vast majority of doctors do not know how steroids work; how to select correct dosages; how to modify dosage on a daily basis; or how or when to increase, decrease, or maintain levels of steroid consumption when a patient's condition worsens. Neither do they know how to normalize natural steroid production, overcome the resulting steroid deficiency, and get the patient off artificial steroids permanently.

Professor Buteyko's discovery includes a thorough understanding of drugs and can help you to both stay alive and enjoy a greater level of freedom in your everyday life. We can show you how not only the dosage but the side effects of steroids can be minimized once your individual and precise needs have been gauged, and we can show you how you can soon stop taking them altogether. These drugs play a very similar role in the life of an asthmatic as insulin does in the life of a diabetic. When the body hyperventilates, it stops producing natural steroids, so manufactured ones are required. But once you have learned not to overbreathe and your own natural steroids are being produced, prescribed medicine becomes redundant. With our help and that of your doctor, this is achievable. During this interim period it is essential to follow Professor Buteyko's principles and to carry on taking your steroids, but only under careful guidance.

The Peak Flow Meter

A peak flow meter is a device used to measure the volume of your forced expiration. The idea is that you blow into it as hard as you can to produce a reading that tells you your ability to blow out air. The higher the reading, the greater the volume of air and the better the result, according to doctors.

This device is familiar to every asthmatic and emphysema sufferer and in our view it is a thoroughly worthless piece of equipment: misleading, harmful, and only good for showing how strongly you can exhale. Even then it gives out imprecise measurements and can, in fact, induce asthmatic symptoms. Few doctors query the usefulness of peak flow meters and they can't explain why they can sometimes trigger an asthma-like effect. Attempts made by doctors and patients alike to maintain good peak flow figures are doomed to fail because trying to increase peak flow figures artificially leads, in every case, to hyperventilation. As we know, hyperventilation leads to asthma, the need for drugs, and a destructive cycle.

When you blow into the device, you blow out a great deal of carbon dioxide, which tells your body to defend itself by constricting the bronchotubes. This is the reason why asthmatics and others with breathing disorders experience wheezing, discomfort, coughing, and tightness of the chest after blowing out air. It is pointless to try to improve your peak flow figures without understanding the reasons for your problem. We know that asthma is caused by hyperventilation, which causes inadequate carbon dioxide to reach the body. A peak flow meter can cause hyperventilation.

Reconditioning and normalizing breathing patterns should be the first goal of every asthmatic—and a peak flow meter does nothing to effect this. We suggest you throw away your peak flow meter—now.

Watchpoints

Asthmatics should take special care to avoid attack in the following situations, particularly before they have reconditioned their breathing by following our program:

• When leaving a warm room for a cold street, or vice versa.

• When showering. Rapid changes in water temperature have been known to trigger attacks.

• Talking for long periods, which can encourage you to take in more air than you need. Schoolteachers, telephone salespeople, and anyone who needs to speak frequently as they work should be especially careful. See page 222 for techniques on breathing correctly when you talk.

• Dusting and making beds. Dust and mites, which can encourage attacks in asthmatics, thrive in even the most carefully laundered duvets and mattresses. Try and get someone else to make the bed or be sure to keep your mouth closed when you do so. Think about buying a special mattress cover or investing in one of the more powerful vacuum cleaners.

• Watch your diet. Asthmatic problems often become worse in cold weather, particularly if you have had colds or flu. Make sure you are getting lots of vitamin C and zinc, which can encourage the health of the immune system, and take the herb Echinacea, which has been proved both to boost immunity and reduce the duration of viral symptoms.

• Take care when you are flying. A pressurized cabin can play havoc with breathing. Concentrate on your breath control for several days before you fly and especially on the day of travel, right up to boarding the plane.

Remember:

• In all situations that can trigger an asthma attack, you must control your breathing. If you experience any asthma symptoms or find yourself hyperventilating, stay calm and concentrate on the breathing exercises.

• Sleep as upright as possible, supporting yourself with several firm pillows. There is always a danger that the pillows might move during a restless night, but begin by propping yourself in the right position, and settled on the left side of the body (see pages 52–53).

• Concentrate on your Breath Connection exercises before you go to bed, particularly if you have had a stressful day or have been in situations that normally trigger an attack. If your breathing is under control, you are much less likely to be wakened by an attack or to suffer one in the morning.

Special Note
Before embarking on the Breath Connection program in this book you should ascertain whether you are suffering from

any of the illnesses and disorders noted in Appendix B (see page 253). Some conditions are too complicated to be addressed without the guidance of a qualified practitioner or specialist. In the Resources section, we tell you how to find a reputable practitioner in your area. Always remember that the Breath Connection techniques, although simple, are very powerful and should only be practiced carefully. Never deviate from the guidelines supplied here and if you are in doubt, or feel uncomfortable at any point, take expert advice.

5

Breath Connection for Mild Asthma

Mild asthma can be as disrupting and distressing as more serious asthma, although it may not hold the same risks for the sufferer. Everything is relative, of course, and it is very likely that while you are in the grip of an attack, your symptoms may seem anything but mild, even if you have been diagnosed with a mild condition. Everyone has a different ability to cope with illness, just as everyone has different pain thresholds. Chances are, whether your asthma is mild or severe, you are suffering a great deal and are unlikely to be relieved or comforted by the fact that your condition is *mild*. We are aware that all asthma causes suffering and can lead to more serious illness. Breath Connection can ease that suffering.

We promise that within a few days you will be less dependent upon medication, and that your breathlessness and wheezing will be reduced if you follow the program for a week. Perhaps the most important result of the program is the fact that you will be able to control your asthma, rather than your asthma controlling you. As your body and your emotional health become stronger, you will begin to feel more in control of your life, and your health and well-being can be improved immeasurably.

We call your asthma mild if you

- Have never had any critical, life-threatening attacks
- Have never been hospitalized for asthma
- Have never used oral steroids, such as Prednisone
- Do not use Severent or a nebulizer
- Experience symptoms less than three or four times a day
- Can gain relief from a single puff of an inhaler

If one or more of these points does not apply to you, we would consider your asthma to be severe.

The importance of the balance between oxygen and carbon dioxide has been made clear. Carbon dioxide beneficially affects almost every organ and system in the body and can help to stop asthma from gaining any ground. If they could, pharmaceutical companies would undoubtedly bottle carbon dioxide, and there would be a large-scale fight for the patent. But carbon dioxide is free, and in order to experience its unique benefits, you need only learn a series of breathing exercises that will allow you to access it. Do your Control Pauses (see page 48) and breathe shallowly, with your mouth closed, to prevent this priceless gas from escaping. You will see results within days.

Another great benefit of the Breath Connection program—which is useful for all asthmatics and emphysemics, as well as everyone concerned about the general state of their health—is that it acts as an invaluable monitor. Your Control Pauses will tell you a great deal about your general state of health and help you to chart your daily progress. This can be enormously comforting for sufferers of any condition. If you are on top of your health and can gauge the results of the program, you will feel in control. You will never again have to fear illness in the same way. You will never again have to ask yourself "Am I really well?" "Am I more vulnerable than others to a life-threatening illness?" "Can I look forward to a long and healthy retirement?"

The Control Pause exercises will let you know in advance when things are wrong and help you to take control before early problems take hold. You will be much more confident and able to deal with health worries effectively.

It's simple! When your CP goes up, it indicates that your health is improving. When it goes down, take note and seek advice before any problem becomes more severe.

Preparing for Breath Connection

Everyone who is mildly asthmatic should prepare for Breath Connection by doing the following:

- Using their inhaler only when they cannot breathe.
- Getting used to breathing through the nose only, even when engaged in sporting activity. If this is impossible, take a break from the sport until your asthma is under control.
- Concentrating on learning how to shallow breathe.
- Making a habit of sitting comfortably and learning to relax.
- Beginning to breathe in more and more shallowly until your breathing is very gentle and quiet.
- Taking heart when things become difficult. It is worth persevering. Poor breathing can be changed much more easily than most bad habits.

The Technique

Each morning before breakfast (do this even if you are not hungry enough to eat any), sit and relax for five minutes. You can accomplish a whole series of breathing exercises while listening to the radio or some music.

1. Check your pulse over one minute and then practice a Control Pause.
2. Start shallow breathing for five minutes, and then do another Control Pause exercise.
3. Take a further five minutes for shallow breathing out.
4. Then, breathe in, breathe out, and hold your breath for the length of your last Control Pause, plus five seconds.
5. Now breathe lightly for five minutes.

Technique for mild asthmatics

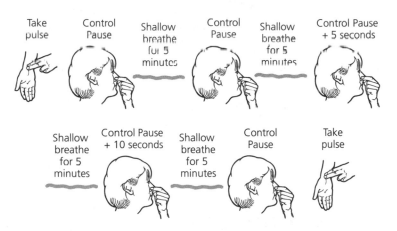

Practice this 3 times per day before meals until your symptoms disappear.

6. Breathe in, breathe out, and hold your breath out for the length of your last Control Pause, plus 10 seconds.
7. Finally, breathe shallowly for five minutes, then check your Control Pause and your pulse.

This type of breathing may have been a little faster than the type of breathing you are used to, but remember that the crucial thing is the reduced volume of air, not the speed at which you breathe. It is healthy and normal for you to feel slightly different to begin with, as your body adjusts to your new habit.

The whole morning exercise will take about 25 minutes, and we recommend that you try to repeat the sequence before lunch and your evening meal.

It's also a good idea to go through this cycle again, about an hour before you go to bed. Try to avoid eating anything for a couple of hours before each short session.

This series of exercises gives you a great start to the day and allows you to end each day feeling relaxed and calm. You can look forward to a peaceful, relaxing sleep.

Don't hesitate to do a course with a Breath Connection practitioner if you have any difficulty understanding these routines or putting them into practice. All counselors have been trained to understand, and be sympathetic toward, the problems of people who are unused to carving out spaces of time in their lives. They will offer encouragement and guidance to allow you to do so.

Key Points

- Get used to breathing less deeply than you are used to breathing.

- Keep your mouth closed, unless you are eating, speaking, or drinking.
- Close your mouth with special micropore tape (see page 51) before sleep or when you are alone at home.
- Keep up with your preventative medication. Don't stop or reduce steroids until your Breath Connection counselor has given you the OK, in consultation with your doctor.
- Practice your exercises regularly—this means three to four times a day for the next five days.
- Don't overeat or oversleep, and try to avoid sleeping on your back. Try to arrange things so that you are propped up to sleep on your left side.
- Refer to the dietary guidelines in Chapter 12, which will enhance your recovery.
- Don't eat a protein meal in the evening (see page 193).
- Don't push your Control Pause over 60.
- When you finish your Control Pause and breathe in again, keep your mouth closed and try not to take in large gulps of air. Control your breathing.

You will soon find that your asthma symptoms are reduced, and you will need to resort less frequently to your bronchodilator. Use the chart on page 243 to document your weekly progress. If or when asthma symptoms reappear, you can take immediate action to overcome the attack (see the following section).

Overcoming Asthma Attacks

Many people have some advance warning of an attack, and it is important that you go through a single set of steps before one can set in. Try the following:

1. Sit down.
2. Take your pulse and do the Control Pause.
3. Shallow breathe for four or five minutes.
4. Repeat the Control Pause.
5. Take your pulse again.

If you are able to overcome the attack with Breath Connection, shallow breathe for another 10 minutes. You will not need to reach for your puffer if your asthma attack has been relieved. However, if it hasn't, use your puffer and continue to breathe shallowly for 10 minutes. You can repeat these exercises as often as you need to, whenever you want to regulate your breathing or stave off an attack.

Diary of a Mild Asthmatic

The following diary gives you an example of what a mild asthmatic might expect during five days on the Breath Connection program. Responses will differ between individuals, and different people will benefit in different ways. Every person will also progress at their own pace, so don't be alarmed if your progress is unlike what we describe here.

Day One
The number of relievers necessary will be reduced, and you can expect to sleep better. You will find it easier to unblock your nose, and there will less breathlessness and fewer asthma symptoms.

Day Two
You will need even less relief from your regular medication. There will be less mucus in the nose. Appetite will have been

stimulated in people who are underweight, and overweight people will experience less hunger. Breathlessness and the ability to overcome symptoms quickly and efficiently will be improved.

Day Three
Your breath control will be noticeably better, and all of the previously mentioned areas will continue to improve. You will be particularly aware of the changes as you walk upstairs. Coughing may be suppressed. Your use of the puffer will have become occasional and your Control Pause will be stronger.

Day Four
There will be a further improvement in your Control Pause and in your overall condition. Your nose should remain unblocked all day. Your weight will begin to stabilize.

Day Five
By now, the overall improvement in, and control of, your asthma will be about 70 percent, with a similar reduction in the number of times you need to use your bronchodilators. You should also see a 70 percent improvement in your ability to prevent many of the symptoms of allergy, asthma, and sinusitis, among other things. Your mouth will remain closed naturally when you are not talking or eating.

In a few weeks' time, your improvement will be dramatic and your Control Pause will be much higher. Your immune system and nervous system will begin to function better and you should experience an increased sense of wellbeing. You will have more control over your emotions and, if you wish, you will be able to take part in nonaggressive sport without the need for drugs. Dependence upon bronchodilator drugs will have been greatly lessened over the weeks on the program. Necessary weight loss or weight gain will have become steady, and your sleep will be improved. Best of all, your sense of well-being will be enhanced and you will, perhaps for the first time in a long, long time, feel in control of your life.

6

Breath Connection for Severe Asthma

For those of you who suffer from severe asthma, one of the most difficult things to overcome is fear. Many of you have been rushed to the hospital in an emergency or have suffered a life-threatening attack, and it is undoubtedly hard to get over the overwhelming emotion that you associate with an asthma attack, and, indeed, your health in general. People who suffer from any known or unknown fear tend to cling to the known and avoid taking chances that could put them in any physical or emotional danger. We know, therefore, that it may be difficult for you to adapt to the program without some reservations. We ask you to trust us and allow us to take you through the exercises that can not only ease your suffering, but help you to shed your fear forever.

First of all, read the preceding chapter aimed at mild asthmatics, because much of the material written there will be helpful for you, too. Your case will differ from that of a mild asthmatic in that you will need to be ready for action at any time, and you may not have the same warning that an attack is imminent.

We do understand that severe asthmatics live in fear that the enemy might strike at any time—during a business meeting, while traveling, during a family celebration, especially if it involves a heavy meal, or even during a quiet period at home. Stress isn't always the trigger for the awful gasping spasms that can send you into the hospital. Extremes of weather may also be worrying for you. Even making a quick dash to answer the telephone, or running upstairs because you feel strong that day, can lead toward the kind of attack that all asthmatics dread.

If every simple little act of everyday life is loaded with potential risk, it is very hard to plan a normal existence. If fear dogs your every breath and step, your quality of life is seriously reduced. Even going into the hospital, itself a stressful experience, can exacerbate things. Many sufferers report that the concern of family and friends heightens their feelings of fear and helplessness, and you may feel that you have no control to change a situation that is continually spiralling in a downward direction. Your current medication may well give you both temporary relief and an illusion of control over things as you struggle to overcome serious attacks, but it is not curing your asthma. In reality, it is restricting your ability to make the most of your potential and to enjoy the full life you deserve.

We call your asthma severe if you answer yes to any of these questions:

- Have you experienced respiratory arrest, clinical death, lung collapse, or a life-threatening asthma attack that you were unable to treat on your own with the drugs that you had on hand?
- Do you have to use nebulizers, Serevent, or take more than three puffs from an inhaler every day?
- Do you need to use oral steroids every day or in a series of courses?
- Is your Control Pause less than 10 seconds?

- Apart from your asthma, do you suffer from any of the following: diabetes, a heart or kidney condition, epilepsy, high blood pressure, hypoglycemia, or emphysema?

A single affirmative answer means that you have what we classify as being *severe* asthma. If you have said yes to more than one, you will have even more to gain from practicing the Breth Connection methods.

JOANNE AND JENNY

Joanne and Jenny, 15-year-old twins, came to us about nine years ago. They had been asthmatic since birth and their condition was then regarded as being severe. They had been robbed of many of the pleasures of childhood and now they were being deprived of most of the freedoms of youth. Unable to attend normal school, they were taught at home. Even a few steps to the family car for an outing sometimes took an agonizing 20 minutes and they had been hospitalized at least 50 times in their short lives.

When they first started at a Breath Connection workshop, the girls couldn't manage the walking exercises that most five-year-olds accomplish very easily, but they had the will to progress and within four or five days they were spurring each other on with the tempting idea that they could soon be attending parties, instead of being trapped at home. Two months later their father, a ship's doctor, returned from a long voyage and found the twins playing volleyball in the back garden. He was astonished but naturally delighted to see how far and how fast they had progressed since he had seen them last.

You really can breathe your way out of this prison of devastating illness. It will take some effort and time but, as many who have already taken part in our program will testify, it is well worth it. Right from the start you will experience an improved sense of well-being that will encourage you to persevere. As your confidence grows, so will your control—until you are the master of this condition. Your need for medication will reduce steadily until the point that you find yourself being categorized as *mildly* asthmatic. As your breathing becomes more balanced your body will no longer depend upon asthma as a defense mechanism against its loss of carbon dioxide. For the first time in your life, perhaps, you will feel free. Progress for some patients is astonishingly fast. Others need a little more time. Don't lose heart—everyone gets there in the end.

The chart on pages 244–245 should be completed regularly and, as the days go by, it will be all the proof you need that your recovery is under way. You will see that by changing your breathing patterns you have the power to influence the severity of your asthma and the tools with which to cure it.

TONY

A successful and dynamic businessman, Tony did not want to admit that the asthma he had suffered since childhood was severe. He considered it mild, even though he was taking up to 20 puffs of Ventolin on bad days. He had been prescribed steroids but didn't bother to take them as he felt they offered no relief and he was, in any case, worried about side effects. He accepted that two puffs of Serevent in the morning and another at night could be helpful but realized that it was only giving symptomatic relief and not getting to the root cause of his asthma. He doubted if any treatment could do that.

Tony's diet was quite sensible: He drank only in moderation, exercised regularly, and didn't smoke. He had once had a severe asthma attack during a business trip abroad, and he dreaded a recurrence, knowing that changes in climate and extra stress could exacerbate things.

During one long flight, a head cold passed to his throat and bronchi and this time countless puffs of Ventolin brought no relief. A heavy restaurant dinner was followed by several frightening hours during which he fought for breath and Tony eventually called an ambulance to his hotel. He made a good recovery after receiving oxygen, nebulizers, IV aminophylline, and steroids but was advised to remain in the hospital under supervision, taking oral steroids because his oxygen level was so low. It was this experience that convinced Tony that his asthma wasn't so mild after all and led him to Breath Connection when he returned to Britain.

He embarked on the program with commitment and enthusiasm and after only three days was using just two puffs of Ventolin and none of his prescribed Serevent. He was advised to get out of the habit of puffing Ventolin automatically before sport, sex, walking upstairs, stressful meetings, or going to bed. He soon learned that he could do everything he normally did without hyperventilating or needing Ventolin. He also learned how to control his asthma by subtly adjusting all aspects of his lifestyle, and he learned how to anticipate the onset of an attack if he lapsed. He discovered that he was most vulnerable when his Control Pause was low and his breathing deep and found that a startling relief of his symptoms took place when he breathed shallowly. Not only did his Control Pause go up, but he felt very much better.

After two weeks Tony no longer needed Ventolin at all and could take four flights of stairs without pausing for breath. He had also realized that it was easy to incorporate Breath Connection exercises into his demanding business schedule and was well worth the small effort that it required.

Preparing for Breath Connection

- Learn how to check your pulse (see pages 53–55).
- Read and fully understand the theoretical parts of this book.
- Breathe through your nose and keep your mouth closed at all times, except when talking, eating, or drinking.
- If you are taking oral steroids now but are engaged in a plan to step down the intake, as described in an earlier chapter, stop doing so. From now on, keep your steroid intake at the same level until your asthma has improved to such a degree that we would describe it as mild and one puff of your bronchodilator is sufficient to alleviate your symptoms.
- Use bronchodilators only when you need to. Don't take them to prevent an attack, and ignore any previous schedule you may have been following.
- Stop using a nebulizer on a regular basis. Use it only if two or three puffs of the inhaler or other form of medication does not work. If you must use a nebulizer, try to limit use to 30 seconds—at the very maximum, no more than three minutes.
- Take only a single puff of your inhaler at any one time.

- Avoid long-lasting, slow-working bronchodilators such as Atrovent or Serevent because you will need faster relief than these can offer.
- Practice shallow breathing. Think of this as being the start of a training course and remember that bad, old habits always take time to unlearn, especially when you are striving to adopt new, good ones at the same time. Within five days there should be a clear improvement noticeable enough to encourage perseverance.
- Remember that dedicated retraining after a lifetime of incorrect breathing may actually take some weeks. This is a little like dieting. You may initially lose a great deal of weight, but you soon reach a plateau, and subsequent changes are less dramatic. Your weight loss may even be more difficult to maintain. Similarly, with the Breath Connection program, some severe asthmatics feel so elated by the immediate results of the first few days that they are discouraged when the dramatic rate of improvement is not maintained over the next stages. Try not to be discouraged. The essential groundwork had been laid and steady, permanent improvement will follow. We do not offer the respiratory equivalent of a crash diet, but we know that our spectacularly fast early results can inspire patients to maintain the discipline.
- You will have learned to try to use your lungs less. Make sure that the amplitude of your chest (full expansion) has been decreased and that the movement of your diaphragm has decreased.
- Remember to tape your mouth shut at night (see pages 51–52).
- Take time to read and follow the dietary guidelines we discuss in Chapter 12, which will enhance recovery.

- Remember never to push your Control Pause beyond the point of comfort, as it will aggravate the risk of hyperventilation.
- Never push your Control Pause above 60.

We cannot overstress the fact that the Breath Connection techniques can have a powerful effect—as powerful as any drugs—and care must be taken to follow the instructions exactly, in order to achieve maximum effect.

CHARLOTTE

Severe asthma can strike at any age. Charlotte was a late developer and did not experience symptoms until her late sixties. Each of the several doctors she consulted prescribed different drugs and she has, over time, absorbed a confusing amount of conflicting advice and information about asthma. Because she bruised easily and had concerns about osteoporosis and stomach problems—all common side effects of steroids—she took only one oral steroid a day. She was unaware that during hospital visits she had been given large doses of steroids. Because many patients are alarmed by the use of steroids, doctors and nurses in hospitals often refer to them euphemistically. For this reason, Charlotte had no reason to believe that she was being given a high dose of a medication that she did not want.

Manufactured steroids can have side effects, but can be useful as a temporary measure on the Breath Connection program. They can help to rebalance the breathing while you retrain. After a short time, the dosage can be reduced under supervision, and your body will begin to produce its own natural steroids.

Having read about us, Charlotte flew from her home in North America to take part in a Breath Connection workshop in London. She claimed that talking helped her to breathe, and she was not at all sure that keeping her mouth closed would work. But she listened and learned and was determined to follow the Breath Connection regime to the letter. We explained to her that properly prescribed steroids have their uses for asthmatics and indeed may well have saved her life on several occasions in the past.

Charlotte found that after one session—which she had not enjoyed in the least!—she could sleep peacefully at night. After three months of faithfully following Breath Connection exercises, Charlotte's asthma had become so mild that she could go for weeks without needing to take more than the occasional puff on a ventilator. Her medication was now just 5 percent of what it was when she came to see us. Only occasionally, to ward off colds or flu, Charlotte takes between half and one tablet of Prednisone. Her hospital visits are now a thing of the past.

The Technique

1. Check your Control Pause and your pulse (see pages 48 and 53–55).
2. Practice shallow breathing (see page 50).
3. Continue to take your pulse, then do the Control Pause and afterward decrease your breathing for two minutes.
4. Do another Control Pause, relax for a few minutes, and then breathe lightly. You may feel slightly heady, but this is perfectly normal and nothing to worry about. You're just experiencing the power of the

Breath Connection techniques and in these early days some sensations may feel strange.

5. Do another Control Pause followed by four minutes of shallow breathing.
6. Do another Control Pause. Rest for a few minutes.
7. Do the Control Pause again but this time shallow breathe for six minutes afterward.
8. Check your Control Pause and take a rest.
9. Check your Control Pause again and this time shallow breathe for eight minutes. Repeat number 6 above.
10. Now do the Control Pause exercise once again, followed by 10 minutes of shallow breathing. Check your CP again and then take your pulse.

The entire exercise should take only about 25 minutes.

As you go through each stage of the CP and pulse checking (see pages 244–245), make a note of the figures. When you study them later, you will see that as the Control Pause figure went up, the pulse rate came down. You will certainly feel better after completing this exercise and should get into the habit of performing it regularly and charting progress so that you can see, week by week, how you have progressed.

Carry on three times a day, two hours before meals, for three or four weeks or until you no longer need to resort to bronchodilators. Stay on your steroids. These should only be reduced under the guidance of a Breath Connection practitioner or a sympathetic doctor.

Some people worry that their GP will be hostile or cynical to the Breath Connection program and it is true that a few of them might be dismissive. If you encounter resistance from your GP, I suggest that you show him or her this book.

Daily technique for overcoming severe asthma

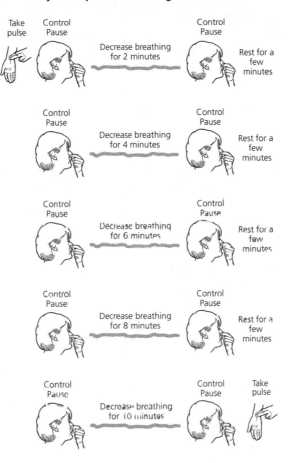

The Breath Connection technique has been associated with Australian research of the highest repute, and your doctor will be more likely to respond to the project if he or she is aware of its authenticity. If your doctor steadfastly refuses to help you to progress via the Breath Connection program, you can, of course, always ask for a second opinion.

If you do not feel any better after a month or so, you may need some individual coaching from a Breath Connection practitioner. Courses are available all over the United Kingdom and the United States. If there isn't a course in your area, you may want to combine a holiday or a business trip with a visit to one of our centers. Above all, don't be discouraged. Failure to respond to the Breath Connection techniques outlined here simply means that you have very individual needs, and they will need to be assessed and dealt with by an expert. We are confident that the technique will work for you, even if it does take more time. Self-help isn't always possible, particularly when a condition is deep rooted.

In the course of following the previously described steps for a few weeks, you might still experience an asthma attack. If so, you will find the following advice helpful.

Overcoming a Severe Asthma Attack

Whenever you experience the onset of an attack, stop whatever you are doing. Then take the following steps:

1. Take your pulse and do a Control Pause.
2. Then shallow breathe for 10 minutes and take another Control Pause.
3. Take your pulse again.
4. If this doesn't work, Professor Buteyko recommends that you take just one puff from your inhaler. Then, if necessary, take another puff five minutes later.
5. If you're still in discomfort, use your nebulizer for one to three minutes. Only if this fails should you use the full nebulizer. The most important thing is that you

allow your body the chance to muster its own resistance before leaning on your familiar props.

Professor Buteyko also points out that if your puffer didn't work, you might need to increase your oral steroids—in consultation with your doctor—because it suggests that your asthma is unstable. In some cases, you may be able to decrease your oral steroids, with your doctor's advice, but only gradually and under the following conditions:

- You don't use your inhaler more than three to four times a day.
- Your control pause is not less than 10 seconds.
- Your pulse is not more than 100 beats per minute.
- Your attacks haven't been sharp or sudden.

This technique for severe asthmatics is a first step toward conquering asthma completely. Steroid use and requirements will vary between individuals and it is impossible to formulate a system that will work for everyone. You will need to work fairly closely with your doctor, and, perhaps, a Breath Connection practitioner to assess your needs on a weekly basis, until the condition has been righted.

Technique for dealing with a severe asthma attack

| Take pulse | Control Pause | | Control Pause | Take pulse |

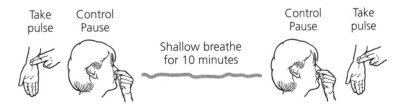

Shallow breathe for 10 minutes

Diary of a Severe Asthmatic

The following diary gives you an example of what a severe asthmatic might expect during five days on the Breath Connection program. Once again, responses will differ between individuals, and different people will benefit in different ways. Every person will also progress at his or her own pace, so don't be alarmed if your progress is unlike what we describe here.

Day One

The severe asthmatic will continue to take steroid medication but will be able to restrict use of puffers and other forms of relief and will usually be able to set aside nebulizers. Quality of sleep will improve and there will be far fewer problems in the early morning.

Day Two

Breath control will have improved and there will be even less need for puffers. Breathlessness will be reduced and appropriate eating patterns for both the underweight and overweight will begin to emerge.

Day Three

There will be a marked improvement in the Control Pause and all other general symptoms. Your overall condition will have improved. There will be further reduction in the need for drugs.

Day Four

This steady improvement in all areas will intensify.

Day Five

Changes will inspire all-around confidence, and you will find it easier to complete the exercises. You will be able to keep your mouth closed without too much conscious effort.

After a few weeks there will be a reduction in your need for medication of about 50 percent, considerable improvement in the Control Pause, and you will be able to endure colds and flu without an automatic trip to the hospital. Asthma attacks and symptoms will have become mild and a single puff on a reliever will be enough to stave off an attack. The quality of your life will have improved enormously, and simple things that nonasthmatics take for granted, such as walking down the street without breathlessness, will become the norm. Coughing fits will be eliminated or greatly shortened, and your weight will have become more balanced—or, at least, well on the way to becoming so. You'll be sleeping much more peacefully, which means that you will function better in every single aspect of your professional and private life.

Key Points to Remember

- Sleep on your left side (see page 52).
- Tape up your mouth (see page 51) before sleep and whenever you are home alone.
- Avoid protein meals in the evening (see page 193), which can take a great deal of oxygen to digest and increase the possibility of suffering an asthma attack in the night or following morning.
- Avoid all dairy foods, which can increase mucus production.

7

Breath Connection for Emphysema and Bronchitis

Emphysema is slow suffocation.

Because it is generally believed that cigarette smoking has intensified, if not caused, the condition, many sufferers will have to endure the unsympathetic attitudes of others who believe that they have only themselves to blame. This can cause feelings of isolation and depression in the sufferer, which can make the condition worse. Asthmatics are, at least, spared the lack of sympathy and indignity of being told that they are the cause of their own illness.

The horrific symptoms of emphysema outweigh the severity of the crime, and no sufferer should be treated with disdain. Emphysema is a frightening, serious illness, and it can take a dramatic course that leaves the sufferer literally gasping for breath on a daily basis.

Naturally, we do advise against cigarette smoking, which is a dangerous habit. Hostile warnings are, however, unlikely to change the habits of a committed smoker and illness should garner sympathy, whatever its cause. Even more controversially, perhaps, we are not convinced that smoking is the cause of emphysema. We do know that emphysemics who smoke will feel markedly better if they follow the Breath Connection program.

The most punishing and cruel aspect of emphysema is the fact that it completely restricts the life of the sufferer. Not only do emphysemics suffer debilitating breathlessness but they experience a crippling reduction in mobility that makes it harder and harder for them to lead a normal life. If you are emphysemic and already struggling with physical restrictions, the Breath Connection program can help to arrest many of your symptoms. If your illness is in its early stages, we can help you to avoid, or certainly delay, the worst symptoms if you start to follow our program now. A normal life, or at least a semblance of one, can be resumed and your life expectancy can be increased.

You will need to set aside some time to follow the Breath Connection program and self-discipline will be required. The chances are that family and friends, anxious about your condition, will do all they can to encourage you and they will be almost as gratified as you will be to observe the improvement in your condition. Every step toward restored mobility can lead to another and then another.

MARIE

Marie was on the waiting list for a double lung transplant, although she had little confidence that even this drastic measure would help her much. At 74, she had severe emphysema and had been confined to a wheelchair for several years. Her massive daily medication included six to eight nebulizers, with up to 25 puffs of Ventolin between doses. She also inhaled steroids (the incredibly powerful Beclomethasone) twice a day and often took oral steroids as well. Moreover, Marie took antibiotics whenever she had a chest infection. While she was waiting for a hospital place, Marie was given courage by her husband to start the Breath Connection program. Because she had been attached to an oxygen supply 24 hours a day, she was, understandably, fearful about taking the pipes out of her nose to do the Control Pause.

Marie used to be a smoker, and although she had stopped some 20 years earlier, she had been told that smoking was the cause of her illness. Her face was ashen, a reflection of the very low oxygen level in her blood, and she often had to sleep in her wheelchair, which meant that she got little proper rest. Rising from it to go to the bathroom at night was a regular nightmare. In short, Marie's life was desperately restricted.

She embarked upon Breath Connection after she had been waiting for her operation for almost a year. She took almost immediate heart when she learned from her Breath Connection practitioner that surgery would probably be unnecessary if she undertook the program. She was also surprised to learn that he did not consider that her old smoking habit was the cause of her current condition.

Her first Control Pause was very low—only five seconds—but after just a few exercises on her first day, she only needed to be attached to her oxygen supply for three hours a day and to use only two nebulizers. On the second day, she only used the nebulizer once, in the morning, and had one oxygen boost in the evening. On day three, she was able to rise from her wheelchair and take some faltering steps. After years in a wheelchair, her leg muscles had atrophied, but this would soon be remedied.

Her Breath Connection practitioner told her to count the number of steps she was able to take every day to see how they increased. She was also advised to shallow breathe upon waking each morning. She was to eat only when she was hungry, which was a considerable challenge for Marie, who had become used to eating heartily five times a day.

By the fifth day of the program, Marie was not using a nebulizer, was down to two or three puffs of Ventolin, and could begin to walk 50 meters four or five times a day. After another five days, she could double that distance and her skin was healthily pink. Three months later, Marie met her GP when she was out shopping—on her feet. His surprise at the sight of her was such that he rather tactlessly told her that, because he hadn't seen her for some time, he had assumed she was dead. Marie was far from dead.

In the past, there was very little hope for emphysemics. Breath Connection can change that. You can work from home as well as with a practitioner and witness steady progress. Carefully document your progress on the charts on pages 246 or 247, and over time you will see results. Initially, results may be slight and sluggish, but continued effort will bring permanent change and the visc of emphysema can first be loosened and then reversed to a significant degree.

Emphysema is a severe respiratory disorder wherein the air sacs (alveoli) in the lungs are permanently enlarged and partially damaged. Lung tissue is usually hardened and rendered inflexible by the loss of blood to essential vessels that nurture this tissue. Lung capacity is decreased and patients experience shortness of breath, especially when walking uphill or even upstairs. Many emphysemics need to use oxygen at night and some have to sit in a wheelchair attached to an oxygen cylinder.

But, until doctors accept that the major cause of emphysema is not smoking, and that double lung transplants are not the only answer, the majority of cases will never be successfully treated.

Emphysema Myths

The facts are complicated and may seem to be contradictory:

• The majority of emphysema patients stopped smoking long before they contracted the illness; indeed, in some cases 20 years have elapsed since the last cigarette, and some patients, including many children, have never smoked at all.

• Most doctors will say that asthma and emphysema are two very different conditions, and yet they prescribe the same drugs to both groups, often in larger amounts to the emphysemics. All emphysemics hyperventilate, in fact, they overbreathe more than asthmatics. Yet doctors continue to tell them that they should breathe more deeply.

• We know that emphysemics breathe somewhere between three and five times the norm, and that this advice is compounding the problem.

• Doctors often prescribe oxygen for emphysema. However, the air we breathe contains 21 percent oxygen, already more than our bodies need. People who live in high altitudes, where oxygen levels are lower, tend to live longer, stronger lives than those at lower elevations, and yet doctors continue to prescribe 100 percent oxygen which is known to be harmful, even toxic.

Not Just a Lung Disorder

The conventional medical profession tends to view emphysema as being simply a lung or breathing problem. Their answer is to replace the faulty part with a new one, much like a car manufacturer would replace a faulty part in an engine that isn't working properly. This is completely at odds with the way we see things at The Hale Clinic. We believe that all conditions should be treated holistically—that is, addressing the mind and the whole body. When one part of the body goes wrong, it is usually a reflection that there is an imbalance in the body, not just in that one part. Going back to the example of the car manufacturer, we would recommend an entire service, not just a replacement part when the engine does not work properly. We believe that all systems are interactive.

Therefore, transplanting lungs in emphysemics is not the answer. The root imbalance will still exist within the body, and a seriously ill person will have the additional trauma of a serious operation. So often emphysema patients remain stricken with disability even after such costly surgery, and there is, of course, a risk of complete failure, as there is with any operation.

The fact is that Professor Buteyko was right when he discovered that emphysema is one of the body's mechanisms to fight hyperventilation. He found that the body reduces lung capacity in order to limit its loss of carbon dioxide and will increase it again when a balanced and quieter breathing pattern is reestablished.

By using the Breath Connection self-care program, emphysema sufferers have found that the advance of their condition has been slowed down or halted, that they have been easily able to reduce their drug intake—both bronchodilators and steroids—and thereby minimizing previous drug-related side effects. Every aspect of their quality of life has improved, from sleep and emotional state of mind to the ability to participate in normal activities such as walking and playing with children and grandchildren. Very often, working under specialist guidance, their visible improvements are so obvious that any previous threat of a lung transplant has been consigned to history.

As always we advise you to undertake our program with care and in consultation with your doctor or under the guidance of a Breath Connection practitioner. Those suffering from emphysema or other bronchial disorders should not undertake self-care, if you are prone to any of the related conditions noted in Appendix B. The extra support and supervision you will receive from an expert can only hasten your recovery.

Mild and Severe Emphysema

Preparing for Breath Connection

• It is essential that emphysemics strive toward a healthy lifestyle that includes physical exercise. For milder conditions, this means walking, swimming, cycling, horseriding, or jogging every day, always with a closed mouth, however great the exertion may seem.

• The most important thing is to enjoy your physical movement—however limited it may be in the beginning—and to remember that by taking on these activities, you are helping yourself to reduce medication, as well as to feel better.

• Emphysemics take two types of drug: steroids—either inhaled or in tablet form—and puffers, Salbutamol, Ventolin, Serevent, and nebulizers. Breathing exercises are essential for their efficacy.

Daily technique for mild to severe emphysema

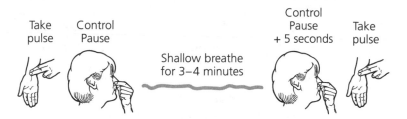

| Take pulse | Control Pause | Shallow breathe for 3–4 minutes | Control Pause + 5 seconds | Take pulse |

Each morning before breakfast, before dinner and an hour before going to sleep do a Control Pause and then shallow breathe for three or four minutes. Then do another Control Pause with an extra five seconds. Charting your progress on a daily and week-by-week basis will help you to monitor your improvement.

Walking Exercises for Moderate to Severe Emphysema

1. For those with moderate to severe emphysema the first thing to learn is how to control your breath while walking. Sit comfortably, check your pulse, do a Control Pause, and begin to shallow breathe.

2. Now stand up and continue to shallow breathe very slowly, listening to your breathing. Begin to take a few steps, walking very carefully round the room for about 20 to 25 paces. You should try and clear your mind of any thoughts so that you are completely relaxed. These exercises are often best practiced somewhere safely familiar such as in your own home.

3. Your breathing now will be deeper than it was when you were sitting down and this is quite normal. You

should feel that your breathing is absolutely under your control.

If you become breathless, feel you are losing control, and have a desire to open your mouth you can do the following:

- Keep walking and try to suppress your overbreathing by attempting to take in less air with each intake of breath.
- Slow down and walk even more slowly.
- Stop, hold your breath, and begin to walk very slowly again.

Your ability to walk without becoming breathless, while keeping your mouth closed, depends on the Control Pause. If this is very low, walking even a few meters will be beyond you. But if you can increase your Control Pause to 40 or 45 seconds you will be able to run—yes, run—upstairs to the third floor without distress.

You should now rest to take your breathing rate down. Then you can start again, walking a little faster this time. Soon, you should be able to walk at the rate of the average person in the street.

Each time, walk for as long as you can, but plan a realistic distance that will not cause you to slow down or to lose control of your breathing. Try 20 meters on first day, gradually increasing to 50 meters by the end of the week. When you're up to 5 kilometers a day, you've reached your goal. It's a great achievement! Not all physically fit people are able to walk that far without effort. Some emphysemics even find that they get so used to the swing of walking quite briskly that they have trouble walking slowly!

The important thing to remember is to keep your mouth closed at all times, whatever your walking speed. Some people find this quite a challenge and say that it increases their breathlessness. You will need to find your own correct pace—the one at which walking and breathing is comfortable and possible without opening the mouth. You might be ambling or positively striding—find what is the right speed for you. The point of this technique is to retrain your breathing; the other benefits of the physical exercise are secondary. Once you have learned to control your breathing, you may want to go on to more challenging activities such as sports, cycling, or going to the gym. If you still find it difficult to keep your mouth closed while taking any form of exercise, keep it shut with tape.

Once again the micropore tape we recommend is light and barely visible: it's not like placing a strip of masking tape across your mouth! If you do feel self-conscious about it, consider that many cyclists and even pedestrians in cities wear masks against pollution. You'll be wearing an adapted form!

So, to remind you

- Do your Control Pause three times a day, before breakfast, lunch, and dinner.
- Shallow breathe for three or four minutes between CPs and add five seconds to the second Control Pause of each session before taking your pulse.
- Don't forget to record your progress on the chart!

Sitting Exercises for Severe Emphysema

If your emphysema is so severe that you are in a wheelchair and attached to an oxygen balloon for long periods, it's obvious that you will not be able to engage in the walking program previously outlined. But being wheelchair-bound doesn't mean that you can't recondition your breathing and make some small physical movements.

Unless you are completely paralyzed, you can work on your breath and retrain your lung muscles. Don't assume that your need for a wheelchair will be infinite. More importantly, don't use it as an excuse. There is no reason why you can't fight to lessen your disabilities. By following the exercises we recommend in the next section, you really have nothing to lose!

As usual, the exercises should be completed at least two hours before mealtimes and an hour before going to bed.

The Technique

Exercise A

1. Control your breathing by taking slow, shallow breaths through the nose. Take off your oxygen straw—don't worry, you will be fine.
2. Check your pulse and measure your Control Pause. Now breathe out gently.
3. Then hold your breath out and at the same time tense the muscles of your hands for up to three seconds.
4. Then relax, breathe in gently, and continue to shallow breathe for a few minutes until you are ready for the next exercise. Keep your mouth closed.

Exercise B

1. Breathe out, hold your breath, and tense the muscles in your legs for up to four seconds.
2. Relax, breathe in gently, and continue to shallow breathe through the nose—as always—for three or four minutes.

Exercise C

1. Breathe out, hold your breath out, and this time tense your whole body for three seconds.
2. Relax, breathe in gently, and continue to shallow breathe for four or five minutes, mouth closed.

Repeat these three exercises as often as you can, always checking your Control Pause before and afterward. Your CP should improve by a second or two each time, your pulse rate will be reduced, and your body will feel warmer afterward. When you have completed each session, replace your oxygen straw only if you feel you must. If you think you can manage without it for some of the day, try to do so. But put the straw back on before going to sleep.

It is particularly important for emphysemics not to push the Control Pause too high. Your body's instincts will be the best monitor here. If you begin to feel uncomfortable during the Control Pause, stop and begin to shallow breathe for a few minutes. Look upon the Breath Connection program as something to be administered in dosages just as you would regard medication prescribed by your doctor. You should never exceed your Control Pause beyond comfortable limits unless you are taking guidance from a Breath Connection practitioner.

Regardless of the severity of your condition as an emphysemic, this is a summary of the basic guidelines:

- Sleep on your left side (see page 52).
- Keep your mouth closed as often as possible.
- Tape your mouth when sleeping or during the day, if alone.
- Avoid dairy foods such as milk, cheese, and yogurt, which can increase mucus buildup, and cut down on

protein, which increases your need for oxygen. Do not eat a protein meal in the evening.

Breath Connection for Bronchitis

Bronchitis may not be as serious a disorder as asthma or emphysema but it can, nonetheless, generate enormous distress and create restrictions in the lives of its victims. It is another condition predicated by a shortage of carbon dioxide and exacerbated by overbreathing.

For those who suffer from it, perhaps the most troubling aspect of this illness is the continual, painful, chest-wracking cough that it brings and, if not properly treated, bronchitis can easily lead to those other, more severe, respiratory disorders. So, bronchitis should never be seen as some relatively minor, seasonal, or merely inconvenient illness. We take it very seriously indeed and regard it as a very unpleasant but useful early warning that the health has begun a dangerous downward spiral. Action now can save all sufferers a future of even more debilitating disease.

Medical reference books define *bronchitis* as an "inflammation of the mucous membrane of the bronchi (the two main airways to the lungs) which often affects the throat, larynx and bronchioles." Chronic bronchitis is normally associated with swelling of the bronchial mucous glands, which are irritated by cigarettes and air pollution. Despite much current thinking, we know that these may be factors in the exacerbation of the condition, but they are not the root cause. The variable and frequently damp climate in Britain has also been held responsible for a number of cases.

It is also commonly believed that bronchitis is caused by infection, like sore throats, head colds, and pneumonia, as it is usually preceded by the sort of bugs that spread rapidly around air-conditioned offices and centrally heated houses. These render us vulnerable to attack from microorganisms which settle in the sinuses and strain our defense mechanisms. Certainly much bronchitis begins this way, but one of the reasons why it becomes a chronic, rather than short-term, condition is the fact that our immune systems are not strong enough to fight infections—and that is often the result of improper breathing. Most smokers never suffer from bronchitis. Yet many people who have never smoked in their lives do develop this disorder. The polluted air in the cities where some of us live can't be the cause; bronchitis afflicts many people who live in clean environments. Smoking and air pollution can exacerbate the problem, but they don't cause it. The cause of bronchitis—like so many other respiratory conditions—remains a mystery.

JAMES

James had chronic bronchitis and he was only seven years old. His father brought the boy to us because he had endured violent coughing fits for nine months and nothing—conventional medicine, a recent course of Chinese herbs, trips to the seaside and mountains— had helped. James's father had been outraged when the family GP suggested that the boy was secretly smoking, and his disillusionment led him to Breath Connection.

When we first met James, he had tonsillitis as well, the most recent of a string of illnesses and infections that had kept him away from school for long periods of time. On only the second day at Breath Connection, James's cough stopped. Over the next five months, having learned to

practice the Breath Connection exercises at home, James
did not suffer from any colds or flu. His personal best!

Antibiotics can sometimes help in cases of pneumonia,
but only if the pneumonia is bacterial. All doctors admit
that antibiotics are useless against viruses of any type, and
many cases of pneumonia are viral. To date, all attempts by
scientists to identify the microorganisms that settle in the
bronchi—causing bronchitis and pneumonia, and proving
resilient to the efforts of the immune system to fight them
off—have failed. The few microorganisms that have been
pinpointed appear to be carried by the majority of us, and
yet few of us go on to contract the illnesses. Whatever bug
is killing us has continued to elude scientists, as is the reason why some people have the capacity to fight it, and
others do not.

Perhaps even more importantly, there is no cure for
bronchitis, because its cause is unknown. Like asthma,
bronchitis is usually treated with drugs to ease or mask the
symptoms.

Hyperventilation and Bronchitis

Professor Buteyko has long maintained that hyperventilation
affects the metabolic responses of every cell in the body,
starting with the nervous system, then affecting the heart,
and third, targeting the lungs and bronchi. He has said that
when the cells of the bronchial "tree" become damaged,
inflammation and swelling occur in the upper part. What we
call bronchitis will follow. When the problems affect the
lower part of the tree, there is danger of a severe condition
known as *bronchioectathis*. This is very difficult to treat.

Any infection, adverse weather condition, cigarette smoke, or even something as innocent as eating ice cream can aggravate this condition. It is also known that it often precipitates asthma, which is yet another reason why we should study it and strive to unravel its mysteries. These two conditions are clearly linked in that patients with a characteristic bronchial cough may suddenly experience breathing difficulty, develop a bronchospasm, and become what is called asthmatic. The correct term should be *asthma with bronchitis*. As Professor Buteyko has explained, when patients begin to develop a pattern of hyperventilation, they lose carbon dioxide. This upsets the metabolic balance of the bronchial cells as they become further inflamed and weakened. By increasing breath intake and further upsetting the oxygen/carbon dioxide mix, the body implements its reserve defense mechanism—a bronchospasm—and the terrible coughing begins.

Fortunately, not everyone with bronchitis will go on to develop asthma. For this to happen, there must first be a predisposition to bronchospasm. People without adequate natural immunity may develop emphysema, or bronchioectathis, which can be far worse. Yet there are others who have stronger defense mechanisms who will suffer bronchial spasm at times, but never develop bronchitis. Asthmatics—in particular, children—may develop bronchitis as well, mainly due to the use of certain inhalants. People who are concerned about wheezing may visit a doctor who has no real way of determining whether he or she should be treating asthma or bronchitis! The truth is that almost no one in authority knows what to do.

Until about 40 years ago, it was common to call such attacks in young children "wheezy bronchitis" or "bronchitis with phlegm," as the word *asthma* was considered to be too frightening. But, at some stage, doctors began to believe

115

that all children thus afflicted were indeed asthmatic, and they prescribed treatment accordingly. Asthma treatments were often mistakenly and heavily prescribed, causing damage to sufferers who did not need them.

If you suffer from bronchitis, we strongly recommend that you follow the Breath Connection technique for bronchitis. A few simple exercises every day will scarcely inconvenience you, yet they could spare you the threat of much worse things to come, as your breathing is rebalanced and your bronchitis recedes. As soon as you see your Control Pause rising on your daily chart you will know that the downward spiral toward serious disease has been arrested.

Please never optimistically assume that because you have a disorder that you can live with, no serious action needs to be taken. Severe, chronic ill health sometimes starts with signals too slight or minor to be registered. Perhaps, therefore, we should be grateful for the unmistakable ways in which bronchitis announces itself. Indeed, all pain could be looked at it in this way—it is a clear warning from our bodies that something is not right. Our bodies are telling us to take action now, before it is too late.

Daily technique for bronchitis

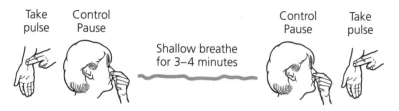

Take pulse Control Pause Shallow breathe for 3–4 minutes Control Pause Take pulse

Repeat this exercise in the morning before breakfast and before you go to bed at night. Monitor your daily progress in the charts for the Weekly Bronchitis Program.

This type of analogy applies to a smoker who ignores a light but persistent cough and thus the stealthy development of lung cancer, or the person with an acute toothache who puts off going to the dentist until it is too late to rescue the tooth. Listen to your body; don't ignore its messages.

It is, naturally, human nature to hope or assume that a problem will go away. Our bodies are far too precious to risk such an optimistic attitude, and we should seek advice at the first sign of something being amiss. It may be an overused cliché, but there is no doubt that prevention is far better than a cure.

Chronic illness is expensive—both personally, and to the taxpayer—and can, in some cases, be very difficult to treat. The longer you leave a health condition, the longer it will take to cure. If you discovered some evidence of dry rot in your home, would you wait until the problem became more extensive before seeking help? Not likely. You'd be worried and possibly annoyed about the expense and nuisance of getting it fixed, but you would be aware that the problem could become worse if you didn't treat it now. Your health is more important than your house—make sure you give it at least the same care. This is why we take illnesses such as bronchitis—and others mentioned in a later chapter—very seriously.

Let's look at the four principal bronchial situations and combinations and consider how to deal with them:

- Bronchitis
- Bronchitis and mild asthma
- Bronchitis and severe asthma
- Bronchitis and emphysema

Typical of the first situation is a cough which can be defined as pure hyperventilation, or overbreathing. But we must not assume that this is just a case of simple bronchitis. There is a very strong chance that other illnesses will emerge and develop in this weakened area of the body. The consistent coughing will have reduced carbon dioxide levels throughout the whole body, and all parts will have been affected. Defense mechanisms, such as asthma, bronchospasm, or the production of excess mucus, will also be evident. Other dangers are pulmonary sclerosis (a hardening of the lung tissue) or fibrosis (the function of the lung is affected when fibrous matter builds up), which can be very serious indeed. Bronchitis can also lead to heart disease, high blood pressure, and a whole host of other conditions stemming from hyperventilation. There is no such thing as "simple" bronchitis.

This chain can be broken, and the first step is to eradicate the bronchitis, so that the danger of other conditions, many of them potentially fatal, is reduced. Throughout this book we are aiming to prove that you have not been saddled with a disease that is unmanageable or irreversible. We can empower you to overcome physical disabilities that can be righted and we urge you to persevere. Take preventive action now, and you can avoid unnecessarily ill health for as long as you live. We are pleased to note that more and more people are seeing a persistent cough as evidence of a problem, rather than just suppressing it with cough medicines or, worse, ignoring it completely. This action could save their lives.

The Anti-Coughing Technique
There is not a finite amount of mucus in your bronchial tubes, as many people imagine. You can cough for days, or

months, or years on end, and your body will still continue to produce mucus, and there will always be something to cough up. The production of mucus is one of your body's defense mechanisms against the loss of carbon dioxide, and mucus is replenished as quickly as it is lost.

Preventing your body from producing too much mucus will stop your cough.

In the grip of an exhausting cough—a common and distressing occurrence for those with bronchitis, asthma, and emphysema—the untrained impulse is to clear your lungs of the mucus that has built up. This sensation is particularly noticeable in the morning. Coughing is the body's natural response to mucus buildup and it is yet another defense mechanism, designed to expel foreign bodies and anything else hampering the breathing process. But these are not normal circumstances. You must learn to resist the urge to cough. Instead, you must learn to control the hyperventilation that has caused the buildup of mucus, and the spasm, in the first place. Medication might help, but not as much as the steps on page 120).

We know that the cough is caused by the damage that hyperventilation has created in the lining of your bronchi. We also know that a spasm of coughing will cause you to overbreathe even more. Coughing spasms can be lengthy and exhausting. Occasionally resorting to a simple over-the-counter cough suppressant may be helpful, but there are more natural means. The anti-cough technique will always bring relief, and you may also be able to avoid coughing spasms entirely by strengthening your immunity to bronchitis. The daily self-care program, which incorporates the Control Pause, will help you do so.

Anti-coughing technique

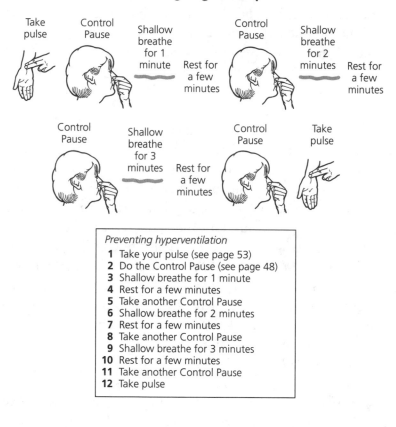

Take pulse — Control Pause — Shallow breathe for 1 minute — Rest for a few minutes — Control Pause — Shallow breathe for 2 minutes — Rest for a few minutes

Control Pause — Shallow breathe for 3 minutes — Rest for a few minutes — Control Pause — Take pulse

Preventing hyperventilation
1 Take your pulse (see page 53)
2 Do the Control Pause (see page 48)
3 Shallow breathe for 1 minute
4 Rest for a few minutes
5 Take another Control Pause
6 Shallow breathe for 2 minutes
7 Rest for a few minutes
8 Take another Control Pause
9 Shallow breathe for 3 minutes
10 Rest for a few minutes
11 Take another Control Pause
12 Take pulse

If you have bronchitis with mild asthma, you can also follow the technique offered on page 79. This technique is useful for asthma symptoms, including coughing.

Bronchitis and severe asthma are the most difficult to treat, and this type of bronchitis must be taken very seriously. Use the anti-coughing technique and refer to the program for severe asthmatics on page 95.

Bronchitis with emphysema is, unhappily, a typical combination. Emphysemics often feel like coughing after the briefest of walks or conversations. This problem takes some time to treat, but it is worth the investment. Start by practicing the anti-coughing technique. Refer also to the sections earlier in this chapter on dealing with emphysema.

You may think that the time spent attempting to relieve a cough is wasteful. We assure you that it is well worth your while. Think of the time and energy spent struggling through coughing fits. Think how they might have impaired your work or affected your colleagues' work. Make this technique a priority, even if it means getting up a little earlier or turning up at work a little bit late.

Use the Anti-Coughing Technique (AT) at the first sign of a cough. It is often easier to stop an asthma attack than it is to arrest and gain control of a coughing fit. In the case of asthma you can always reach for medication, but nothing, except this technique, will stop your coughing. Be patient. Eventually you will be in control.

For existing mucus, you way wonder whether it is better to cough it up or swallow it. We suggest coughing it out, but only when it is comfortable for you to do so. Don't force it, and never use expectorants or any other cough medicines, including herbal remedies, when participating in the Breath Connection program. Try to release your mucus in a single, easy motion, or you will risk further hyperventilation and overbreathing.

8

Breath Connection for Panic Attacks and Stress

Thousands of people who would not describe themselves as being asthmatic endure frightening panic attacks without realizing that hyperventilation—the same cause of asthma— is at the root of their condition. Panic attacks can be incredibly debilitating, and because there is no instant remedy in the form of an inhaler as there is during an asthma attack, it can be even more frightening. Conventional doctors tend to regard panic attacks as brief and physiologically normal responses to stressful situations, and they are largely regarded as being harmless.

Stressful situations can, of course, induce an attack, and an attack is most certainly a natural response by the body to fear or panic. However, for some people, normal, everyday activities can cause an attack. Shopping, using public transportation, taking an elevator, or even just walking into a party can trigger an alarming series of physical responses. Moreover, the fear of an attack can generate serious, deeper psychological debility.

During a panic attack, there may be dizziness, palpitations, chest constriction, and muscle fatigue. For some there are blackouts, a feeling of near suffocation, and even a fear of a heart attack. The attack may pass quickly, and some sufferers may be able to calm themselves by constantly reassuring themselves that they will be all right. But the fact is, the condition that caused the attack—hidden hyperventilation—remains even after the attack has passed. Permanent avoidance of panic attacks can be achieved by following the Breath Connection program.

The urge to take deep breaths at the onset of an attack can be overwhelming, and certainly in the past, doctors and psychologists recommended just that action. One established remedy has been to breathe into a paper bag, and then to inhale from it—a surprising confirmation that during hyperventilation our bodies need carbon dioxide, not great gulps of oxygen.

Counseling, abdominal breathing exercises, and relaxation techniques have often been suggested for the treatment of panic attacks. However, when we hyperventilate, the blood vessels throughout the body—including those feeding the brain and heart—are constricted, and the nervous system is affected. It is unlikely that soothing words, however well-learned, will be of much use to someone fighting for breath in the grip of a sudden attack.

This particular form of what is called hidden hyperventilation and the overbreathing which exists between attacks can be simply addressed by Breath Connection. It is important to realize that a foundation for a severe panic attack is being laid if shallow breathing is not practiced on a day-to-day basis (see exercise on p. 134). As we have said earlier, attacks of this nature are often more worrying and more difficult to deal with than the kind of spasm endured by known asthmatics, who will probably have some form of relief on hand.

Technique for panic attacks

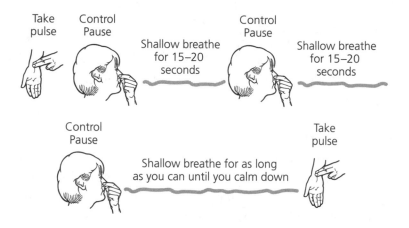

The Technique

1. If you are suffering a panic attack, stop and do the Control Pause three times. Shallow breathe for 15 to 20 seconds between each pause.
2. After the final Control Pause, shallow breathe for as long as you can manage or until you calm down. This can be anything from 5–60 minutes.
3. Do this before entering any situation in which fear might induce an attack, whether it is walking into a room full of strangers or simply facing a crowded street.

This exercise will boost your carbon dioxide level and stave off panic. However frightening it may seem, this sort of problem is normally a mild one. Gaining the confidence to know that you can overcome it will certainly help you to deal with other, more severe problems you may face.

If you cannot stop to practice this technique in the throes

of an attack, keep your mouth closed and try to shallow breathe through your nose.

Before embarking on the Breath Connection exercises in this chapter, you should ascertain whether you are suffering from any of the illnesses in Appendix B. If you do, it will be necessary for you to practice the Breath Connection program under the guidance of a qualified practitioner.

Stress

While panic can sometimes seem, and indeed may be, irrational, most of us have experienced stress and can understand the complicated chain of symptoms that accompany it. Demanding jobs, moving home, family life, relationships, financial problems, emotional pressure, and even joyful events such as Christmas, a wedding, childbirth, or a holiday can burden us with stress. For obvious reasons, divorce or bereavement can be even worse. Many people seek short-term relief with alcohol, nicotine, other drugs, or even food, but all of these can be avoided by following the Breath Connection program.

What Happens When We Are Stressed?

The stress reaction is a natural response to fear. It prepares the body for "fight or flight" by tensing the muscles and constricting the blood vessels. However, because most of the stressful experiences we encounter today do not require us to fight or flee, the body is left in a state of physical tension, which can result in a lowering of immunity, rendering us more susceptible to disease. There are literally dozens of common ailments associated with stress, including recurrent headaches, dizziness, rashes, colds and infections, panic attacks, aches and pains, loss of appetite, compulsive eating, irritability, fatigue, tearfulness, sleep problems, and lack of concentration. As you know from our earlier discussions, Breath Connection has been successful in helping almost all of these conditions. Most importantly, Breath Connection can help you to cope with stress in general.

The Technique

Try to control stress using the Control Pause technique (see page 48), in the following sequence, when you awake in the morning, before lunch, and before going to bed at night.

Daily technique for reducing stress generally

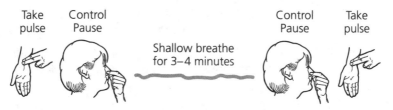

| Take pulse | Control Pause | Shallow breathe for 3–4 minutes | Control Pause | Take pulse |

Try this in the morning (before breakfast), before lunch, and before going to sleep.

If you are confronted with a potentially stressful situation at any other time of the day, a quick Control Pause and some shallow breathing will calm you down and enable you to deal with the situation more effectively. You can still rush to your meeting—only minutes later!

1. Do three Control Pauses, followed by 5-, 10- and then 15- or 20-second intervals.
2. Practice shallow breathing for two to three minutes.
3. Repeat if you do not feel calmer.

Calming technique for dealing with an immediate stressful situation

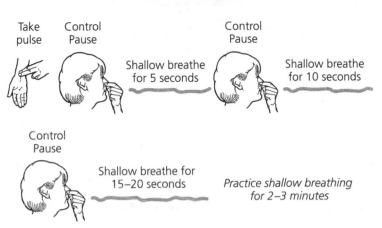

Take pulse

Control Pause

Shallow breathe for 5 seconds

Control Pause

Shallow breathe for 10 seconds

Control Pause

Shallow breathe for 15–20 seconds

Practice shallow breathing for 2–3 minutes

Meditation in the morning or at night can be enormously helpful, and we strongly recommend it. It is, however, seldom practical to meditate in the middle of a busy day. The preceding technique offers one of the best and fastest methods for stress relief that we know. We all live in a world and an environment complicated by choices that would have been unimaginable even to our parents' generation. Ever advancing technology does not, ironically, seem to have simplified our lives. But we can teach ourselves to adapt and cope with stresses and panics in the most natural way. Once again, you can breathe your problems away.

9

Holistic Self-Care for General Well-Being

We may appear to be healthy—with bright eyes, clear skin, shining hair, and strong limbs. We may play tennis or run, work hard all day yet still feel ready to go dancing all night. . . . How appealing the idea of perfect health is. A lucky few do have it—and, sadly, they are just a few! Luck it may seem, but in reality a good deal of subtle self-discipline may underpin that image of effortless total health.

Even if you are one of the lucky ones, don't become over-confident. However well you look, seem, and feel, you can fall prey to illness and it can come as a total shock. The best gymnasiums, cosmetic treatments, and the finest clothes may all contribute to a glorious illusion if, beneath the skin, some-thing is going wrong. The increased stress of modern life, particularly in cities where no one can avoid breathing in toxic fumes, can take an insidious toll. The elimination sys-tem—that complex network which includes the kidneys, liver, and skin as well as the bowel itself—is put under a great deal of pressure in our society, with pollution, food additives and preservatives, increased alcohol intake and smoking, not to mention the number of chemicals that are used to grow even the freshest, healthiest-looking foods. We tend to brush off minor ailments as the result of being rundown or in need of a holiday. Even if we exercise and eat carefully, we can become ill.

Whether you feel healthy now, or suffer from common, niggling health problems, Breath Connection can make a huge difference in the way you look and feel—on and below the surface. Before you embark on a self-care program, check to ensure that you don't suffer from one of the illnesses listed in Appendix B.

DELIA

Delia had never been ill before she contracted a rare form of gland cancer. She was 45 years old. Her husband had been extremely supportive as she experimented with numerous alternative as well as conventional approaches to her disease. They even traveled to the Philippines, where they had read healers could perform miracles with cancer patients. Sadly, nothing worked for her. When Delia first came to us she could not walk to the second floor of our clinic. She was barely sleeping, her hair had all but dropped out, and she was so stressed and emotional that she was constantly tearful. Her tumor, she had been told, was the size of a fist. As well as affecting her hair, the chemotherapy and radiation had made Delia look like a woman of 60 instead of one in her prime.

After three months of working with Breath Connection on a special anticancer program Delia's tumor vanished. She regained her appetite and energy and slept well again. Soon she was ready to enjoy a proper holiday. Her previous doctors could only say that they must have been mistaken in their earlier diagnosis.

Tragically, two years later, when she was still feeling fit and well, and perhaps against her better judgment, she was persuaded to undergo a different course of treatment and she died soon afterward.

In almost all cases of cancer, patients are already in terminal stages of their illness when they come to us. However, the Breath Connection program can extend their lives by up to two years and also enhance the quality of that remaining time. All Breath Connection practitioners wish that patients would seek to recondition their breathing much sooner and thus reduce the danger of serious illness taking a fatal grip.

Monitoring Your Health

The importance of regularly monitoring your state of health via the Breath Connection program cannot be overstated. It will reflect the actual state of your health (which may differ from how well you think you are). If your Control Pause (see page 48) drops suddenly, you have been given a very clear signal that preventative measures are required. If you suspect this change might be stress-related, turn at once to the program for stress on page 125. The importance of this monitoring system cannot be overstated. You can put to rest any fears that terrible illness might be lurking round the corner by changing and maintaining your Control Pause. Checked regularly, it is an extremely accurate guide to your physical condition. If your Control Pause reaches and remains at 50 or 60, you will not suffer from degenerative disease. It's that simple.

This might seem like a very bold assertion, but it is based on Professor Buteyko's research in Russia involving literally millions of cases. He found that no single person with a CP of 50 to 60 had degenerative illness. This statistic, based on years of research, is enormously reassuring.

But our self-care program is not just about prevention. It has been devised to help well people to improve their health further, which will allow them to get even more out of life.

With a 50 to 60 Control Pause, all of your body systems—immune, hormonal, digestive, elimination, respiratory, cardiovascular, and the others—will be functioning properly. You will have more energy, need less sleep, and find your natural weight. The glowing good looks that often accompany such a state are a happy bonus. By following our program, your health will no longer be a vague area of mystery, confusion, and contradiction but something that you understand and experience, and it is measurable!

What Your Control Pause Tells You

Most people have long been aware that exercise and a well-balanced diet—with plenty of fresh fruit and vegetables and clean water—make a huge difference to health and well-being. But we are only just beginning to understand how incorrect breathing can negate the benefits of other sensible habits. If you find that your Control Pause is lower than 50, you should correct things by following the basic Breath Connection program. If—to your surprise and alarm—it is down toward 20, you should start immediate preventative measures to avert the risk of some form of degenerative disease taking hold later.

If you find you have a low Control Pause, don't panic. The problem will probably be rooted in your weakest target area. All of us have weak points or systems in our bodies, the result, usually, of genetic inheritance. During the course of your life this weakness can be exacerbated by poor nutrition, overbreathing, stress, overwork, or a variety of other factors. Genetic research increasingly shows that there is such a thing as a cystic fibrosis gene, or a cancer gene. If you are born with such a gene, you will always have a vulnerability where that particular disease is concerned, although it is by no means inevitable that you will come to suffer from it. However, something such as poor nutrition could activate the program for that gene. Similarly, if your area of weakness is your circulatory system, or heart, stress or hyperventilation could cause you to suffer from a related illness. But, if you eat sensibly, exercise, manage your stress levels, and avoid hyperventilation, the danger of heart disease is dramatically diminished. The reverse is also true.

If your Control Pause is as low as 10 to 15, it is likely that you already suffer from some illness, although it may, at present, be hidden. Such conditions as diabetes, low blood pressure, tuberculosis, and even tumors can lie silent and dormant for a long time before something, perhaps a general malaise, alerts you that something is wrong. You may even have experienced some specific symptoms, without realizing what they indicated. In a few cases—that of motor neurone disease and some cancers, for example—by the time you experience symptoms and seek advice it will be too late for conventional medical help. The sad truth is that some people can have a CP as low as 15 and still feel energetic and well. It is vitally important to remember that good health goes beyond surface performance. You need to learn to listen to your body, and to pay attention to any change in normal performance or function, such as sudden headaches, recurrent breathing problems, pain of any description, or even just a general malaise. And the best measure of what is going on beneath the skin is the Control Pause technique.

Professor Buteyko says that there are almost no exceptions to the link between a person's CP and his or her general health. A person might be apparently strong, muscular, and young, but if that person's Control Pause is only 10 or 12, he or she is very ill in some way. Alarming as this truth might seem, it has to be considered.

Once again, a very low Control Pause is not cause for panic. Instead it is a welcome warning that action—immediate action—is required. The cause of your hidden hyperventilation can be reversed and we are here to show you how. You can make great strides with this book alone, but seeking guidance from a Breath Connection expert will probably hasten the reversal of your symptoms. Everyone responds better with individual help and encouragement. Dieters tend to be much more successful with group support or counseling, just as most of us feel more inspired to exercise with the help of a personal trainer, who can tailor our programs to suit our needs. Complementary medicine has always focused on the special needs of the individual, and we have seen how effective this approach can be.

With a healthy Control Pause of 50 to 60, you have perfect balanced breathing and you can relax, knowing that you are in no danger of asthma, emphysema, bronchitis, allergies, cancers, or any of the other conditions that the Breath Connection can deal with. But things can change, particularly if there is a tendency within your family to fall prey to certain types of illness, so it is wise to be watchful and have your health checked from time to time, and regularly monitor your control pause.

People with a Control Pause between 20 and 40 seconds may have already developed some of the lesser defense mechanisms against overbreathing, such as a blocked nose, susceptibility to colds and flu, snoring, and weight gain. This means you already have moderate hyperventilation and a few simple exercises will help to remedy this.

Daily technique for self-care program for healthy people

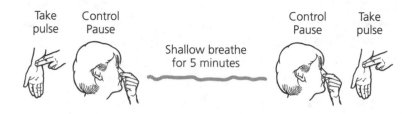

The Technique

1. As a general technique, take your pulse (see page 53) and do the Control Pause.
2. Shallow breathe for five minutes before doing another CP and then take your pulse again. Do this first thing in the morning and before going to bed.
3. Create a weekly self-care chart for yourself (see pages 243–252 for examples). It will guide you through the program and you will find it helpful to document your progress and note your improvement.

Another exercise is particularly helpful when you under stress, mentally tired, or have spent too long in front of a computer screen.

Technique to relieve a stressful situation

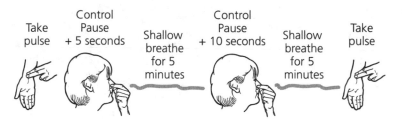

1. Take your pulse (see page 53).
2. Do the Control Pause, plus five seconds.
3. Shallow breathe for five minutes.
4. Take another CP, plus 10 seconds.
5. Shallow breathe for a further five minutes.
6. Take your pulse again.

A slightly longer exercise is recommended when you have a cold, hayfever, or flu. Do this three times a day before meals. For some people it may be advisable to reduce food intake by as much as half—but see Chapter 12. Clearly these measures would not be appropriate for an anorexic, or someone with blood sugar problems, but most people—particularly if they have a cold or flu—will benefit from eating smaller amounts without actually skipping meals. A light and simple diet puts much less strain on a network of systems already working hard to overcome a temporary disorder. Your body needs all available energy to fight illness, and you don't want to waste this precious energy on digesting a heavy meal.

1. Take your pulse.
2. Do the Control Pause.

Technique for colds, flu, and hayfever

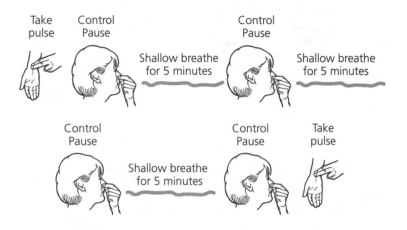

Take pulse | Control Pause | Shallow breathe for 5 minutes | Control Pause | Shallow breathe for 5 minutes

Control Pause | Shallow breathe for 5 minutes | Control Pause | Take pulse

3. Shallow breathe for five minutes.
4. Another Control Pause.
5. Shallow breathe for five minutes.
6. Do another Control Pause.
7. Shallow breathe for another five minutes.
8. Do the Control Pause.
9. Take your pulse.

Before any sport, aerobics, working out in the gym, or other physical exercise, you should take your pulse, do a Control Pause, shallow breathe for five minutes, and then repeat the exercise after physical exercise and sport.

Keep your mouth closed throughout and, if necessary, find ways of reminding yourself to do so. Some people find it helpful to place little messages or even tape up posters in places where they practice the exercises, rather like those who are trying to lose weight tape pictures of obese people to

Technique for before and after physical exercise and sport

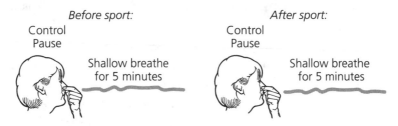

Before sport:
Control
Pause

Shallow breathe
for 5 minutes

After sport:
Control
Pause

Shallow breathe
for 5 minutes

the fridge door, or write stern little deterrents where they know they will see them.

Points to Remember

• These points apply to all of the exercises and techniques in the self-care program.

• Always keep your mouth closed at night, particularly if you snore. This will lead to a better quality of sleep. Keep it sealed with tape at work, in the car, when exercising, when you are alone, or whenever you can manage it. Affix tape vertically rather than horizontally if the latter feels too restricting.

• Put up reminder messages or stickers wherever these may be helpful. Don't feel embarrassed—tell people that you are fighting a respiratory condition, or otherwise improving your health. You may start a trend!

• Sleep in your left side (see page 52).

• Don't go to bed unless you are tired.

• Avoid dairy foods and too much protein, junk food, tea, coffee, and sugar, all of which put strain on the excretory system and can encourage the production of mucus, or encourage hyperventilation.

- Do not eat a protein meal at night
- Eat only when you are hungry, not just because it is a certain time of day (see page 189).
- Increase physical activity. While you are on the Breath Connection program, take the stairs instead of the elevator, for example, and walk to the shops instead of driving. Gardening, jogging, and even housework are all beneficial forms of exercise. Golfers should walk rather than take a golf cart.
- Almost all sport is recommended. Simply remember to check your Control Pause first and 15 minutes after you have finished and to keep your mouth closed. A lower CP after exercise indicates that you have lost too much carbon dioxide through overbreathing, so you should reduce your pace or the duration of your sporting activity until you have reconditioned your breath. Once you have learned to breathe the Breath Connection way, you will enjoy your sport or exercise much more. Swimmers, in particular, should remember to breathe through the nose only. If you want to go faster, hold your face under water long enough to take more strokes. Just don't open your mouth when you breathe.
- After driving for any distance, reading, watching TV, walking—whether on the street, field, or pitch—in fact, after any activity, get into the habit of checking your Control Pause at regular intervals so that you can see if a pattern emerges. It is helpful to see which activities cause it to rise, and which cause it to lower. It's a simple habit of self-monitoring to get into, and an instant health check.

Finally, the Breath Connection program involves the following:

- Breathing in less air than you have been used to in the past.
- Keeping your mouth closed all the time, except when eating, drinking, or talking. Tape up your mouth as often as you can and certainly when alone.
- Continuing to use steroid medication if you are using it, and retaining your preventer. Don't cease or decrease your medication until you get the OK from your Breath Connection practitioner and your own doctor.
- Avoiding overeating, oversleeping, or sleeping on your back. Get into the habit of sleeping on your left side and practice Breath Connection exercises regularly. If you are using a bronchodilator, you will reach a point where you will have no symptoms and no longer require it.

10

Breath Connection for Asthmatic Children

Any parent whose child suffers from asthma will tell you that the sight and sound of his or her small son or daughter straining to overcome an asthma attack is the most frightening and distressing experience there is.

Your child is in pain, and virtually beyond the reach of the comfort of your hands, arms, or voice, and your sense of helplessness may be compounded by sorrow if you are aware that asthma is an inherited condition. Worst of all, your child's life is in danger.

You might not suffer from asthma, but perhaps a parent or grandparent did. Many of us carry the gene that predisposes people to asthma. If you suffer from asthma, your child has a 50 percent chance of inheriting the condition. If both you and your partner are asthmatic, this figure soars to 90 percent. But inheriting the gene does not mean that your child will go on to suffer with asthma. With diet and lifestyle management, asthma can be prevented.

Not all children suffer from severe asthma. If they are lucky, they may suffer from the odd mild asthma attack, or some of the related conditions, such as eczema or hay fever. Severe asthma is quite different. Children with severe asthma may have been doomed to a lifetime of restricted physical activity, a constant fear of a sudden attack, general breath-lessness, drug dependency, social unease, and a general inability to embrace life's potential.

Professor Buteyko asserts that, whatever their genetic inheritance, all asthmatics hyperventilate. The sooner that parents can train their children not to do so, the fewer asth-matics there will be. Even if your child has severe asthma, a little concentrated work—which most children find fun—and some easy adjustments to your family lifestyle can pre-vent your child from enduring the many deprivations of an asthmatic life. Once your child has stopped hyperventilation and has become accustomed to a safe and sensible diet, he or she will be much safer. High stress levels, or bouts of flu, may bring occasional relapses, but breath control will enable bal-ance to be restored quickly. Asthma is a defense mechanism against the body's loss of carbon dioxide. If there is a correct balance of oxygen and carbon dioxide in the blood, geneti-cally weakened areas will become stronger and less suscepti-ble to problems.

Breath Connection for Children

Many children, happily, grow out of asthma, particularly after they have learned not to hyperventilate. But this is no reason for them, or you, to endure the worries and panics that asthma can bring. If your child suffers from regular, seri-ous asthma attacks, the constant hyperventilation may have led to more serious illness, such as diabetes, epilepsy, or can-cer. The earlier you begin Breath Connection for your child, the more chance you have of preventing these conditions from developing. If your child managed to fight asthma at a relatively young age, the Breath Connection program should still be undertaken to ensure that the rest of the body is in a balanced, healthy state. Furthermore, and less seriously, training your children early will help to prevent problems such as chronic blocked noses and snoring. On a more positive note, Breath Connection will enhance your child's powers of concentration, which will help him or her to cope with stress and pressure in the future.

Is It Safe?

Parents who are concerned that their child might be troubled or traumatized by the Breath Connection program can rest assured that the vast majority of children find it great fun. Children are even more receptive than adults to the retraining methods, not surprising, perhaps, in light of the fact that their bad habits have had a shorter period of time in which to develop. Children tend to be un-self-conscious about learning techniques and treat them as a new game. The program offers parents a wonderful opportunity to create strong foundations for their child's health by training them to breathe correctly.

In the past, many doctors diagnosed any child with the slightest wheeze or touch of bronchitis as asthmatic. Drugs to treat the condition were duly prescribed. Soon, these children really did become asthmatic, as their breathing deepened, and drug intake necessarily increased. Professor Buteyko maintains that if your child is wheezy, you should not attempt to deal with the situation by giving him or her drugs. You need to train your child to breathe correctly. The wheeze itself is not dangerous—in fact, it acts as a message from the body that something might be wrong. Only when there is obvious and serious breathing difficulty should your child be given asthma medication.

Sometimes the body switches to another defense mechanism, such as eczema, one of the same family of diseases that includes asthma and a number of other allergic conditions. Some children grow out of these conditions, but it is not a good idea to wait until they do so. Professor Buteyko observed that a whole host of conditions are linked to hyperventilation, and the longer your child suffers from asthma or another problem that indicates deep, incorrect breathing, the more likely he or she is to develop one. Asthma can kill, but it can also be contained.

BARRY

On rare occasions, our advice is not enough, and we admit to feeling deep frustration and despair when this occurs. Barry was a 15-year-old with severe asthma. Before his mother brought him to us, he had been under the care of one of the country's leading respiratory specialists, but this had not prevented a frightening respiratory arrest in a hospital bathroom one night. This attack marked Barry's fourth serious crisis in four years.

Barry's mother, Sonia, had ensured that he had all the nebulizers he needed at home, in her car, and in his schoolbag, but none of these precautions comforted her much. Barry was very overweight, was bullied at school, and was unable to take part in sports or games. He was a sluggish and understandably unhappy young man. Sonia came to us without consulting Barry's existing doctors because she feared that they would be discouraging about and skeptical of Breath Connection. But Barry made extremely good progress and soon stopped needing nebulizers, taking only two or three puffs of an inhaler each day. But he simply refused to take oral steroids because he was under the impression that they were the cause of his obesity.

The irony is that he would have needed to take only two or three tablets each day, rather than the 40 or so a day that he had been given on his many emergency hospital admissions. If he had taken small doses of steroids, Barry could have coped with respiratory problems, such as a slight cough or the flu, with ease. Instead, he was hospitalized time and again for these problems, and at the hospital he was forced to take very high doses.

During one of his hospital visits, Barry told his specialist about Breath Connection. His consultant's response was to tell Barry about a wonder drug that would soon be available to deal with all of his problems. It was a drug that would have all the advantages of steroids, but no side effects. Barry was so keen to believe this, just as he had been keen to believe that he would grow out of his asthma, that he refused to take part in Breath Connection exercises from that moment onward.

He was no longer a small child, and Sonia felt unable to force him to continue. So, Barry returned to using his nebulizer four or five times a day and went back to his routine of regular hospital visits. We had not been able to convince him that small doses of correctly administered steroids would help him, and that he would, eventually, have no dependency on them as his asthma symptoms disappeared. Nor could we convince him that every aspect of his life—both now and in the future—would improve if he stuck with us.

The wonder drug on which Barry pinned his hopes never had the desired effect and he remains severely asthmatic and severely overweight—an unhappy exis-

tence for an unhappy young man. This sad story under-
lines how important it is to take asthmatic children to
Breath Connection as soon as possible.

The Breath Connection program can significantly reduce symptoms of asthma in children and offer guidance for parents in order to help them cope. If parents are asthmatic themselves, there is even more reason to attend. Our program can train children from an early age to balance their breathing and to reduce the likelihood of developing disease in later life.

All parents want the best for their children—a good education, friends, holidays, toys, and nice clothes—but your greatest gift to your child is a foundation of good health. Without this, every aspect of a child's later life will be restricted. Elderly people may expect to have illness or disability of one form or another and, although we at Breath Connection would never advise it, it seems somehow more acceptable to allow an unhealthy state to continue. But for children who are ill, the prospect of a lifetime of ill health and disability is tragic. You as a parent can do a great deal to prevent this situation from developing, and we can show you how.

Keeping Informed
Correct information is always a good start. If, until now, your asthmatic child has been given steroids and bronchodilators, his or her symptoms may be quite minor. Don't be fooled. Your child is not free from asthma, the symptoms of the condition have merely been suppressed. The asthma exists, and its root cause, hyperventilation, must be addressed

before real progress can be achieved. More asthma medication is prescribed today than it was 50 years ago, and yet the incidence of childhood asthma has soared. If your child does grow out of asthma attacks, but continues to overbreathe, his or her body will find another way of coping with the reduced levels of carbon dioxide, possibly by contracting a more serious illness. Even mild asthmatics should be encouraged to take part in a program of counterattack. The fact that your child already has asthma means that his or her health is on a slippery downward slope. Its cause is hyperventilation.

But this condition can be reversed. Your child will be able to participate fully in school life, with friends, with family, and all of the systems of his or her body will function properly. The danger of more serious illness later in life will be removed or reduced dramatically. You, in turn, will be able to relax and stop worrying about your child's future health—and you'll probably become a more relaxed and efficient parent. Whenever you are worried, you can monitor your child's progress by participating in the STEPS program (see page 149).

At the Hale Clinic, we have felt a great sense of fulfillment to see children helped by the Breath Connection program. Somehow, seeing childhood disorders corrected is one of the most exciting aspects of Breath Connection.

Children who have been diagnosed as being asthmatic should follow the subsequent program. Those with a cough and bronchitis should practice the shallow breathing exercises and a STEPS program (see page 149). We will try to make all of these activities fun, and you can do so at home as well. Charts can be filled in with colored markers or stars to record progress, and small rewards for a job well done will appeal to most children's sense of competition.

For simplicity, we have described the child as "he," but the guidelines do, obviously, apply to girls as well!

Here's how you should begin:

- Make sure your child uses his medication correctly. He should only use a bronchodilator if he his having difficulty breathing. Ensure that steroids are being taken correctly (see page 67).
- Learn as much as you can about the drugs that your child has been prescribed (see pages 59–72). If you still have questions, don't be afraid to ask your doctor to explain things further.
- Teach your child to do the Control Pause. Make it into a game.
- Stop using a peak flow meter. To assess your child's condition at any time, use the Control Pause. Listen to him when he tells you how he is feeling.
- Teach your child to keep his mouth closed when he breathes, and to keep it shut unless he is talking, eating, or drinking. Tape his mouth at night. Tape yours, too, if it helps to inspire him!
- Reduce or eliminate chocolate, cola drinks, ice cream, dairy products, and junk foods. Apart from the fact they can ruin teeth and lead to weight problems, they often have little or no nutrition and can be hard to digest. Any foods that are difficult to digest increase the body's need for carbon dioxide. Furthermore, fizzy drinks create "wind," and a further loss of carbon dioxide. Don't allow a high-protein meal within two or three hours of bedtime.
- Encourage him to sleep on his left side. If necessary, prop him up with pillows to prevent him from turning. Check that all is well several times during the night.

147

STEPS

STEPS should only be undertaken by children suffering from asthma or bronchitis. If, in addition to these problems, they have any of the conditions asterisked in Appendix B, they should be taken to see a Breath Connection expert rather than relying on a self-care program. A Breath Connection practitioner will be able to advise on complications and will be able to help your child to achieve excellent results. Any children with diseases other than asthma and bronchitis should be taken to see a Breath Connection expert rather than relying on a self-care program. Always check with us first, to see if we can be of assistance. There is every chance that we can help with existing illnesses, and we should certainly be able to help reduce the need for drugs. If your child suffers from a condition that involves unavoidable medication, we can provide a form of treatment to run alongside.

If your child is younger than five, it is best to attend a Breath Connection course to learn what you can do to help him. Then explain why he is doing the exercises. Try to help him to understand that taking in too much air is making him ill. It may be hard for such a young child to grasp the idea, but it is important that it is carefully explained. Never force or push a young child if he is hesitant. Instead, make it into a game, and try to ensure that he sees the exercises as a form of play. Tape the mouths of the whole family, and cut silly shapes for each family member. If the whole family is involved in the process, it is unlikely that your child will feel that he is being singled out for some kind of strange treatment.

Problems for your older child can be dealt with by following STEPS. Remember that asthma-related problems, such as a blocked nose, a cough, or shortness of breath, can cause your child to tire easily. Don't push him too far. Be gentle and patient, and the results will soon be evident.

The Technique

1. Start by taking your child's pulse. Don't worry if it seems to be a little high. Children often have higher pulses than adults.
2. Ask him to stand with his mouth closed. If his nose is blocked, ask him to breathe using a corner of his mouth only.
3. Ask him to breathe out through his nose if possible. He should hold his breath out and pinch his nose between his thumb and forefinger.
4. Ask your child to pretend that he is walking underwater, with his mouth and nose closed, and to do this for as long as he can. Count his steps and make a note of it for his chart. Encourage him as he walks.
5. As soon as your child starts to feel uncomfortable, he should begin to breathe in again shallowly. Tell him to resist the temptation to gulp when he releases his nose. Join in with him if you think it would be helpful.
6. Once he has completed his steps, he should continue to breathe shallowly with his mouth shut. Any child who began this exercise with a blocked nose will probably find that it is becoming less congested.
7. Ask your child to sit still and breathe gently—like a small mouse—for three or four minutes. To check that he is doing this correctly, put a finger under his nose to feel the airflow. It should feel very, very light. Teach your child to do this at the first sign of any asthma problem.

8. Take his pulse at the end of the STEPS program and look at his chart so that you can monitor his progress.

STEPS program for asthmatic children

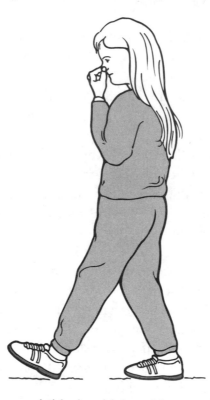

Ideally, your child should be able to take 120 steps, which is the equivalent of a Control Pause of 50 to 60 seconds. One hundred twenty steps means that he is unlikely to suffer from asthma. Don't worry unduly if he is well below that ideal 120 steps. With gentle perseverance, he can reach that figure. It is a good idea to do one daily Control Pause with your child as another way of measuring to see if his asthma is clearing or becoming worse.

Now let's imagine the day of a typical parent with a typically asthmatic child who has woken with asthma symptoms. The STEPS exercises should be performed before resorting to a bronchodilator, although this can be offered if STEPS does not work to relieve the symptoms. If it does work, congratulate your child—and yourself!

Repeat the exercise two or more times throughout the day. Quite soon, your child should be able to manage by himself if you are busy, but remind him to note or remember the number of steps he took so that these can be added to the chart. It is good for him to learn to take responsibility for his health. When your child goes to school, make sure that he has taken the required dose of steroids, if appropriate. But remind him to use his inhaler or bronchodilator only if he cannot control his symptoms with correct breathing. Ask him to keep his mouth closed whenever possible. Naturally, you will need to speak to his teachers at school to explain his problems and to enlist their support.

It is unlikely that your child will be embarrassed about his asthma. So many children suffer from it these days that at playtime children often line up for their puffers, which have been entrusted to the teacher at the start of the day. Some puffers are even designed in the shapes of animals and footballs to make them more user-friendly. We don't know whether to be heartened or discouraged by this! It all helps to reduce the stigma of asthma, but it does show that a whole industry has grown up around the manufacture of a device that should not be necessary in the first place. However, at this point in time, as many as one in four children uses a puffer or is developing asthma symptoms.

A welcome upshot of this is that few children have problems keeping their mouths closed, using tape or puffers, or otherwise following their programs in public places. Not only are there so many of them in the same boat, but they will do almost anything to be able to rush around the playground normally. Adults are far more likely to feel awkward.

After school, your child should perform the next exercise. Ask him to walk across the largest room in the house, or around the garden, if possible. His mouth should be closed. He should walk slowly at first, and then gradually increase his pace over two or three minutes. This will help him to get into the habit of walking—and, ultimately, running—with his mouth closed. Repeat the exercise two to four times, gradually increasing the time your child spends on it until he can actually run fast for 20 or 30 seconds without breathlessness. After each STEPS exercise, your child should be able to increase the time he spends walking or running, even if it is only by a few seconds. Whenever possible, stay near your child so that you can observe and note his progress.

Do the STEPS program with your child two or three times, about an hour before he goes to bed. Then tape his mouth and ensure that he falls asleep in the correct position. When you check on him during the night, replace the tape if it has been loosened. Gently close his mouth if it has fallen open.

If he has moved onto his back, slip him back onto his left side. If your child has had a history of having asthma problems at a particular time of the night, set your alarm so that you can be there with him just before that old danger point. Wake him gently if he is wheezy or if his breathing is too heavy and deep. It may sound unkind—and not much fun for you, either—but this will stop him from being violently wakened by an asthma attack. Settle your child back to sleep, cuddle him, and wait with him until he is sleeping calmly again.

The STEPS program can be adapted to fit in with whatever interest your child has. If he enjoys computer games, tell him that his asthma is an invader that has to be zapped. He could even put his daily chart onto his computer and fill it in himself on screen. A younger child could be encouraged to think of his asthma as a naughty elf who came to visit, but must now go home. Do whatever you know to be appropriate for your particular child, and do so at the earliest possible age and stage. It is important he understands that by taking part in the exercises and other aspects of the program, he is taking control of the unwelcome illness that upsets his body and stops him from doing the things he enjoys best in life.

Maintenance for Asthmatic Children

Once your child has reached 120 steps, continue practicing regularly two to three times per day for a few months. Then practice once a day for a few months and then practice once a week indefinitely.

This will enable you to monitor your child's health on a weekly basis using the STEPS program. If the number of steps starts to decrease significantly, then temporarily increase the steps program to two to three times per day until your child can reach 120 steps again.

Preventative Self-Care for Well-Being

Even if you have no reason to suppose that your child has inherited the asthma gene, and even if he suffers from no obvious respiratory illness, you will likely want to do everything in your power to encourage the kind of good health that will set him in good stead for the rest of his life. You can start by involving him in a program of preventive measures and exercise from about the age of five.

Unlike most adults, children are learning all the time—sometimes unconsciously, and sometimes with an infectious sense of wonder and enthusiasm. So take little notice if they grizzle briefly when you introduce the new routines. All children soon get used to them and usually enjoy the novelty of a new way of doing things. It is much easier to reeducate a child to breathe properly than it is to change the habits of an adult. You don't have to overstress the health angle if you feel that this aspect of the program may be a turnoff for your young Mister or Miss Cool.

Hyperventilation can affect any child at any age, and it can program a child to be vulnerable to many serious illnesses later in life. We cannot make this point too often, or too emphatically. We heartily recommend that you begin the program to protect your child's future.

The Technique

Here is the basic plan:

- Encourage him to keep his mouth closed unless speaking, eating, or drinking.
- Tape his mouth at night. As we mentioned earlier, there are now tapes with animal faces and all manner of devices that make this simple step an unthreatening game. If it's fun, your child will take part. Encourage him to sleep on the left side.
- Keep dairy foods off the table, and avoid carbonated drinks and sugar, especially early in the morning. Find deli-

cious, healthy substitutes for treats. There are many sources of calcium, other than dairy products, and you should encourage your child to eat plenty of them (see page 192).

• Encourage your child to keep his mouth closed during sports or games. If this proves difficult, try to steer him toward less strenuous outdoor activity until he is able to do so.

• Keep a close watch on all your child's breathing patterns.

• Do the Control Pause (see page 48) with him at least three or four times a day, even after he has become used to performing it by himself. It will be useful for you to observe any fluctuations, and when his levels drop, you will be alerted to take him to a Breath Connection practitioner.

• All of these measures will help your child to perform better at school, and be happier, as well as healthier. You'll be pushing at an open door as he sees for himself how much more he is enjoying every aspect of his life.

• Please note that the STEPS program is just for children with asthma or bronchitis.

Mouth Taping

A word here about the issue of mouth taping, which some parents consider to be a controversial technique. Some parents need to be persuaded to follow this advice and have to be disabused of the idea that they are being cruel to be kind. Mouth taping is not cruel. There is no pain whatsoever involved in the gentle application of a light tape. Furthermore, it is lifted off, rather than fiercely pulled, like an adhesive strip on an elbow or a grazed knee. Children tend not to be restricted by it, particularly if they have been used to wearing it at home during the day and see that their parents have also placed a strip across their own lips. Tape should always be placed vertically rather than horizontally, so that you child can easily remove it if he feels uncomfortable.

If you feel like you are imprisoning your child by using the micropore tape as he sleeps, just remember that your child can easily remove it for himself if he feels uncomfortable. Chances are that he will slip quickly into a calm and restorative sleep, and the tape will be in place the next morning. Some parents wait until their child has drifted into sleep before applying the little strip to close their mouths. That, too, is just fine.

CARL

Carl was 13 and crazy about surfing. He was determined not to let his asthma prevent him from enjoying it. He carried three Bricanol inhalers whenever he was near the waves—one strung around his neck, one in a pocket of his swimming trunks, and one taped to his surfboard. After two weeks of customized and strenuous Breath Connection exercises designed to build up his carbon dioxide levels and beat hyperventilation, Carl was able to give up all of his medication. His father, a businessman, gave a lunch party for all of the members of his staff who wanted to learn more about the balanced breathing techniques that had saved his son.

The Severely Asthmatic Child

Severely asthmatic children will have had to be hospitalized at least once because of their asthma. Undoubtedly, you were frightened by any attack that led to hospitalization and are determined that such an attack will never occur again. This is what you must do.

First of all, ask yourself why it happened. Think carefully. Was it hyperventilation? A lack of steroids, particularly as your child's condition became critical? Almost certainly your child was given massive doses of bronchodilator drugs (nebulizers) and put on oxygen for some time after his admission. When you were with him, did you have the correct information and the right drugs on hand so that you could insist that the dosage was correct for him?

No one wants to be pessimistic, but if an emergency does occur, we do feel that you should be there to inform his carers about his previous conditions and actually insist that you have a small dose of oral steroids ready for him to take when the need arises. You need to be in charge and should not have to wait for well-meaning, but possibly misinformed, doctors to decide your child's fate. Doctors normally respect the health records that diabetics carry with them, and the same should apply to asthmatics. A smaller dose of steroids, regularly administered, is likely to be much more effective than huge, emergency doses for any asthmatic—adult or child.

Here is an example of the same type of concept. Sunlight can, in moderation, be very beneficial. Too much of it, too quickly, can be extremely harmful. Steroids are much the same. A little, moderate dose is fine. Too much, and it puts enormous strain on the system.

Be firm and insist on supervising the drugs that your child is given during an emergency, and the rate at which the dosage is administered. Oral steroids should only be necessary if a single puff of Ventolin does not bring relief. One tablet, chewed, with a drink of warm water, should help. Don't allow another one to be administered for an hour or two. Then keep going until the child is clearly more comfortable. Don't worry too much about oxygen. The air around you has enough, and he will not need to be given any more. Later, ensure that your child only takes steroids when there is obvious distress. Seeing that his breathing is regulated is the main thing, so don't let yourself be bamboozled into agreeing to large doses of unnecessary drugs.

When your child is safely back at home, try to keep to your normal routine. Stick to his exercises, and make sure that his diet is sensible. Don't push him to eat if he has no appetite, and don't be tempted to put rewards such as chocolate bars in his school lunchbox. You are likely to feel so relieved he is on the mend that you will give into any demand, but be firm! Apples, bananas, honey, cereal bars, and other such things can be just as delicious.

When he is ready to begin school, continue with your discipline and remind him to stick to the "mouth-closed" routines. This shouldn't be a contentious request, since the very recent memory of his crisis will still be fresh in his mind and he will want to do anything to avoid that trauma again. Quietly tell his teachers about the attack so that they can be particularly observant. Remind them that however plaintive he might be, he should not be allowed to participate in sports or organized games quite yet. He may also need his teacher's encouragement and reminders to keep his mouth shut. He should be allowed to keep his puffer in his pocket at this time, rather than hand it over to a teacher. You will have told him when and how to use it.

Remind your child to take his bronchodilator when he needs it—not when anyone else tells him to. Ensure that he has one or two tablets of oral steroids in his bag, and remind him how and when to use them.

After school, collect your child in the usual way and make sure that you behave as if things were quite normal again. Subtly, however, you should encourage him to continue with his breathing exercises, and not feed him until he is hungry. Without making a great deal of fuss, you must spend extra time with him, especially before he goes to bed at night, to note his changing condition. Open the window as he gets sleepy, and make sure that his mouth is taped and that he is in the right position for restful sleep. Check on him up to five times during the night while he is still in recovery from a severe attack.

Refuse any offers of antiflu vaccines or any other conventional safeguards for the time being. You are doing well enough, and he does not need a vaccine that might weaken his immune system and trigger a further attack. Dismiss any offers of techniques that are based upon increasing the lung capacity of your child or methods that claim to clear mucus. By now, you know that mucus is a friendly defense mechanism.

We are in the process of converting your child's severe asthma to mild asthma. You've been through and weathered a crisis. You are on course, and it's important that you don't let anyone misdirect you.

Summary for All Parents

- Introduce the Breath Connection program as a game, which will help your child to take control of his condition.
- Where appropriate, do the STEPS exercise three times a day with your child, especially before bed.
- Ensure that your child's mouth is closed when he sleeps. Use micropore tape (see page 51), if necessary.

See that he sleeps correctly, propped up on his left-hand side.

- Avoid giving foods that we have warned against (see page 191).
- Follow the self-care program so that your child can learn the best habits in the best possible environment— the family home.
- Congratulate yourself—you are doing wonderful work!

11

Breath of Life

By now you are aware of the dangers of taking in too much air, or hyperventilating. In this chapter, we go a little deeper into the thinking behind this central, essential principle. We explain in more detail why unbalanced breathing can be so harmful and why it sets the stage for a whole host of health problems.

In some circumstances, Professor Buteyko was able to offer a clear explanation of how overbreathing damages specific bodily functions and systems, why it becomes the vehicle or channel for certain disorders. In other cases, the professor noted an empirical link between hyperventilation and illness, in that when a patient's breathing became balanced, the disease disappeared even though there was no precise physiological explanation for this.

The idea that carbon dioxide is at best a waste gas and at worst a poisonous one has become so fixed that until now minimal research into its uses and importance has taken place. One of our great hopes is that this book will inspire further research into the role that this natural gas can play in alleviating a huge range of disorders. Some readers may still wonder how something as simple and automatic as breathing could possibly be at the root of so many illnesses. While it is fairly obvious how incorrect breathing can affect respiratory disorders, you may find it hard to see how carbon dioxide deprivation can account for a raft of other conditions, ranging from angina to varicose veins.

Think of it in this way: Our planet's atmosphere is made up of many gases, primarily carbon dioxide and oxygen. Changes in the balance of these gases over the centuries have led to huge environmental disruption. Humans have also evolved and developed over the centuries, and not always at the same pace as the radical environmental changes. Shifts in the balance of these important gases in the environment affect us all. It is a great pity that more medical research has not been devoted to addressing the importance of the way we breathe and the relationship between the two key gases that we require to do so. There has been a huge lack of research into the way that our body systems respond to these gases and how our changing environment may have affected our overall health. Breathing, oxygen, and carbon dioxide hold the answers to many of the illnesses that have baffled doctors and scientists for many years.

Those of you who already suffer from asthma, emphysema, bronchitis, or any of the other disorders listed in Appendix B may only be interested in dealing with your diagnosed disease. But the Breath Connection program can also help you to avoid falling prey to new illnesses and can help you to avoid a huge range of nonrespiratory illnesses. We cannot stress too strongly how a deprivation of carbon dioxide influences many, many body functions, as well as our body's performance and its ability to react to hostile circumstances.

Although every physiology is unique, we can confidently make some generalizations that apply to everyone.

There is a common, modern belief that our capacity for good or poor health is genetically predicated and that there is little we can do to change our destiny. At Breath Connection, we believe that every individual has the power to overcome a huge number of genetic disadvantages, if and when he or she needs to. Many of our weak, genetically inherited areas can be identified by a cool review of lifestyle and may be positively changed where necessary. We can't change the color of our eyes, gender, basic shape, hair color, personality, or IQ— at least not without varying degrees of effort and artifice. But in many cases, we can improve our health naturally and, in some cases, with very little effort.

Our Genetic Legacy

Our genes have bestowed one legacy, but, with the benefit of modern science, we have, today, more flexibility than ever before. We now have the wherewithal to counter many of the inherited factors that we cannot live with. Many of us can reduce the risks that genetics play with our health, regardless of our priorities. Whether you want to live longer, or better, or whether you want to slow down the physical signs of aging, help is at hand. This book isn't about beauty or cosmetic issues, but we do appreciate that this may be a factor for some readers. The Breath Connection program improves health on all levels and makes a very noticeable improvement in the way you look and feel.

There is little that we can do about the environment that we live in; all of us can play a small part in helping to green our lifestyles, but we are, in the end, stuck with existing pollution, food additives, and other factors that influence our health. There are, however, many things that we can do, on an individual basis, to minimize the effects of our environment. Lifestyle changes can reduce the overall burden on the body and make it easier for our bodies to cope with the demands placed upon it.

As an individual, you can stop smoking, reduce your alcohol consumption, especially spirits, and cut down on red meat and other proteins. Seek quality rather than quantity when you are choosing foods, and avoid those that have been processed and altered with additives and other modifications. Get more regular exercise. This advice is basic for anyone who has ever taken steps to improve health, but it cannot be stressed too often. What may not be clear is the fact that you can strengthen any genetic weaknesses by creating a lifestyle that is conducive to good health. And, even better, you can strengthen your body even further by reconditioning your breathing.

As you know, illness of many kinds is often the result of a carbon dioxide deficiency. In this chapter, we look at the way that this deprivation can affect a series of essential bodily functions, including the cardiovascular, digestive, eliminatory, hormonal, and immune systems, as well as brain and respiratory function. We show how the efficiency of each of these systems relies not merely upon balanced breathing, but upon complete and harmonious interaction between all the systems. This is the basis of holistic treatment, for whole health.

A Holistic Approach

Many of our doctors hold the view that illness needs only to be treated when it occurs. When illness strikes, the affected part or system is treated, but the rest of the body, including emotional factors, is generally ignored. We believe that illness is part of an overall process and the result of an imbalance within the body itself. There is no point in treating only one part, when the cause is an overall imbalance. Taking the example of a car manufacturer once again, doctors are happy to change tires, replace spark plugs, or tune a faulty engine, but they aren't happy to recommend a complete engine check or a broadscale service. We believe that all of the parts work in tandem and are inextricably linked. The health of one system undoubtedly affects the health of every other system in the body. Once again, this is the basis of holistic medicine. Breath Connection offers holistic treatment. It aims to provide an optimum level of carbon dioxide so that all your vital organs and systems are oxygenated and all-around health is achieved.

As we look at each of the physiological systems in turn, try to think of them as interconnecting cogs. When they are all running smoothly, your body functions well. A blockage or something out of sync in any of these cogs can affect all of the other cogs and trigger disease, usually in the area in which you are genetically predisposed to be weak.

Conditions ranging from angina to epilepsy are caused by hyperventilation. What we call *disease* can often simply be a manifestation of carbon dioxide deprivation.

In each section, we explain the role that carbon dioxide plays and what illnesses could manifest in your body when you have a weakness in that area. We also give you an idea of what to expect when things have been righted. Never forget that your own will has a major part to play in all this and participating in the Breath Connection program is part of your choice to take control of a longer and more fulfilling life. As a bonus, reconditioning your breathing may well

enhance the quality of the genes you pass on to future generations. We know that if we damage our cellular structure and
produce dysfunctional genetic changes through, for example,
what we eat (many food additives have been found to be
mutative, tending to affect the genetic pattern that is passed
on to unborn children), we can be creating genetic problems
in our children and our children's children. By improving the
quality of what we eat and drink, by ensuring that our bodies are working at optimum levels, by aiming for a balanced
mental condition, and by eschewing smoking, drinking,
recreational drugs, and too much ultraviolet light, we are
safeguarding our genetic template not just for ourselves but
for our present and future families.

Even if you do not suffer from illness in any of the specific areas we cover, remember that hyperventilation creates
an environment within the body for disease to take hold.
Although you may be experiencing good health at present,
the stage will have been set for illness, in whichever part of
the body you have a weakness. Breath Connection is preventative medicine; you can reduce your chances of suffering
from illness at a later date by creating a healthy body environment now.

As you learn to recondition your breathing, you will
notice an improvement in many bodily functions. Your
metabolism will probably speed up so that you will absorb
nutrients such as vitamins and minerals more rapidly, and,
although you will have more energy, you will be inclined to
eat less if you are overweight. Anorexics will recover some of
their appetite. Most allergies will disappear as you create the
correct acid-alkaline (pH) balance, and your elimination system will improve dramatically. In fact, a major detoxification
of the body will begin and you will become less vulnerable to

the minor infections and diseases that are environmental hazards for us all.

The test of any theory is "does it work in practice?" Many people in the United Kingdom and in Australia have already enjoyed huge benefits from taking part in the Breath Connection program, particularly with respiratory conditions such as asthma, emphysema, and bronchitis. Many others conditions, listed in Appendix B, have been relieved significantly.

Learning to recondition the breathing is a major part of preventative health care, as important as nutrition and exercise. This system represents nothing less than the birth of a new medical system, which heralds one of the most exciting, important, and far-reaching medical breakthroughs of the century.

Respiration

ASSOCIATED DYSFUNCTIONAL CONDITIONS:
ASTHMA, EMPHYSEMA, BRONCHITIS, BREATHLESSNESS, CHRONIC FATIGUE, SNORING, INSOMNIA, SLEEP APNEA, CYSTIC FIBROSIS, BLOCKED NOSE, SINUSITIS

We have learned that respiratory illness is not caused by getting too little air, but by inhaling too much. In fact, some sufferers inhale as much as eight times more than the healthy norm. Hyperventilation reduces the carbon dioxide stored in the alveoli of the lungs, and one way the body copes with this is to close down the airways. The tragedy of taking drugs such as those contained in bronchodilators is that they unnaturally dilate the bronchial tubes to facilitate breathing, yet dilated air passages are the cause of the attack in the first place. Not only are such manufactured drugs addressing only symptoms and responses, but they fail to deal with the cause of the problem and actually make it much, much worse. While drugs may offer brief relief in the short term, in the long term, they suppress symptoms and aggravate the condition.

Carbon dioxide is nature's own bronchodilator. When the level of carbon dioxide in the lungs is maintained, the body does not need to go into spasm to reduce the intake of breath. One exercise for children (see pages 150–155) instantly boosts the level of carbon dioxide in the body and can be used instead of drugs to give instant relief from the spasms, wheezing, dizziness, and coughing associated with respiratory disorders. More important, by completely reconditioning the breathing, the original problems can be circumvented and fewer, if any, attacks will be experienced in the future.

Take Care

Almost 4 million people in the United Kingdom suffer from asthma, and about a third of those cases are serious. We know that the condition kills about 2,000 people every year, a figure that triples in the United States. Despite being linked with atmospheric pollution and other external factors (such as allergens, pollen, house dust, animal hair, mold, fungi spores, climate, temperature, and stress), asthma was comparatively rare even 75 years ago, when parts of the world were arguably more polluted.

Asthma has been recognized by physicians for hundreds of years, and it has not been considered to be a serious illness until the 1930s. While no statistics on the death rate of asthmatics in the distant past are available, we can certainly see a general trend emerging in the twentieth century. As the century nears its end, it is clear, beyond all doubt, that asthma is a very significant cause of premature death. It's time we took it more seriously. Here's a brief history of our approach to asthmatic disease:

- In 1794, the distinguished Edinburgh physician Cullen wrote: "The asthma, though often threatening immediate death, seldom occasions it, and many persons have lived long under this disease." Sir William Osler wrote: "Death during the attack is unknown." (Young J. Pentland, 1892)
- A nineteenth-century dictionary of medicine includes the following entry: "Patients rarely, if ever, die of spasmodic asthma. Though death may ensue from some of its complications and sequels, and the disease being a functional one, cannot be said to have any morbid anatomy."
- J.J. Conybeare's 1929 textbook (Livingstone) states: "It is doubtful whether death has ever been caused by uncomplicated asthma [asthma without emphysema]. Nor does asthma tend necessarily to shorten life. Asthma is compatible with long life, and many chronic asthmatic patients live to a good old age and die of some other ailment at the last."
- In his 1930 volume, *The Treatment of Asthma* (M.K. Lewis), Dr. A. H. Douthwaite wrote: "The prognosis of bronchial asthma is one of the greatest difficulty. So far as longevity is concerned, the outlook is not necessarily adversely affected. Many asthmatics live well past middle age, for they seem to be less prone to other diseases which are apt to rise in the fifth decade. Family longevity is a point to be borne in regard to the future."
- Dr. W. Fox, a general practitioner since 1931, and author of the book *Asthma* (Robert Hale, 1995), was one of the first doctors to raise the alarm. He said: "What is going on here? Here we are, in 1992, in the grip of a worldwide

epidemic of asthma deaths and only a few years ago our clinical ancestors were calmly saying that it never happened. Were they all blind? It seems hardly likely since death from asthma suffocation is a particularly horrifying spectacle, and the medical giants of the past were so impressed by the curious benignity of asthma that they all mentioned it."

• In an uncanny representation of Professor Buteyko's own thinking, Dr. Fox continued: "The physicians' approach —if effective—must inevitably cause deaths, and the apparent harmlessness of asthma up to the recent past is because the medicines used in those days were ineffective."

• Opinions down the ages seem to support our view that asthma need not be a killer. Yet Dr. Douthwaite was writing at a time when Britain's cities were frequently cloaked in filthy industrial smog and many, if not most, of today's wonder drugs had yet to be developed. Ironically, the dramatic increase in asthma in the Western world—to near epidemic levels—comes at a time when the amount of asthma medications being prescribed is at an all-time high. We have to ask the question: Why, today, with the millions being spent on asthma research both in the United Kingdom and United States, is asthma getting worse, not better?

• In 1997, Dr. Richard Norton observed in *Wheeze of the World* that while Ethiopian peasants don't get asthma, wealthy Europeans do. Prior to unification, asthma was far more prevalent in West Germany than in East Germany, despite the fact that the East had much greater pollution problems and its inhabitants had severely limited access to medication. This paradox remains: The more we learn about it, the less able we, in the West, seem to be able to control asthma. Researchers come up with many theories about asthma's causes and subdivide these into reasons behind different types of asthma—allergic, nonallergic, emotional, environmental, and so on. They have, however, sought in vain to identify the actual root cause.

Overbreathing

Breathing through your mouth, as many people with respiratory disorders habitually do, involves inhaling larger quantities of air than is necessary. Apart from detrimentally affecting your carbon dioxide levels and increasing the risk of breathing in allergens, mouth-inhaled air can irritate the airways, resulting in inflammation, constriction, and excessive mucus production, often leading to a blocked nose and sinusitis. When the airways are narrowed, breathing becomes labored. This can lead to a panic attack, which causes you to gasp for air and compound the situation. Furthermore, the low carbon dioxide levels found in asthmatics reduce the body's ability to produce the natural form of the hormone cortisone and this can leave the body vulnerable to allergic responses.

Chronic Fatigue Syndrome (CFS)

Another disease of the respiratory system is chronic fatigue, but sufferers are seldom aware that they are overbreathing. Due to the Verigo/Bohr effect (see page 240), sufferers feel tired when their muscles do not receive enough oxygen. Fit people will feel healthily tired after exercise because they have used up oxygen stored in the muscles, but this is quickly replenished with rest. If you have chronic fatigue syndrome, your muscles are losing oxygen because of incorrect breathing, not through physical exertion. Hyperventilation can also prevent blood flow to the brain, leading to dizziness and loss of concentration and memory. Other symptoms include weakness, exhaustion, sleep disturbance, breathlessness, heartburn, cramps, and pins and needles.

Chronic fatigue syndrome

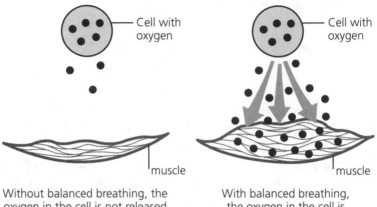

Without balanced breathing, the oxygen in the cell is not released into the muscle, causing the muscle tiredness of chronic fatigue.

With balanced breathing, the oxygen in the cell is released into the muscle.

The diagram shows how oxygen feeds the muscles. With CFS, the oxygen becomes tied to the hemoglobin due to the Verigo/Bohr effect (see page 240) and is not released into the cells. The large circle containing smaller ones shows how oxygen is unable to reach the muscles.

Sleep Disorders

Snoring, insomnia, and loss of breath during sleep are also symptomatic of malfunction in the respiratory center of the brain and are caused by hyperventilation. We know that snorers are more likely to develop high blood pressure and heart problems than nonsnorers and snoring can be the first stage of sleep apnea, a condition in which episodes of temporary cessation of breathing, lasting 10 seconds or longer, occur during sleep. This condition requires you to sleep with a special machine in your bedroom and kills more people than asthma does. It is vital that all snorers tape up their mouths, sleep on their left sides, and follow the Breath Connection program, first, to stop their snoring but also to prevent the later development of much more serious conditions.

GORDON

Gordon was 43, married, and a senior executive in a multinational computer company. He suffered from one of the most terrifying of the respiratory conditions— sleep apnea. In this condition, people unaccountably stop breathing while asleep. If they don't wake, they will die. Many sufferers are so frightened by the conse- quences of this condition that they are unable to sleep at night and get by with short naps throughout the day.

Gordon was becoming something of a social embar- rassment, falling asleep at social events and even at the dinner table. His snoring had already caused his wife to sleep in another room and being alone at night had probably increased his fear of suffering an attack of sleep apnea. He was puffy and overweight and had more or less given up on his condition, after years of quick-fix diets. He had slept with a sleep apnea rescue machine in his room for two years, but when he gave up on this too, his daytime lapses into sleep became much worse.

Gordon had a very low Control Pause when he first came to Breath Connection. During his first week he learned how to breathe with a closed mouth. After a few days he had learned how to sleep comfortably for a few hours each night, without his machine, and this soon increased to half the night. Five weeks after beginning the course, Gordon could sleep through the night without his machine and his sleep apnea had begun to improve. His weight began to decrease, and he lost about 14 pounds during the first week of the course. After three months, he had shed nearly 55 pounds.

His Control Pause rose to 24, and, feeling rested, slimmer, and altogether better, he set about improving his health even further.

To summarize, it has been estimated that only 10 percent of the population naturally breathe in the correct way. Breathing correctly means breathing slowly and shallowly. As with any habit, particularly one acquired over a lifetime, training yourself to breathe differently may feel awkward at first. The breath reduction exercises you will learn during the five-day Breath Connection program will introduce you to a new way of breathing that will not only reduce any existing respiratory problems but have a hugely beneficial effect on other areas of your body.

In neither Papua New Guinea nor Ethiopia do people deep breathe. They have, moreover, no word for asthma. We in the "civilized" West have been inured with the idea that deep breathing is both natural and healthy despite the fact that there has never been any scientific evidence to suggest this is the case. Professor Buteyko sees asthma as a disease of so-called civilization.

Cardiovascular Conditions

ASSOCIATED DYSFUNCTIONAL CONDITIONS:
ANGINA, HEART FAILURE, PALPITATIONS, HIGH AND LOW BLOOD PRESSURE, MIGRAINE, IMPOTENCE

Shortage of carbon dioxide constricts the cardiovascular vessels. Although it is not as visibly obvious as it is with respiratory diseases, a shortage of carbon dioxide reduces circulation in the arterial vessels (the heart, brain, liver, and kidneys) and expands the vein vessels. Depending on where your weakest areas are, this can result in conditions such as a blocked nose, hemorrhoids, or varicose veins as well as more serious threats to health. It can lead to problems with circulation, which in itself is responsible for a whole host of other conditions. When the blood circulation malfunctions due to a need for more carbon dioxide, a strong spasm of the brain vessels can occur, particularly if other factors such as loud noises, particular foods, and a lack of sleep are involved. For some people the result is a migraine headache.

The Hyperventilation Syndrome
In common with those who researched Viagra, we at Breath Connection regard impotence as a vascular problem. By breathing correctly, the blood circulation to the penis is improved, thereby sustaining and lengthening the duration of erection. Often, patients with diabetes, heart problems, and blood pressure also suffer from impotence. All of these conditions are linked to hyperventilation.

Angina is another example of an illness affected by this malfunction of blood vessels due to carbon dioxide deficiency, as are heart palpitations. According to Professor Buteyko, most heart surgery could be avoided if patients were trained not to overbreathe. Moreover, if someone has already had a heart operation, learning to breathe the right way can prevent new heart problems from occurring.

High blood pressure is also linked to a carbon dioxide deficiency in the cardiovascular system. Overbreathing constricts or narrows the brain vessels, as Professor Gavin Andrews of St. Vincent's Hospital in Australia confirms:

> The body has to increase the blood pressure to secure normal oxygenation of the brain. Your doctor then measures your blood pressure and prescribes tablets for high blood pressure for the rest of your life. Ironically the body wants to keep your blood pressure high in order to get oxygen to the brain yet these pills will lower your blood pressure and do the opposite of what your body really needs. However, unless the condition is recognized as being caused by hyperventilation/overbreathing, it is necessary to take such pills in order to prevent a stroke or heart attack. Such medication may make a person look healthy by lowering their blood pressure, but they are not really healthy because the root cause has not been addressed. By retraining the breathing the blood pressure will return to normal and proper oxygenation of the brain will re-occur so the medication can be reduced in consultation with your doctor.

According to statistics, low blood pressure causes more heart attacks and strokes than high blood pressure and is another symptom of overbreathing. When following the Breath Connection program, all blood pressure or heart conditions must be supervised by an experienced and qualified Breath Connection practitioner.

The program can actually help to prevent strokes. People who have suffered a stroke in the past will often breathe with their mouths open, a sign of hyperventilation. And during a stroke, the person suffers from lack of oxygen to the brain. Subsequent Breath Connection exercises bring that oxygen back to the parts of the brain not permanently damaged by the stroke, so that in many cases the patient is able to regain mobility and speech.

The Digestive System

ASSOCIATED DYSFUNCTIONAL CONDITIONS:
IRRITABLE BOWEL SYNDROME, CONSTIPATION, FLATULENCE, BLOATING OF THE STOMACH, BELCHING, HEARTBURN, ULCERS, ACIDOSIS ALKALOSIS

When carbon dioxide is dissolved in water (of which our bodies comprise over 70 percent), it is converted into carbonic acid. This splits into bicarbonate ions and hydrogen ions and affects the delicate acid-alkali (pH) balance of the blood. This balance profoundly affects every chemical reaction and process in the body. All areas of the body have distinct pH levels that need to be controlled. These levels range from the extremely acidic (pH = 2) fluids in the stomach to the alkaline juices (pH = 7.5 to 8.8) in the pancreas. The pH of the blood is slightly alkaline and even a very slight shift in its balance can have dire consequences. No one can live more than a few hours if this balance shifts significantly.

Bicarbonates formed from dissolved carbon dioxide act as buffers within the body and help to neutralize acids and maintain the body's optimally alkaline state, which is very important for digestion. A balanced pH level in the blood is maintained through respiration. It is particularly affected by carbon dioxide levels. Hyperventilation causes us to breathe out more carbon dioxide than we should and is responsible for a corresponding shift in the blood's pH value to a more allergic state. Oxygen is alkaline and carbon dioxide is acidic. The essential balance between these two is needed for the digestive system to work properly. A low level of carbon dioxide in the lungs leads to respirator alkalosis, meaning an excess of alkaline reserves in the blood. This makes the body much more susceptible to viruses, allergies, cramps, and convulsions and explains why people with this area of weakness are more prone to colds and flu than others are. No one is quite sure why, but it is thought that this alkaline blood leads to inflammation and swelling of the lung lining.

It also results in spasms within the bronchial tubes and an imbalance of the metabolic processes—leading to the condition that we call asthma. A drop in the blood's carbon dioxide content of just 3 percent can upset the pH balance to such a level that death is the result. The link between respiration and health is critical, and carbon dioxide plays a crucial role in the balance.

Once the pH of your body is upset, your entire immune system is affected. A weakened immune system allows adverse conditions, such as colds and cancer, to thrive. We cannot claim to cure cancer, but following the Breath Connection program can often lead to a substantial extension of life span and improve the quality of life as well. Even in the terminal stages of cancer, the program offers pain relief without resort to such drugs as morphine. This leads to a more peaceful passing.

The Excretory (Elimination) System

ASSOCIATED DYSFUNCTIONAL CONDITIONS:
CONSTIPATION, DIARRHEA, FLATULENCE, BLOATING OF THE STOMACH

Our human waste-disposal and detoxification systems are especially important today, when our bodies are likely to be assaulted by chemicals and pesticides in the food chain and water supply however carefully we try to avoid them. This century, we have been introduced to 70,000 new chemicals in the environment. Much of our food is processed, especially junk food, and the poisons it creates need to be eliminated properly. You have only to look at a friend (or yourself) after a monitored fast or a stay at a health farm where a detoxification program has been followed to see the difference. Bloating has disappeared and weight has been reduced. The skin will have a healthier glow and there will be much more visible as well as invisible energy. A detox can be a vital part of treatments for a range of conditions from common colds to serious cancers.

However, when we hyperventilate we prevent our liver and kidneys—the organs responsible for flushing out toxic waste—from functioning properly. Lack of carbon dioxide, leading to unbalanced pH, makes it very difficult for cells in these purification machines to regenerate. Apart from contributing to many disorders of the nervous system and to the development of some cancers, this leads also to premature aging of the body.

The Breath Connection program has a major detoxing affect and greatly speeds up the elimination process. Many people with asthma who embark on the program find that they have diarrhea initially or that their feces loosen up considerably during the first days of the course. This is perfectly natural. Often our feces are not properly eliminated and stick to the walls of the colon, slowly spreading toxins throughout the body. This can lead to gastrointestinal and autoimmunity disorders including celiac disease, ulcerative colitis, Crohn's disease, and headaches. By balancing your breathing, the unwanted substances that trigger such problems are effectively flushed out of the body.

Where serious poisoning derives from external factors such as the tragic and dramatic fallout from the radiation spill at Chernobyl and the chemical warfare conducted during the Gulf War, the Breath Connection program can also assist recovery. Professor Buteyko's methods have been used in Chernobyl and received official recognition for results from the Russian government. We believe that similar results could be achieved with Gulf War Syndrome patients.

The former Soviet Union's Institute for Cosmic Medicine also embraced new ideas that have been proven to work. It focuses on the best medical care for its astronauts and Professor Buteyko's breathing methods are taught for application during space travel.

The Nervous System

ASSOCIATED DYSFUNCTIONAL CONDITIONS:
DIZZINESS, LACK OF COORDINATION, INSOMNIA, STRESS, IRRITABILITY, ALLERGIES, EPILEPSY

Carbon dioxide is used to tranquilize humans and animals. Air containing 10 percent CO_2 would make you feel distinctly dizzy. If that level was doubled, you would probably lose consciousness. At more than 20 percent, you might die. Your body is extremely sensitive to changes in the level of carbon dioxide that it inhales—much less so with oxygen. On average, each breath that you take contains about 20 percent oxygen, but even if that were to be increased by 400 percent, you probably wouldn't notice it. Only when the level dropped to below 15 percent in high altitudes would you experience distress.

As your body is 50 times more sensitive to carbon dioxide than it is to oxygen it is important that you learn about the effects that it has on all the essential systems. A decreased level of just 0.1 percent can cause dizziness, palpitations, wheezing, and a blocked nose—in short, an asthma attack. A similar increase would reverse the process.

Carbon dioxide, therefore, helps to regulate the nervous system's activity. This is why people in primitive cultures have practiced overbreathing for centuries in order to produce the heightened excitement required during certain rituals and states of altered consciousness. As an occasional activity, this probably does no long-term harm, but habitual overbreathing results in the malfunctions previously noted.

When considering the nervous system—that which affects the brain, spinal cord, peripheral nerves, and sensory organs—it is worth considering the words written by consultant chest physician L. Lum in the *Chest, Heart and Stroke Journal* (Chest, Heart, and Stroke Association): "Carbon dioxide is not just a waste gas. It plays an important function in governing bodily functions." In his book, *Epilepsy* (Oxford University Press, 1981), Anthony Hopkins states that hyperventilation is frequently used as a test procedure in treating epilepsy by inducing an epileptic fit through deliberately overbreathing. Hopkins also remarks that hyperventilation is a "trade name" for stress.

Neurological Function
- Is the principal regulator of the internal pH balance of the sensory and motor neurons of the brain
- Influences the transmission of nervous impulses at the

synapses (the junction between the neurons or their contact with a muscle cell or gland cell)

• Affects the amount of activity in the automatic nervous system and thus controls the state of balance between sympathetic and hostile activity—our "flight or fight" responses

The Hormonal (Endocrine) System

ASSOCIATED DYSFUNCTIONAL CONDITIONS:
PREMENSTRUAL SYNDROME (INCLUDING TENSION), ALLERGIES, INFERTILITY, AND MENOPAUSAL, THYROID, AND GYNECOLOGICAL PROBLEMS

Hormones are special chemicals that are secreted through the bloodstream by the endocrine glands. These include the pituitary gland, which regulates our growth, and the thyroid, which, as well as regulating our metabolic rates, governs the testes and ovaries that produce our sex hormones. Professor Buteyko found that balancing the breath was good for infertility and contributed to treatment of menstrual, pregnancy, menopausal, postmenopausal, and postnatal problems.

SARAH AND JANINE

Sarah attended a Breath Connection course because of severe and frequent migraines. She did not even mention to her practitioner that she was having trouble conceiving. Within three weeks of starting to balance her breath she found that she was pregnant, after eight years of trying.

Similarly, Janine had been drawn to Breath Connection because of panic attacks. She was so badly affected

by traffic that she kept her eyes tightly shut as her husband drove her to the clinic. In social situations, she would
freeze, and she often felt like crying in public. This forced
her to give up her job. Even simple activities such as shopping and pleasurable ones such as outings to the theater
or eating in restaurants were ordeals for Janine. Like
Sarah, she did not mention her infertility problem when
she came to see us. When she found that she was pregnant, just weeks into her regime, she had the added
happy bonus of finding she was able to go shopping for
all the things she would need for the baby.

Just a small secretion of natural chemicals from the
endocrine glands can produce a dramatic response in the target cells with which they are compatible. As with all other
systems in the body, hormonal activity is part of a balanced
and interdependent control system. When we consider the
link between the hormonal system and carbon dioxide, we
should bear in mind what Yale University's Professor Y.
Henderson had to say: "Carbon dioxide is the chief hormone
of the entire body; it is the only one that is produced by every
tissue and that probably acts on every organ."

Through the effects of increased CO_2 on the hormonal
system, the pancreas functions more efficiently, therefore the
metabolism speeds up, food is absorbed much better and the
appetite is considerably reduced, leading to weight loss in
overweight and obese people as their food cravings diminish.
As we noted earlier, the Breath Connection program has the
miraculous effect of stimulating appetite in anorexics as their
balance is restored by correct breathing.

The Immune System

ASSOCIATED DYSFUNCTIONAL CONDITIONS:
ALLERGIES, AIDS, CHRONIC FATIGUE SYNDROME (CFS), SKIN
DISEASES

The body is incredibly well designed and under normal circumstances can efficiently rally its own defenses against infections, viruses, and other invaders. However, our immune system can be severely challenged if we are breathing incorrectly and, as we learned from looking at the digestive system, when the body's pH balance is upset and the immune system is weakened, it becomes harder for the body to fight off disease. A weakened body is also more susceptible to allergies, among other things.

Many allergy tests show that many people have a sensitivity to a wide range of foods and substances, including wheat, dairy foods, chocolate, and fruit, as well as grass, pollens, and even fabric softeners. But, although these triggers may cause symptoms, they are not, in fact, the cause of the allergy. An allergy exists when the immune system is weakened. We believe that a weakened immune system is a result of hyperventilation.

When your immune system is working under par, it creates a fertile ground for allergies to develop. This explains why people with strong immune activity are able to eat and drink common allergens without any problems. It also explains why even healthy, typically nonallergic people can experience reactions to foods and substances when they are run-down—following a bout of flu, for example.

Immunity is a subject that is gathering huge scientific

184

attention of late, and there are many theories regarding its function and dysfunction. For example, HIV and AIDS have continued to flummox the medical profession, as has chronic fatigue syndrome and ME. What we do know, however, is that AIDS sufferers and people who are HIV positive have immune systems that have been seriously damaged.

For anyone who suffers from an immune-related condition, well-being can be vastly improved by following the Breath Connection program in conjunction with other treatments.

Brain Function

ASSOCIATED DYSFUNCTIONAL CONDITIONS:
ANXIETY, PANIC ATTACKS, INSOMNIA, DIZZINESS, MEMORY LOSS, CONCENTRATION PROBLEMS, DEPRESSION, STRESS

Carbon dioxide controls the flow of blood to the brain. When there is a low level of carbon dioxide in the blood—a condition called *hypocarbia*—blood flow is reduced, causing constriction of the blood vessels. This can lead to a whole range of conditions, including dizziness, memory loss, and lack of concentration. Former world chess champion Anatoly Karpov used Professor Buteyko's breathing method to prepare for international chess tournaments. It worked for him by enhancing his concentration.

Panic attacks (see pages 122–125) are severely aggravated by hyperventilation. Reactions can be triggered by activities that sufferers would normally take in their strides, such as crowds, heavy traffic, a congested elevator, or even normal human contact. When you start to panic, you overbreathe even more. This further reduces the oxygen supply to the brain, which in turn increases the panic. Another vicious cycle sets in.

Anxiety, anger, stress, depression, and even agoraphobia (fear of open spaces) are all manifestations of hyperventilation. There may be other, psychological causes behind these states, but overbreathing is an important factor in their severity and recurrence. In many, many cases, physical illnesses disappear when the patient's breathing is rebalanced, and emotional conditions are also righted.

It is important to note that during the Breath Connection program, a few people experience dysfunctional mental states, including anger, irritability, and depression for a short period. This occurs because the body is working hard to rebalance itself. Many therapists would consider this a good sign—in that suppressed emotions are coming out, leaving a clean slate behind. If you feel uncomfortable, or if it becomes a problem, stop the exercises for a few days and start again.

Key Points

- We have learned in this chapter that breathing is not something that only affects our respiratory system, but has an impact on the workings of the entire body.
- Whether or not you suffer from any of the illnesses that can be successfully and directly treated by the Breath Connection program, you can benefit from reconditioned breathing.

Now we are ready to look at how the Breath Connection program can be integrated into every aspect of your daily life.

12

Feeding Your Health

O f all the controversial, almost revolutionary, principles embraced by Breath Connection, those concerning food and diet initiate the most surprise. What we advocate overturns many of the beliefs central to the philosophies of most traditional dieticians and nutritionists, although it is in line with some practices in complementary medicine.

At Breath Connection, we don't even discuss diet with our patients until the second or third day of the program, by which time they will have learned a great deal about how to control their hyperventilation. You can, however, start observing our dietary guidelines from day one.

The system we advise almost always results in a steady balancing of your weight, until your optimum or ideal weight is achieved. That's a happy bonus, as we do not set out to help people slim down or put on much-needed weight. Overweight people invariably lose pounds while following the Breath Connection program. Equally, anorexics and even the slightly underweight find that by following the Breath Connection dietary guidelines as well as the breathing exercises, a correct level of appetite is restored. Some anorexics find that they want to eat small amounts as often as six times a day! By obeying the reeducated calls of a faster metabolism, the body digests food more quickly and more efficiently.

Don't worry about references to timing, such as undertaking exercises before breakfast. If breakfast for you is a cup of herbal tea, that's fine. And don't panic if you have to eat out in a restaurant. Read on to see the wide range of foods you can choose from the menu. Italian, Middle-Eastern, and Indian restaurants may offer the most enticing choices, and they are all within the limits of your program.

It is normally best to stick to vegetarian options in the evening, having your protein meal earlier in the day (see page 191). Be very careful about dairy ingredients that might be included in sauces. Above all, don't feel forced to eat more than you really want, or to try a little taste. For some people, it might be best to avoid eating out during the first few days of the program. This gives the body a chance to adjust to some new habits and nutritional changes.

If the idea of making a dietary change daunts you, have a nice little daydream about something to which you'll treat yourself when the program is complete. Maybe a new piece of clothing in a smaller size? This time next week you can buy it and wear it.

We realize that some individuals may require a customized diet plan and may need to supplement their diets with certain vitamins and minerals. Your Breath Connection practitioner can provide you with a program that will suit your individual needs. The guidelines presented in this section are general ones; if you feel you must adapt them to make it work for you, we suggest you come along to see one of our practitioners, who can give you some good advice.

vegetables—especially green vegetables—and whole grains, such as brown rice. If you are desperate for something milky, try rice milk. Potatoes are also OK in moderation.

If this sounds dreary, you will be heartened to know that Professor Buteyko advocates the use of seasonings such as black pepper, mustard, herbs, onions, and garlic. Use olive oil in cooking, rather than butter, and choose whole-grain bread over processed white or brown. Eat plenty of fresh fruit.

You can eat lamb, chicken, pulses, and fish in moderation, but learn to ditch the notion that a meal isn't proper if it doesn't include protein. Nutritionists agree that an adult should consume an average 20 grams of protein a day, with children and athletes requiring a larger quantity. Those with certain medical conditions may also require a higher amount of protein.

Foods that are high in calcium can also aid sleep and stave off conditions such as osteoporosis. Natural sources include kelp, turnip greens, rhubarb, broccoli, lamb's kidneys, tofu, tinned salmon with bones, baked beans, halibut, fortified oatmeal and other cereals, molasses, all leafy green vegetables, and kale. Don't be fooled into thinking that a glass of milk at mealtimes is necessary; you can get more calcium from other sources than you can from any dairy product.

Mealtime Guidelines

- Try to plan breakfasts consisting of fresh fruit or juices; porridge made with water and served with running honey or pure maple syrup; cereals with rice milk; toast with an olive oil spread; a bowl of mixed seeds, nuts, and dried fruit; or a cereal bar.
- Lunch could consist of a small amount of lamb, chicken, or fish, with a salad and some lightly cooked veg-

Mealtimes

Our most important rule is that you should eat only when and if you are hungry. Never eat because it is a certain time of the day; because the people you are with are eating; or because your mother, partner, diet book, or doctor says you should eat. Eat because, and only because, your body tells you it wants food.

Despite its perfect logic, this may not be easy to accept. Most of us were brought up to believe that regular mealtimes were an essential part of good health. We were taught that breakfast is the most important meal of the day, and that skipping it would damage our mental and physical energy. In the first instance, our mothers, shortly followed by endless books and articles on nutrition, stressed that regular fuel was necessary for our bodies to function—particularly while we are young and growing. Apart from anything else, the idea of sitting down with friends and family, and merely sipping water or a fruit drink while they are enjoying a full meal, may not be appealing. It is, however, an essential habit to learn.

Fixed mealtimes have become fixtures, and they were not always devised for our convenience, as anyone who has been roused at 6 A.M. for a hospital breakfast or served an airline lunch at 11 will testify. Don't let other people's schedules dictate yours. Don't eat to please your mother, hostess, or spouse. Listen to your body, and feed it when it tells you that it needs food. If your appetite is fierce at four o'clock in the afternoon, have a proper meal, not just a snack. Arrange things so that you are near a source of good, nutritious food if you are away from home, or pack a suitable picnic in anticipation. Don't feel you need to build yourself up if you are unwell. At such times, your body needs its energy to aid your recovery, not to digest food, particularly if it is the wrong kind of food.

Central to all of this is the fact that eating without hunger makes you hyperventilate and the symptoms of respiratory illness will be aggravated. The very fact that you are opening your mouth and taking in air that way is, of course, a contributing factor.

Good and Bad Foods

We have all been indoctrinated to the fact that we should not eat junk food. It is low in nutrients and normally contains additives, preservatives, sugar, and other chemicals that are all detrimental to good health. These chemicals are toxic and can cause your body to hyperventilate in order to get rid of them. Of course, many natural foods contain toxic substances, but they are in much smaller amounts. Junk food is not to be confused with fast food. You can make delicious and nutritious snacks and meals as quickly as waiting for a pizza delivery to arrive, and you might even save some money. Vegetables, grains, and cereals are inexpensive compared to ready-made foods.

Overeating many foods, such as animal proteins (which include meat, fish, eggs, and milk), increases our intake of breath per minute. Our bodies cannot utilize proteins without first breaking them down into their constituent amino acids. The extra energy required to perform this task—in the form of oxygen—is similar to that needed for a brisk walk of some duration. That's why, after eating a high-protein meal, your breathing becomes labored as your body struggles to digest it. It's also the reason why so many people are sapped of energy after a heavy meal.

190

As the day progresses, include less and less protein in you diet. It's not a new theory that heavy meals should be avoided late in the evening, but we go a step further. We suggest that not only should you avoid late-night eating, but you should cut down or cut out protein completely in your last meal of the day. A near-certain way to a poor night's sleep—and, of course, hyperventilation—is to eat heavily and unwisely before going to bed. A late protein meal is not only hard on your stomach, which has to work overtime to digest it while you and your body's other systems are trying to rest, but it encourages deep breathing, the very thing we are trying to prevent.

Another received wisdom is that it is good for you to drink as many as eight glasses of water a day. According to Professor Buteyko, you should drink as much water as it takes to quench your thirst. The amounts will vary from person to person.

We do, of course, have a blacklist of forbidden foods. These include such high-protein foods as cheese and other dairy foods, especially milk, yogurt, crème fraîche, goat's cheese, and goat's milk. Apart from being high in protein, dairy foods encourage mucus production, which can be dangerous for an asthmatic. Soy-based foods, chicken, red meat, and fish should also be limited. You (and your child) can obtain calcium from many food sources other than the familiar dairy ones (see page 192). We also advise strongly against the use of table salt, although natural sea salt crystals are fine for seasoning. Steer clear of foods that contain caffeine—and that includes tea, cola drinks, chocolate and cocoa, as well as coffee.

Professor Buteyko found that the foods that contribute to the elimination of asthma and other respiratory illnesses are

191

etables. You could choose a baked potato or rice with vegetables very sparingly drizzled with virgin olive oil. For dessert, try a fresh fruit sorbet or some nondairy cake. Fruit salad (without cream, of course!) is ideal.

- At dinnertime (or, indeed, earlier in the day), you could have some pasta or noodles with a tomato or pesto sauce, or any of the nonprotein options that were offered for your previous meal. Roast or steamed Mediterranean vegetables can be delicious, and they are extremely healthy.
- Follow the rules of any responsible diet and cut out processed foods. Alcohol is also a toxin, and should, if possible, be avoided in the early stages of the program.
- Try to eat slowly, chewing properly, with your mouth closed.
- Leave food on the side of your plate when you have had enough.
- Shop thoughtfully and study labels for additives and hidden sugars.
- Eat organic, which is much healthier—and tastier!
- If you can, buy as much as possible from health and whole-food shops. It may prove to be a little more expensive, but you can eat and enjoy your meal with confidence.
- It is also better to shop ahead, so you won't be tempted to grab something unsuitable from the nearest outlet when hunger strikes. It's a good idea to have some healthy cereal snacks on hand at all times.

Diet Checklist
- Eat only when you are hungry.
- Do not overeat.
- Try to avoid high-protein foods.
- Avoid caffeine.

- Reduce your sugar intake.
- Avoid milk in any form, except rice milk.
- Avoid cheese, yogurt, and other dairy products.
- Eat plenty of whole grains and fresh green vegetables.
- Use natural sea salt, not table salt.
- Drink water when you are thirsty, but not unless you are.
- Listen to your body's demands and don't be bullied into eating by other people.

No significant dietary change is easy. It may be even harder to change a child's eating habits. Be positive, and tell your child that it won't be long before he or she experiences the benefits of an altered diet. Children adapt easily, and they soon forget old routines. Before long, the new program will be the norm, and your child may well prefer it to the old one. Tears at mealtimes are easier to cope with than asthma attacks in the night, so bear that in mind when your child objects to the fact that creamy chocolate sponge cake is no longer on the menu.

Your own progress and that of your children will advance almost exponentially if you all follow the dietary guidelines we have outlined here.

13

Planning and Preparation

Any major life change has the potential to be energizing and exciting. It makes sense, however, to anticipate the doubts, worries, and even fears that naturally accompany any break from the familiar. It often takes a great leap of faith, and considerable confidence, to make permanent changes in our lives, whether those changes affect our relationships, our work, or our home life. Changes to our health can be positive, but it is not unusual for people to feel hesitant about committing to a new lifestyle, particularly if they felt confident and secure in the old one.

In this chapter, we show you how choosing to adopt the Breath Connection way of life is easy. With a little thought and planning, it can be so enjoyable, you may wonder why you ever delayed.

At times, all of us cling to the security blanket of our bad habits, or even illnesses. Habits and states of mind and health supply us with part of our identity. It is an interesting phenomenon that human beings tend to set themselves up for failure, no matter how much the results are coveted. Although we may realize, intellectually, that a change is for the best—whether it involves changing the way we look, how much we weigh, our overall health, or all three—it is often difficult to put that longing for change into action. You know the feeling: Perhaps you have tried lots of self-improvement courses or treatments, such as diets, skincare regimes, exercise routines, only to have failed to commit to or fulfill your ambitions. Perhaps you dread the challenge of new opportunities that a new and improved self might have to face.

It's important to remind yourself—and do so constantly—that there is never really any new self. That healthier and more confident person is still you, and you are someone who can now familiarize yourself with your new potential.

There are a few logical preliminaries to consider before embarking on the Breath Connection program. Being realistic and honest with yourself will help to make the program work for you—and with you. Here is some practical advice:

• Make practical preparations. Arrange a conducive environment for your exercises. If you can't designate a separate room where you can be alone for short periods throughout the day, screen off a corner of the bedroom or a seldom-used room such as a dining room, if you have one.

• Elicit outside support. Tell everyone who interacts with you on a daily basis what you are doing and why. Anyone who cares about you is bound to be encouraging. Moreover, it is undoubtedly more difficult to lapse, let alone fail, if you have stated your aims. A sense of pride, or the feeling that you are letting others down, can help to keep you motivated.

• Develop a positive mental attitude. You can motivate yourself by the promise of a treat or a night out with friends, if you keep to the program for a week. Promise another, special, reward for when you reach your goal.

• Anticipate obstacles in advance, and plan for them. Have a contingency plan for days when you can't seem to find time to be alone, or you just couldn't exercise as you'd planned. This isn't being negative, just pragmatic.

• Be realistic and recognize that it is human nature to procrastinate. This doesn't give you carte blanche to do so, but you won't feel so discouraged when the temptation to put things off is at its most appealing.

• It is also human nature to want results without having to work for them. Don't castigate yourself for giving in to such thoughts. Not *very* deep down you know that little is achieved in any field without some effort and discipline. Just remind yourself that any major change involves time, energy, and a little bit of enthusiasm. In your case, it may also involve the sacrifice of some favorite foods or giving up the habit of eating a late dinner. Remind yourself that these small losses will soon be dismissed as you learn new and better habits. Visualize the healthy, freer life you will have when you complete the course. If that visualization includes an improved appearance, so much the better. Visualize yourself having the energy to participate in games with your children, to play a sport, or to dance with your friends in a way that has been restricted until now. Visualize yourself free from artificial drugs, allowing your body to heal itself with its own natural resources. All of these images should not only be very motivating, but, in their way, self-perpetuating. There is no doubt that people with a positive outlook attract positive energies in life, and the reverse is also true. You can make it happen. These positive affirmations and mental rehearsals can strengthen your resolve. The Breath Connection exercises are not so lengthy or strenuous that much steely resolve should be necessary. Results are quick and effective, and you will, in turn, be motivated by the speed at which you see change.

• Don't be ill any longer than you have to be. You should be aware that you will receive the care, attention, and sympathy of your loved ones whether you are healthy or not. Friends and family will be so delighted by your recovery that you will receive just as much attention. Their attention may be a little less deferential and solicitous, but it will be based on an equal footing, rather than a carer-to-invalid relationship. Isn't that preferable?

Deciding that you want to change your health, your habits, and, through that, your life, is the first vital leg of the Breath Connection voyage. It does, however, need to be supported by a practical strategy, something that has been designed to work for you and your individual circumstances. This is partly why we keep stressing that although we believe that all readers can gain and learn from our book, sometimes the special attention of a qualified practitioner can make the little bit of difference that can push you that extra half mile.

The following practical preparations are for the average reader and should work in the majority of cases. Take care to read and work through them all. They are likely to meet all of your particular needs, especially if you tweak things a little here and there to allow them to fit your lifestyle.

If you can, check your schedule before embarking on the course and try to block off short times of the day or evening, two, three, or four times a day. Many people respond well to the discipline of fulfilling commitments that have been arranged. Make a date with yourself to practice Breath Connection, and reserve that time as yours. Give this date the same priority that you would any engagement, and don't break it unless you have to.

Practical Preparation

The Breath Connection program should initially be followed two to four times a day for a minimum of five days. Different sections of this book address the treatment of various ailments, and offer specific advice on how often, and for how long, you can expect to exercise. Do bear in mind that regularity and consistency are important when following the program, and if you earmark special times of the day for your exercises, it will make a substantial difference. This means advance planning. Where are you going to exercise? At home, in the office, in the gym? Think about the week you have selected to start the Breath Connection program and plan accordingly, postponing nonessential dates if necessary. Remember that you will only need a few minutes for each session, which should, ideally, take place first thing in the morning, just before lunch, before your evening meal, and just before bed. If you find it difficult to fit it all in, start your program in a quieter, less socially demanding week in the near future. Once you have your program in place, you'll find it easier to find time to fit it in—particularly since you will have seen the results and feel more motivated.

If you need to make new arrangements, always fit them in around your Breath Connection commitments. Remember that you have made an appointment with yourself and it is your priority. We are aware that people with demanding jobs, in the office or in a household with children, for example, may find it difficult to make and keep to commitments. Many of us are used to putting ourselves second, or even third, while we cope with busy jobs or family life. In order for you to experience good health, you need to take care of yourself. That means learning to put yourself first and ensuring that your priorities are right. You always have time for the things you put first.

It's equally important that people with less demanding lifestyles make a date and stick to it. If you have a long, empty day stretching ahead of you, it's easy to rationalize that you have all the time in the world, and that you will fit in your exercises at some point. Chances are, however, that the day will slip by and you won't ever get to them. Make an appointment with yourself and treat it as a priority.

Environment

The place where you practice your Breath Connection exercise should, ideally, be quiet, private, comfortable, and warm. If there is a telephone nearby, disconnect it for those few minutes and enjoy the added luxury of silence. If your household is a bustling one, you might like to hang a "do not disturb" sign on the door of your chosen place, for the short duration of the exercises. Explain to your family what you are doing, and request a few moments' peace.

We know that some people have become so captivated by the Breath Connection process that they have redecorated the rooms in which they practice in tranquil colors to suit the mood. Excellent! Of course, we realize that this is not practical for everyone, but it does help to practice in an inspiring environment. Some people have created an environment in which they will work best by surrounding themselves with a few favorite objects or pictures. Make your space as positive and inspiring as you possibly can. You should never feel that you are shoved into a corner. This is your time, and your space. You want to feel comfortable and relaxed. This is quality time, aimed at improving your health on every level. Make sure you create an atmosphere that is conducive to that.

Time-Keeping

You will need an accurate clock, with a second hand. Better still, invest in a stopwatch to count your Control Pause with accuracy. Purchase some micropore tape (see page 51), and keep it on hand for use when you are alone in the house.

Diet

Plan your meals for the week and shop in advance, ensuring that there are no forbidden foods in the refrigerator to tempt you during moments of weakness. We talk more about diet in Chapter 12 (see pages 190–194). Buy a few healthy but delicious snacks from health food shops if you fear the odd emergency. Inform your family or partner of your new routine, and ask him or her for support. The main idea is to eat only when you are hungry. Others may have to get used to you being at the table without eating.

Try to avoid a high-protein meal in the evening (see page 191), and avoid foods with additives, or anything that has been processed. Dairy foods are also not recommended, so you will need to create delicious and nutritious meals based on fruits, vegetables, and a wonderful range of carbohydrates. Eat fish, meat, and pulses only in moderation.

If you must travel for business or pleasure while you are following the Breath Connection program, phone the airline and order a vegetarian or vegan meal. This is particularly important for diagnosed asthmatics or emphysemics, as a heavy protein meal in cabin conditions will aggravate breathing difficulties.

If you forget to book a meal in advance, pack your own snack or drink water on the journey and save your appetite for your arrival at your destination. It can be difficult to avoid, particularly if you are traveling on business, or even pleasure, but try not to eat out during the first few days of your course. If it is unavoidable, tell friends that you are on a restricted diet and explain why you are doing so. Most restaurants have fresh salads and delicious vegetarian options. Stick with these while you are eating out. Try to remember Professor Buteyko's advice about eating only when you are hungry and not because it is mealtime. You can socialize perfectly well at a dinner as you pick at a suitable salad.

The best thing you can eat late at night is a plate of vegetables, and some complex carbohydrates, such as a whole grain or brown rice or potatoes. It can be difficult to watch friends or family digging into steaming and fragrant heaps of your favorite foods, but try to remember that this regime will not continue indefinitely. Perhaps you can persuade some like-minded friends to join you in your special diet.

Replace ordinary salt with crunchier mineral salt. Tea and coffee are not villains, but try to drink them as infrequently as possible, and without milk or cream. Herbal teas are particularly refreshing, or try something such as roasted dandelion root coffee, which is naturally creamy and much healthier. If you feel frustrated, inspire yourself with the promise of a special treat—such as an evening out, or a new piece of clothing—at the end of the program. Try to make yourself feel pampered and not deprived. Buy a book that you have been longing for, or invest in a new CD. Surround yourself with special treats and you won't feel the bite of change.

It is also important to cut down on alcohol during the Breath Connection program. Although it will, at first, help you shallow breathe, it eventually leads to overbreathing. You might be interested to know that this is one of the main causes of hangovers. It can be difficult to resist alcohol when you are socializing, which is why it is important to begin the program during a quiet week. Some people enjoy a drink at the end of the day, to help them to relax or sleep. If you fall into this category, try to keep yourself busy so that you are tired enough to want to turn in and sleep when you get home.

Your body will adapt to the revised eating plan very quickly, and, in a short time, will not expect to be fueled at the old, regular times.

Exercise

For those of you who have exercise or other sports commitments, it may be unnecessary to make some changes to your regular routine while on the Breath Connection program. Just remember to keep your mouth closed, and be aware of the way you breathe as you exercise. This is particularly important for swimmers. Remember not to open your mouth to take in air when you reach the surface. Breathe through your nose at all times. Do a Control Pause before and after exercise, and if your score is less than 20 seconds, give yourself a break from that particular sport until your breath is regulated.

Never deep breathe after any type of exercise. This may seem like an impossibility now, but once you have started the Breath Connection program, you will find it easier and easier to achieve. Once you have taught yourself to breathe shallowly as an automatic response, you will not find it hard to continue breathing in this way, even after strenuous activity.

Asthmatics should be careful to avoid any activity for which they currently use a bronchodilator. This indicates that there is body resistance to the exercise, and you should listen to the message that your body is giving you. Remember that you are in brief and life-changing training for a short period of time, and you should do your best to be in prime condition before beginning the Breath Connection program.

Eliciting Outside Support

The power and support of friends, family, and organized groups cannot be overstated. Gamblers and Alcoholics Anonymous and Weight Watchers, among others, all testify to the role that caring people can play in helping someone break a bad habit or addiction. The first step is often the most difficult one—that of telling people that you have a problem and would like their encouragement as you set about solving it. Women are, in general, more likely to enlist outside support than men, but everyone on the Breath Connection program should have someone with whom they can talk things through. Don't be afraid to ask for help.

Cancer patients have had their life expectancies doubled when they have support groups to lean on, or even one special person to help share the strain. Heart bypass patients have also been shown to benefit from talking things through with groups of fellow sufferers, particularly if there is a measure of good humor involved.

Fortunately, with Breath Connection there is no stigma to overcome. People are not, in general, judgmental, and you will find that your determination to make changes will inspire encouragement. If necessary, ask your employer to be understanding and to tolerate occasional late arrivals in the morning, and short periods of the day when you will need to concentrate on your exercises. By overcoming any respiratory illness, and encouraging your body to work at peak level, your professional performance will be enhanced—a fact that can't hesitate to win over even the most skeptical boss.

Show this book to friends and colleagues, and explain what you want to achieve. Tell them that you are going to follow the Breath Connection program and ask for their encouragement. Don't be daunted if a few people are negative or even amused. We are used to cynicism here, and there will always be people who scoff at the idea that it is possible to make broad-scale health changes by altering the way you breathe. You may even find people who provide you with tales of the importance of deep breathing. Turn away from these doubters and be strong in your conviction. Follow the good instincts that led you to Breath Connection in the first place.

In the first week, try to avoid all who have been negative or unsupportive. If this isn't possible, ask them to respect what you are trying to do, just as you can respect their differing views. You need to be able to focus your energy on the program and should avoid anyone or any situation that threatens your wholehearted commitment.

Most important, remember that in five days your results will speak for themselves. If you do have any lingering doubts about embarking on the program, be positive with yourself and play up the potential gains more than the challenges. After all, what have you got to lose? By investing only five days to begin with, you will experience changes that can transform the way you think and feel.

It is particularly helpful to begin the program with someone else. Naturally, your partner or friend is unlikely to have exactly the same health conditions that you do, but your partner is bound to benefit from the program even if he or she feels completely well. It is more fun to have a friend to compare notes with, and it's important that there is someone to offer strong support if you feel like giving up.

Positive Mental Attitude

Are you someone who sees a glass as being half full or half empty? Are you a pessimist or an optimist? We encourage optimism and believe that concentrating on the potential gains of following the program rather than the negative aspects—giving up a favorite food, for example—will make a huge difference to your overall success. Dietary changes are a drawback for a number of people who begin the program, but we can assure you that the changes you need to make are minor. You will be eating well, and as much as you want to. You won't be sacrificing much at all. Be positive about your commitment and you will reap the rewards.

The decision you made to commit to the Breath Connection program was an enormous stride in the right direction. Some people find it helpful to see visual reminders of the healthy outcome of their course—pictures of people enjoying the pleasures of life, such as taking a long walk in the country, or playing an active sport with friends. Try to choose a picture of an activity in which you see yourself participating when the program is complete. If you are hoping to lose some weight, pin up a picture of an article of clothing that you want to fit into when your weight is regulated. If you suffer from disturbed sleep, find a photograph of someone enjoying a deep and peaceful sleep. Your motivation will be unique to you, and you will need to decide what will work best.

Some people respond to spoken motivation. Tapes offering calm, steady encouragement are available for you to listen to in the comfort of your home. We don't recommend that you play them while driving, as you need to remain alert while you are behind the wheel.

We know that the mind has a very powerful role to play in all self-healing situations. The mind-body relationship is a strong one, and literally hundreds of studies have proven that fact. When you feel good emotionally, you are more likely to feel well physically. Sports professionals psyche themselves up before major competitions, and allow their positive attitude to improve their performance. You can aid your own success by telling yourself, or showing yourself, how much better things will be when you complete the course. Our minds do not differentiate between an activity that is actually taking place and one that is simply and realistically imagined. Take advantage of the powers of mental rehearsal by visualizing your body as strong, healthy, and less drug-dependent.

Make a list of all the positive results you expect to achieve by the end of the five-day course. Make a collage with pictures and words cut from magazines, if they make a contribution to the picture you have of yourself when you are at your best. Perhaps you still have a photograph of yourself, taken when you were in peak health, to remind you. Indulge in a little fantasy of a dream holiday. Go on imaginary shopping sprees. Remind yourself that you might just be a little closer to your wish list if you persevere with the Breath Connection course.

Working Out Obstacles

One of the best ways to overcome obstacles is to anticipate them, and to plan how they will be confronted or circumvented. However carefully you have prepared for the course, and however firm your intentions are, you will undoubtedly face a setback at some stage. The important thing is not to be discouraged. Don't imagine that you are the first or only person to experience a glitch in your program. So you didn't meet your Control Pause target one day? It's not a tragedy, and you shouldn't even consider giving up.

Note down things that might go wrong. Maybe one day you will be interrupted in midexercise and will not have the time to start again. How will you deal with that? Perhaps you gave in to sleeping on your right side because you have always found that position more natural and more comfortable. Maybe you couldn't resist a big, frothy cappuccino. Think back to situations when you have broken your resolve in the past—early in the New Year, for example. Try to remember why you lapsed. Chances are that you weren't ready to change your bad habit. Now you are. You have committed to the Breath Connection course, and the very fact that you mind so much about a small setback proves that you are still committed to it.

If you fall off the horse, climb back on. Don't chastise yourself for slips. Accept that it is human nature to give in every now and then, and congratulate yourself for starting again, with a renewed effort.

Above all, be fair to yourself. Remember that you have embarked on a program of huge change. To reduce your drug intake in only five days is an enormous achievement, especially if you are a severe asthmatic. Congratulate yourself for the progress you have made, and avoid tormenting yourself for any imperfections. Years of being instructed to breathe deeply mean that some people may take longer than five days to achieve the target. That doesn't mean you have failed.

Take your time, think of something inspirational, and get back to work.

Sometimes we call inspiration a compelling outcome, and there can be any number of these, such as better digestion, improved sleep, freedom from drugs, social confidence, ideal weight, freedom from the fear of an attack, or even just an enhanced sense of well-being. Just thinking about any one of these goals should help to get you back on track. It is admirable to have high standards, but setting your sights too high means that you have further to fall when things do not go according to plan. Be realistic, and don't let your disappointment lead to dejection. Remember that you are doing amazingly well, considering what you have had to overcome.

The Appeal of Procrastination

Most people who habitually procrastinate abominate this tendency in themselves. A lucky few genuinely embrace the *mañana* philosophy of life, and actually believe that troubles will disappear if you ignore them for long enough. But the majority of procrastinators are guilt-ridden perfectionists who know perfectly well that tiresome tasks are best faced sooner rather than later, but who delay for a variety of reasons. One common reason for procrastination is the fear of success. Many people fear that they will not accomplish a task as well as their standards demand, and rather than suffer the indignity or disappointment of failure, they do not even begin.

If you have been thinking about the Breath Connection program but continue to put it off, just remember how empowering, how triumphant it feels to address a project over which you have been dithering. Tell other people what you plan. You are more likely to stick with something that you have made grand pronouncements about. Not many of us will suffer the loss of face involved in publicly giving up. The more people you tell, the harder it will be to quit. But be realistic, and don't book yourself onto a course that you will find difficult to complete. If you are changing jobs, having a baby, getting married, or moving to another house, you might want to delay things until your life is a little more settled.

If you continue to put off the Breath Connection program, even though intellectually and in every other way you know it makes sense, perhaps you should consider whether you are clinging to your illness, or present state of being, because its familiarity makes you feel secure. Your physical and emotional conditions are part of your identity, and it isn't always easy to change something so fundamental. Look hard at yourself. If you think the reasons for your failure to begin are linked with this type of attitude, accept them and use that self-knowledge to spur you on. If you are worried about the new challenges that life will impose on you when you are strong and healthy again, think positively. This is going to be the start of a fantastic adventure, something that will soon seem much more appealing than the comfortable cocoon of fearful habit. Acknowledging your fear is the first step to overcoming it, and we can help you do that.

Wanting Results Without Work

Another common human trait is our tendency to want something for nothing. We want results without effort. In our daydreams, we may have perfect looks, perfect health, perfect homes, jobs, and lives. . . . These are healthy inspirational images, and you should hang on to them when you start the Breath Connection program. Just bear in mind that only so much is realistic. We are sure you know very few people who have all of the preceding, and if they do, it is likely that they have worked very hard to achieve that status. Don't expect to gain anything without giving it some effort. Commit yourself to the program, and welcome the change it brings. The certainty is that you will be nearer to achieving what you want when your breathing has been reconditioned.

This is the reality: It is going to take some effort. Stay where you are, with your daydreams and your deteriorating health, or take control and make some effort to effect permanent change. Athletes who want to break records need dedication. So do students who want to achieve the highest honors. If you truly want to experience the benefits of balanced breathing, and the changes that this will bring, you have to work at it. We promise that the effort will soon become second nature and, as such, effortless.

Never say that you don't have time. All of us can make time for the things that matter, and as we said earlier, we always have time for the things we put first. Breath Connection involves committing to just a few minutes, three or four times a day. Your renewed zest for life will allow you to do things more quickly and efficiently, and you will sleep better, and for shorter periods, as a result. Spending a little time now will actually buy you some time later. And time wasted in doctors' or hospital waiting rooms will be a thing of the past. The Breath Connection program will be giving you more time—years and years of it.

Remember the old adage: You need to speculate to accumulate. By investing time today in the Breath Connection program, you will have achieved more than you could ever have imagined. That means a longer, healthier, freer life. Isn't it worth it?

14

The Maintenance Plan

Our plan begins with five days of your time. Not every hour of five days, but a few minutes, every so often. In this extraordinarily short space of time, an entire lifetime of harmful breathing can be adjusted and reconditioned. The path toward health and well-being can be paved.

You have already invested your time and effort, and even if you were to stop right now, your enterprise would have been well worthwhile. The changes that you will have already observed in your breathing, sleeping, susceptibility to asthma, and other attacks are remarkable. But now that your engine has been so thoroughly overhauled, and its performance is so dramatically better, don't you want to keep up the momentum and continue to improve? Aren't you keen to build on your achievement? At the very least, it makes sense to embark on a maintenance plan that will ensure your new energy is sustained.

Some Breath Connection patients are confident enough to enter the next phases of their lives without fear of relapse. Others continue to follow the self-care program we supply. Still others, those with more severe conditions, benefit from the continued supervision of a Breath Connection practitioner. It would be tragic if any of the good work achieved during those first, crucial five days were wasted, so we continue to offer encouragement when it is needed.

If you are concerned that you might not be disciplined enough to keep up the good work, you might need to continue to monitor your breathing habits after the five-day course. For all Breath Connection practitioners, retrained shallow breathing is second nature, so they do not need to set aside time for Control Pauses and pulse readings, unless they happen to be feeling unwell. For you to reach this level of confidence, you should continue with the exercises for a little while after the course. Eventually, shallow, retrained breathing will become completely automatic. If a stressful period comes along, and you think you may lapse into hyperventilating, it is reassuring to know that you can deal with it by reverting to the regular and, by now, familiar exercises. Emphysemic, bronchial, or asthmatic attacks can be a thing of the past.

The fast and dramatic improvements that all patients experience over the five-day course are, of course, a great incentive to keep going. For people with severe respiratory or other health problems, the success achieved in those first days will be all the motivation they need to continue. Expert help at the outset will always be useful for more seriously ill patients to look after themselves in the future.

Our maintenance program has been designed to fit into most people's modern lifestyles. It is also based on a sort of bond of trust. We assume that patients are not going to slip immediately back into the bad habits that lead them to us in the first place. Equally, we know that you do not expect us to make you instantly well after a lapse, a stressful period, or an illness, and you are aware that Breath Connection is not a miracle pill or a wonder drug. What we can do is improve your overall health to such a degree that illness is quickly and efficiently dealt with.

It's important to remember that you should never push yourself beyond comfortable limits. This program isn't about competition, even with yourself. However delighted you may be to see your Control Pause reach 60, and however much you may be feeling the benefits of correct breathing, you do not need to continue to push beyond that point. You have achieved a personal best! If you wish to develop your Control Pause above 60, this must be done under the supervision of a Breath Connection practitioner. This method is very powerful and you will need expert guidance if you wish to improve your breathing performance further.

Take stock after completing your five-day course and do the following:

- Recognize how much more healthy you feel.
- Continue to eliminate some of the physical threats in your life by maintaining your retrained breathing, sleeping, and eating patterns.
- Do all you can to prevent or remove triggers that may cause future illness.
- Build on what you have already achieved to expand your potential for good health.

Practical Advice

The most essential thing is to keep up your shallow breathing. If you need to be reminded, put notes around your home or office. It should, however, be more natural by now, and you should still continue to be aware of your breathing patterns throughout the day. If you start breathing deeply again, immediately change to shallow breathing.

Keep your mouth shut unless you are talking, eating, or drinking—wherever you are. Keep up the habit of placing tape on your mouth before you go to sleep at night. This practice can be discontinued if you are absolutely certain that you are no longer breathing through your mouth while asleep, but until that time, the tape is a good safeguard. Be especially watchful if you find you are snoring again, or if your mouth is dry in the morning.

Continue to sleep on your left side propped up by pillows, to ensure that you do not lose too much carbon dioxide. It's impossible to offer a reason why this works, but years of empirical research by Professor Buteyko have confirmed that sleeping upright, propped up against pillows on your left-hand side, can help to ensure the proper balance of carbon dioxide and oxygen in your body.

Stick to the diet recommended in Chapter 12. Above all, don't eat a heavy protein meal at night (see page 191). Keep dairy foods and sugars to a minimum, and continue to avoid processed and junk foods as much as possible. By now you may have lost your craving for them. Many people will have found that they want to eat much less at mealtimes. Keep up the good work!

Exercise as much as is practical and sensible, and remember to keep your mouth closed when doing so. Remember that the mechanism for your breathing is located in your brain, and the more you practice shallow breathing, the more automatic it will become. Any new behavior or action needs to be practiced consciously before it becomes an unconscious act, and it is particularly vital that you practice until it does become instinctive. You will prevent a lifetime of suffering and disease and feel better than you would ever have believed possible as a result.

Check your pulse and Control Pause every single day, in order to monitor your breathing progress as well as your overall health. If you can, try to see a Breath Connection practitioner from time to time in order to get expert advice if your health has changed in any way. Never try to push your Control Pause when you are on your own. This is a powerful treatment, and it must not be done for too long. Just as you would take no more than a couple of pain relievers when you have a headache, you must treat the Control Pause with respect.

Now that you are working on your own, try not to become overconfident or reckless with your exercises. On the other hand, don't feel that you have failed in any way if you need to see a practitioner for guidance.

Maintenance Suggestions for Mild Asthma
Carry on with the self-care program (see page 79) until you are able to manage without bronchodilators. Maintain your Control Pause at the level it was when you stopped using these drugs. Never, ever push it beyond comfortable limits in the interest of getting a result. This is both counterproductive and dangerous. Your reduced steroid intake should be supervised by your doctor in conjunction with a Breath Connection expert. Don't stop taking your steroids altogether, or you risk a relapse. If you are eventually able to cut them out entirely, it will only be after a slow and steady withdrawal.

Maintenance Suggestions for Severe Asthma
Follow the self-care program on page 93 on a daily basis, but adapt it when your severe asthma becomes mild. Then follow the guidelines recommended for steroid intake (see pages 67–72).

Maintenance Guidelines for Emphysema and Bronchitis
Emphysemics should continue with the program indefinitely. Those with bronchitis should follow it until the bronchitis disappears. If you still feel there is cause for concern, don't hesitate to see your Breath Connection counselor again. Then, continue with self-care.

Maintenance Guidelines for Sports Maintenance
Check your Control Pause before and after any sporting activity and keep your mouth closed for its duration. Before exercise, practice a Control Pause followed by five minutes of shallow breathing. After your exercise, do a Control Pause, followed by five minutes of shallow breathing. Repeat.

There are special chapters in this book offering advice for readers who seek more detailed information about maintenance plans for asthmatic children (see page 149), people prone to panic attacks (see page 124), and for overall, holistic good health (see page 134).

Do I Really Want to Feel Well Again?
Of course you do. All of us would like to experience the type of good health that others take for granted. Perhaps, however, something is holding you back from building upon the good work you have achieved over the five-day course. Perhaps you are under stress, and adhering to our guidelines seems like one more pressure. Many people suffering from stress find it difficult to make changes; clinging to what they perceive to be the few rocks of certainty in their lives is one way to feel more secure. In order to get well, however, things have to change. Don't be tempted to stick with a situation that is making you stressed. Think of your situation as a rut out of which you can climb. You need to make changes to

climb out, and you need determination. Just as you need the will to be well.

Lacking Motivation?

When you embarked on the Breath Connection program, you had the determination to make change. You can recover that will, even if a state of helplessness, which certainly requires less energy, has its appeal. Use your considerable will to help you to get back on course, and to climb out of that rut.

Remember how frightening asthma attacks were—that pain in your chest and the struggle for every breath? Either you continue to make changes in your life or you face going back to that. If you are in a stressful situation and find it difficult, think positively. Use friends and family for support and advice. Draw on others for motivation, and use as many positive affirmations as you can to keep things moving.

If you are feeling stressed and finding it difficult to motivate yourself, there are some excellent tapes that you can listen to in a quiet, calm place.

Again, don't castigate yourself for a brief loss of purpose. Visualize your ultimate aim and, if you must, visualize yourself at your most damaged state in the past. These visualizations will inspire you again.

15

Question Time

The fact that we are asked some questions over and over again confirms the fact that certain issues and aspects of the Breath Connection program consistently baffle a range of people. We don't like confusion, and we certainly don't mind addressing your questions as many times as it takes for the program to become clear. Here are the most frequently asked questions and the answers we always give.

How should we breathe—from the top of the lungs, the middle, or the bottom?
    The way you breathe is less important than the amount of air you take in, as this is what affects the balance of oxygen and carbon dioxide in the lungs. We recommend shallow breathing from the top of the lungs, as this is the best way to avoid hyperventilation.

How many times should I practice the exercises each day?
    We advise three to four times a day: early in the morning before breakfast (perform them even if you don't eat breakfast), before lunch, and again before dinner. Do them again about an hour before bed, if you can manage it. If you have regular colds or flu, you can step that up to five or more times

a day. Or, if you have a good Control Pause of 30 seconds or more, once or twice a day will be enough.

Why do some people have a low Control Pause but no asthma?

If you hyperventilate and have a low Control Pause, it may be that your body simply chooses to exhibit another defense mechanism to stop you from exhaling too much carbon dioxide. Some of the common diseases associated with hyperventilation include epilepsy, emphysema, diabetes, heart problems, cancer, and other fatal illnesses. Less seriously, snoring and a chronically blocked nose are common symptoms. The fact that your target area is the respiratory system, resulting in asthma, indicates that things are not as bad as they might be. The strain of hyperventilation will always be expressed in the body's weakest area or system. If you have been genetically bestowed with a strong respiratory system, you will not have asthma even if you overbreathe. But if your digestive system is weak, you will experience digestive complaints. If your immune system is weak, you will be more prone to infection.

Do all asthmatics hyperventilate and have a low Control Pause?

Yes. The more severe your asthma, the lower your Control Pause.

What is Salbutamol?

Salbutamol is the generic name for Ventolin.

Why do yoga teachers recommend deep breathing?

Yoga teaches breath control and some exercises might involve either deep or shallow breathing, or holding the breath for a designated period of time. Therefore, Yogic breathing does not always involve hyperventilation. Some yoga teachers have embraced the Western view that deep breathing is good for you. We do not agree with that. The diagram below compares balanced breathing, with lung ventilation of about five liters a minute, with full Yogic breathing. In this type of breathing, very deep, slow breaths are taken and held before exhalation. The person is not taking in huge quantities of air because the breath is drawn so slowly,

Yogic breathing

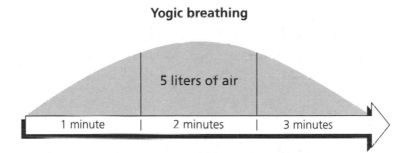

5 liters of air breathed over 3 minutes.

Asthmatic breathing

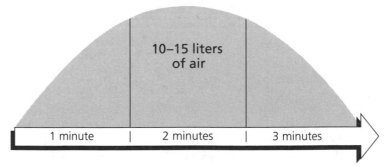

10–15 liters of air breathed over 3 minutes.

221

with the mouth closed. Yoga has helped some asthmatics, but the results tend to be slow.

I am a yoga teacher and I have mild asthma. What should I do?

Stop deep breathing during yoga exercises and tell your pupils you have done so. Ancient yogis did not have a word for *oxygen* and did recommend breath control, but not as a life pattern, only as an exercise. Deep breathing would not be recommended for asthmatics. In fact, your deep breathing may have caused your asthma. Remember that deep breathing has only ever been a part of a yogic program, not something to practice constantly, any more than you would follow another yogic exercise such as remaining balanced on your head for 24 hours a day.

I am a telephonist/teacher with moderate asthma and I have to talk a lot at work. What should I do?

Follow the Breath Connection program and improve your Control Pause. The lower your Control Pause, the more you will find it difficult to talk and the more you will hyperventilate. Learn to talk from your lips only, not taking deep breaths before you begin. Moderate your breath between pauses. You will probably have to take a little more time to relay your message.

I am an extremely busy businessperson, and I have severe asthma. What steps should I take?

You should try to get away from your professional stresses for a week or two. Work on making your asthma mild. If you can take an even longer break, your asthma will become extremely mild if you follow the Breath Connection program. If neither of these options is realistic—although you should think carefully about the ultimate value of your health, and remember that you will be no good to your company if you become seriously debilitated—discuss things with an enlightened doctor, increase your oral steroids in consultation with your doctor, get better exercise, and practice shallow breathing in the airplane or in the back of your car, and during meetings. Steroids could be increased before difficult meetings, during bad weather, and before travel, but do not forget to normalize the dosage when you feel better. Learn how to control your breath when you give talks and presentations (see above). Sleep less, with your mouth taped, so that you will have more time for the exercises. Cut back on alcohol and eat less at business lunches. Have a light, nonprotein meal for business dinners. If you suddenly feel stressed during the day, do a Control Pause and shallow breathe for about three minutes. Smoke less.

I'm a stay-at-home mom with mild asthma, and I have a family of young children. What can I do?

You probably don't think you have time for the Breath Connection exercises, but you do. Like the preceding businessperson, you can make time. When you are enjoying much more restful sleep, it will become easier and easier to do so. Think of all the other things that you struggle to find the time and energy to complete—shopping, cleaning, cooking, collecting children, school activities. You have to breathe, no matter what, so there is no reason not to do it properly. There must be times when you have a few moments to relax and concentrate on your exercises and Control Pause. At the hairdresser? While your children are watching a video? When you are sitting in the garden? In a traffic jam? In the bath? At the very least, train yourself to be aware of your breathing at all times throughout the day.

When we are measuring the Control Pause, why do we empty the lungs rather than hold the breath after breathing in?

It is very important to hold your breath only after you have breathed out. This is particularly important for people with asthma, emphysema, and bronchitis. After you breathe out, your bronchial tubes expand. After breathing in, they narrow. By holding your breath after breathing in, you could develop emphysema through overstretching your lung tissue, and the condition could become aggravated if you already have it. The Control Pause should only ever be measured after breathing out. Holding your breath after breathing in only focuses on your lung capacity, not your degree of overbreathing—and that is what we are aiming to measure.

Do the health conditions you have outlined for the length of the Control Pause apply to both adults and children?

Yes. Age, height, or body size have no effect on the Control Pause. Lung capacity is not an issue.

Why do we need such large lungs if we are supposed to breathe shallowly?

We have a large stomach capacity, even though it isn't strictly necessary. It helps our digestive system to function well. The stomach does not need to be stuffed for this, and it should not be. The stomach was once a reservoir for food when we were hunters. Evolution has outstripped some of the functions of a large stomach, but it still handles the digestive system pretty well. Perhaps we needed that extra capacity for air in our lungs, long ago when people needed more air for the lives they led. Why do we still have the redundant appendix? In a few million years, this organ will probably disappear. It took a long time for humans, whose ancestors came from the sea, to lose their gills. A very few people still have them!

With the self-care program, what kind of improvement can the average asthmatic hope to achieve?

We estimate that the average improvement is about 60 percent reduction in the need for medication, a significant alleviation of asthma symptoms, and a correspondingly more comfortable and enjoyable life. Remember that this is an average figure. If your original situation was desperate, it may take time to reach that level of improvement. If it was only mild or average, the gain could be much, much higher.

Why don't doctors give carbon dioxide, rather than oxygen? Why don't they issue carbon dioxide inhalers?

Quite simply, the reason is that doctors have not been trained to understand the importance and benefits of carbon dioxide. Ironically, about 40 years ago, some doctors did administer small amounts of carbon dioxide to asthmatics and emphysemics. But with the development of steroid drugs came the conviction that the new wonder drugs would always come to the rescue. Carbon dioxide use was discontinued.

Why should we sleep on the left side?

Although the lung capacity is slightly larger on one side than the other, there is no scientific evidence to explain why sleeping on the left side is better. Professor Buteyko simply observed over many years and work with tens of thousands of patients that those who slept on their left sides lost much less carbon dioxide than the others. The results are conclusive enough to make us urge you to arrange your pillow so that you sleep on your left side. You will certainly make up your own mind about this once you have experienced less hyperventilation during sleep.

Is the Breath Connection program helpful for those with degenerative conditions such as arthritis, rheumatism, and heart disease?

Certainly. Check the list of disorders that Breath Connection can help with, in Appendix B.

Should I do the Breath Connection program if I am pregnant?

Yes, the program is very helpful, and it can be especially useful if you suffer from antenatal sickness and postnatal depression. Reconditioning your breathing is beneficial to your developing baby, which is likely to be bigger and healthier as a result.

I have a young baby. What can I do for her?

Attend a Breath Connection workshop if you can, in order to learn how to help your baby. If you can't, read this book carefully and make notes for yourself if you think that would be helpful. Refer especially to the chapter on asthma and childhood. Obviously, placing tape over a baby's mouth as it sleeps is not always going to be a practical option. Do, however, try to close your baby's mouth with your finger when you see her breathing with an open mouth.

Asthma is very difficult to diagnose in young infants. If you know or suspect that you or your partner carry the gene that makes you more susceptible to asthma, be particularly watchful until your baby is old enough to be diagnosed. In the meantime, take practical measures such as reducing dairy foods, taking care to substitute other forms of calcium (see page 192).

Isn't carbon dioxide meant to be poisonous?

Our air contains about 200 times less carbon dioxide than we need to function effectively. That's why the alveoli of the lungs work so hard to make up this deficit by producing enough carbon dioxide for us. It is a myth that it is a damaging waste gas.

Which illnesses cannot be treated by Breath Connection?

At the end of Appendix B, you'll find a short list of conditions that don't, sadly, respond to the Breath Connection treatment because they are not caused by hyperventilation. Ninety percent of the illnesses to which we are prey can be alleviated by the Breath Connection techniques.

Do the Breathing Exercises prevent common colds and flu?

Yes, because they boost your immune system, which means that you will be less susceptible to infection. If you had flu or a cold before embarking on the Breath Connection program, we suggest that you take extra vitamin C, the herb Echinacea, and the mineral zinc. Your doctor or Breath Connection practitioner, who is aware of your personal profile, may offer more specific advice.

Some self-help/relaxation books recommend "retention breath," in which you breathe in, hold it, and then breathe out for a specified number of seconds. What do you think?

This may relax you, but it isn't helping your breathing or your health. If your Control Pause is 50 to 60 seconds, it doesn't matter how you breathe. With the Breath Connection method, the less time you take to breathe in the better, but it doesn't matter how long you take to breathe out.

Is it harmful for me to play the flute or sing?

If you are already hyperventilating and have a low Control Pause, we are sorry to say that it is harmful. As singing and playing wind instruments usually increase your rate of breathing, they are not recommended for anyone with a hyperventilation problem. You should, however, be fine if your Control Pause is high, and you have been balancing your breathing for a while. It is, really, only a question of setting aside your music for a short time. After getting the balance right, you can return to it and your carbon dioxide levels won't be affected enough to worry about. Of course, if you are a professional musician who needs to practice as well as perform under pressure, you may need to seek more specific advice.

What's wrong with the old-fashioned method of breathing into a brown paper bag, and then inhaling to reabsorb the carbon dioxide, especially if I am having a panic attack?

Nothing at all, and many asthmatics have also found it useful during attacks. Some hospitals also use the technique. Remember, however, that it is a quick fix—no more and no less. It will not deal with the root of your problem—hyperventilation.

Once I have learned the Breath Connection methods, will I be able to teach them to others?

No. Don't be misled by the apparent simplicity of our courses. Breath Connection practitioners all have a very sophisticated understanding of every complexity of breathing and its functions. All of our practitioners have been personally trained by Professor Buteyko and have up to 15 to 20 years of experience in teaching his methods.

Can I, as an asthmatic, go scuba diving or go in for other water sports that involve oxygen masks?

You need to check with a Breath Connection practitioner, or your doctor. It depends entirely on your Control Pause.

What are the dangers of developing osteoporosis if I cut down on dairy products, including milk?

See our section on diet and nutrition (page 187). Many other foods offer lots of calcium, including leafy green vegetables, cereals, some fruit, offal, pulses, and tofu.

When can I stop taking steroids?

Only when your Breath Connection practitioner and doctor recommend it.

Are the side effects of steroids reversible?

Yes. Following the Breath Connection program has a profound effect on all of your body systems and can lead to a reversal of all steroid side effects.

What about alcohol on the program?

Avoid it completely, if possible. Remember that the original course is only five days! If that's difficult, cut back to a maximum of two glasses of wine a day with meals. Remember that the Breath Connection program is essentially a holistic one, and you will obtain the greatest range of benefits if you undertake it with your whole health in mind. Aim for positive change all around.

Does that mean I should stop smoking?

You should not smoke while you are involved with the program and, in fact, Breath Connection offers an ideal kick start to a delayed resolve to quit. But we are not judgmental, and we realize that for many people the stress of giving up smoking leads them to overbreathe even more. Focusing on shallow breathing will certainly help you, but you may find hypnosis or acupuncture useful if you want to stop smoking.

Will Breath Connection help with my depression?

Absolutely, yes. It is not just your physical health that the program addresses. Your brain function, emotional and mental states, and instabilities are all addressed. Apart from anything else, you now know that you have taken control, and you have been empowered to do so. This action is almost always uplifting and self-affirming. However, remember that depression is a very complex illness and for some people specialist psychological or psychiatric help may be necessary.

Are the breathing exercises a form of stress management, then?

If you like, yes. Do the Control Pause for a few minutes and your shallow breathing will counteract any negative stress responses that your body produces. Use the Control Pause as a regular basic health and stress-level check.

Does Breath Connection work for genetic disorders?
Sometimes it can, as in the case of cystic fibrosis, for example. Refer to Appendix B.

Is it all right to sleep with plants and flowers in the room?
It's best if you don't. Plants and flowers eat carbon dioxide at night.

Is fasting a good idea?
In general, yes. Think of it as giving your body a holiday from the hard work of digestion, so that it can concentrate on eliminating toxins. Toxins are excreted through the pores of the skin, as well as through the bowel and in the urine. Over the centuries, many advanced societies have advocated occasional fasting. Some claim that the head is cleared and lightened (or enlightened!) as the body rests and clears itself. If you do fast, drink lots of water and organic carrot and beetroot juice. If you merely want to reduce your intake of solids, keep to a diet of light salads without oil, and fruit and vegetables. Raw vegetables are best. You can, if you wish, simply eat boiled rice.

As the body flushes away its waste, you may find that you get headaches, some mild diarrhea, and your breath may smell bad. These are all normal symptoms and act as evidence of the fact that your body is detoxifying. Drink plenty of water to flush the toxins, and try colonic irrigation, which also speeds up the process.

It is generally advised that you discuss any proposed fast with your doctor, particularly if you intend to fast for more than one or two days. If you have certain physical or emotional problems, it might be best to wait until you are stronger. No diabetic or hypoglycemic, for example, should ever fast. Other people should only do so when they have been advised that it is the right time, or optimal point, to embark on this useful cleansing exercise.

Can I be really tiresome and ask you to spell out for me, one more time, how I, as an asthmatic, should program my day?

Your question isn't tiresome at all. We encourage people to be at ease and confident about what they are undertaking with Breath Connection.

- Just after waking, hold your breath and sit up. Breathe gently through the nose and resist any desire to clear the chest by coughing. Try to retain your phlegm and release it in one go later. A violent coughing fit could lead to a full-blown asthma attack. Use the anticoughing techniques if necessary (see page 120).
- Whatever you used to do first in the morning, do it second. Your breathing comes first. An asthmatic's Control Pause is at its lowest, and the danger of hyperventilation is at its height, early in the morning.
- Do your breathing exercises and note down the figures. Allow 20 to 30 minutes for this.
- Take your medication (steroids) but avoid bronchodilators. It could be the mistake of your life—literally—to take relievers without immediate need. Many people—including athletes—do this, but it can worsen the situation in the long term.
- Do not use your peak flow meter. It is merely a register of symptoms.
- Don't eat breakfast unless you are hungry. You risk hyperventilation if you do so. Remember that food is also a reliever, and you should only take it if you need relief from hunger.

- Try to breathe shallowly on the way to work, whether you walk, ride, or drive.
- Do your Breath Connection exercises before lunch. Many people hyperventilate at mealtimes, not because of what or how much they eat, but how they do so.
- Check your Control Pause several times a day.
- Use your spare time—in the car, on a bus, in a restaurant, between meetings, while cooking—to shallow breathe. If you do hyperventilate, it will be easier to control. You could check that your breathing is appropriately light by holding the flame of a lighter beneath your nose. It should barely flicker.
- For those of you who ask which part of the lung you should use for breathing, the answer is the tip of your nose! Imagine that you don't have lungs at all. That way, ironically, they will function well.
- When going out into the cold from a warm room, or vice versa, breathe out just before opening the door, and then take five or 10 steps without breathing at all. Then breathe shallowly. This exercise will help you to avoid an asthma attack.
- If you enjoy sports and exercise, treat yourself! An active lifestyle—even for asthmatics—is far better than an overprotected one. But make sensible preparations. Exercising early in the morning is a good start to the day.
- Do your Breath Connection exercises before dinner.
- Before you sleep, do a Control Pause. Tape up your mouth, settle yourself on your left side, and enjoy the best sleep you've had in years.

16

Science and History

Now that you know Breath Connection works, you might like to learn a little more about why it works and how it was developed.

You know that over 200 illnesses and disorders can be successfully treated by Breath Connection. You know that results are fast, techniques are simple and inexpensive, and seldom drug-dependent. You know that the reconditioning of your breathing and a proper understanding of the vital importance of carbon dioxide is crucial to your health. But how did Professor Buteyko know this when he first began to develop his research in Russia just after the Second World War?

Early in 1960, having endured years when his work was underfunded, if not dismissed outright, Professor Buteyko announced his findings to a forum at the Institute of Experimental Biology and Medicine at the Siberian branch of the then USSR's Academy of Science. Despite encountering initial skepticism, he was allowed to continue with his work and is fully recognized today by his government.

Studies across Russia and in Australia have shown anyone following the Buteyko techniques will benefit and that 90 percent of asthmatics reduce their drug dependency. Both frequency and severity of asthmatic attacks are diminished by natural means. His methods have proved to be a near-infallible way of monitoring general health and of improving quality of all-around health. To date, over a million asthmatics in Russia have benefited from his techniques. And most of them are no longer dependent upon medication of any kind.

Despite vast amounts of money thrown at research into respiratory and other illnesses, few conventional Western approaches have come close to dealing so effectively with asthma, cancers, arthritis, and other degenerative diseases. Symptomatic relief, which requires continued use of new drugs, has been developed but the fundamental problems of asthma and other respiratory disorders have not been addressed. We may be living longer and even have the material comforts that should allow us to enjoy comfortable old age, but for many people their final years—even their middle age—are severely limited by a degenerative disease.

As yet, most of us only seek medical advice when we know we are ill. Then we may be prescribed drugs that we may be expected to take for the rest of our lives. The Breath Connection methods turn this whole idea on its head. Why wait until something goes wrong or breaks down before looking after your body? It's simple. All you need to do is learn to breathe properly.

So why has it taken so long for Professor Buteyko's principles to be embraced here in the West? We tentatively offer an analogy with Copernicus (1473–1543). Before his time, even the most brilliant of Renaissance thinkers believed that the sun and the other planets revolved around the earth. A century later, Galileo, who advanced Copernicus's pioneering theories, was similarly pilloried. In the West today, our understanding of respiratory medicine is still very limited: Few orthodox practitioners realize that so many disorders are connected to incorrect breathing, not simply the obvious illnesses of the breathing tracts and lungs.

At Breath Connection, we operate from scientific foundations. Konstantin Buteyko is a professor of conventional medicine and trained within rigorous scientific disciplines. While recognizing the importance of complementary and alternative medicine, we don't reject established understandings of the way the human body works. It is our hope and belief that the Buteyko principles themselves will soon be regarded as conventional. Bear in mind that Professor Buteyko's work was conducted at a time when the dissemination of ideas from East to West was slower than it is today. It first came to attention outside Russia when one of the professor's chief associates began to demonstrate the importance of Professor Buteyko's ideas and methods in the Western world.

Hyperventilation, or overbreathing as it was known in the nineteenth century, is the simple cause of a huge raft of illnesses. We hope that our book has overturned that raft and shown that shallow breathing, rather than taking deep breaths, is a first principle for permanent good health—whatever your age when you begin to practice it. Hyperventilation is the cause of illness, not a result of it. Be spare with your air. Deep breaths can lead to deep trouble. We respect the other elements—fire, water, and earth—rather more than we have hitherto respected the fourth, air. Just as fire can comfort and help to nourish us but also damage us if it is not controlled, and just as we know that a deprivation of sunlight can cause SAD (Seasonal Affective Disorder) in some people, we should be aware that our consumption of air should also be controlled. Too much air breathed in can be as damaging as, or more damaging than, too much ultraviolet light. We know that we can survive, if we must, without food or water for long periods. Yogis have used deprivation to heighten spiritual experiences. But we are mistaken if we ignore or neglect to monitor the amount of the air we take in and underestimate the value of carbon dioxide.

The regime we offer is not merely about common sense and personal responsibility, however. It is about choice. There is usually a hard way and an easy way to confront every one of life's dilemmas. We hope that we will have shown you that the 'helpful' discipline of Breath Connection pays an immediate dividend. Your life will become easier. You can stop fearing allergies, panic attacks, and insomnia, chronic fatigue, and arthritis as well as conditions most often associated with a disorder of the breathing apparatus.

And all this is due to work and research doggedly pursued by Professor Buteyko years before he had any real hope of his findings being accepted.

Breath control was actually understood over 3,000 years ago in Tibet, where they believed that death entered a person through the mouth. Much later the Romans employed the same word for *breath* and *spirit.* In Sanskrit, *prana* means not only breath but universal life force. Recently, here in the West, it has been observed that creatures, such as mice, who breathe rapidly have shorter life spans than those, such as elephants, who breathe slowly. Such findings have contributed to a universal and timeless debate about how the very act of breathing influences how we expend an allotted life force. These same findings have also served to confuse as they tend to correlate slow breathing with deep breathing and a long, healthy life.

Regulating our breathing conditions all the body's systems, as we have shown, and is a basic form of meditation which can reduce stress as well as beneficially affect physical disorder. But meditation as such should not be confused with the Breath Connection program. Although it can be generally helpful, it does not offer specific help in dealing with disease, as Breath Connection does. We embrace the mind-body holistic principles alongside practical and designated aims and techniques for patients who are or may become ill. We are not in the business of restoring inner calm, in the same way that a meditational program might be.

A hundred years ago, two Austrian scientists, Breyer and Gering, discovered that humans were the only species on earth who had not developed a correct way to breathe. Not much happened after this pioneering finding. Fast-forward several decades to the earliest findings of Professor Buteyko, who began to see that most humans were taking in up to 4 to 10 times more air than they needed and, moreover, saw the link between overbreathing and a huge list of diseases that many before him had seen as being not only chronic and debilitating, but incurable. With generous and proper respect, he acknowledged the pioneering work of Verigo and Bohr (see page 240).

This had helped him to see that when too much air was drawn deep into the lungs, carbon dioxide was then being exhaled in great quantity rather than being retained to facilitate the oxygen's work. Professor Buteyko began to encounter the old chestnut about oxygen being good for us—and so the more the better, please—and carbon dioxide being a poisonous waste gas.

When the human biological system was developing, aeons ago, the air contained a percentage of CO_2 at least a hundred times higher than it is today. But this level has been steadily depleted by the natural development of the environment, including the culture of trees and plants which absorb carbon dioxide. The percentage of CO_2 in today's air is less than one-half of 1 percent. In the months we spend awaiting birth in the womb, we get used to absorbing a gaseous mix which contains seven to eight percent carbon dioxide. What a shock to be born into such a differently balanced gaseous environment and how unnecessary it has been to routinely smack the newborn's bottom, causing him or her to gulp in a lungful of alien air.

The alveoli in the lungs have adapted resourcefully to this situation, as we have seen, and create an environment of 6.5 percent carbon dioxide within the body, but we still need to breathe correctly to maintain this level, and asthmatics and those people with some other illnesses find this difficult. When the carbon dioxide level in the body sinks below 3.5 percent, palpitations, dizziness, and wheezing occur. Breath Connection simply teaches you to normalize the carbon dioxide levels up to about 6 percent, which is our human physiological norm.

Science, as we understand the word, didn't exist as a discipline for study until the early eighteenth century. Until then, ideas about the world's mysteries were largely influenced by religious and spiritual beliefs. Many of these still prevail. Breathing used to be considered a means of cooling the blood. The ideas of the French chemist, Antoine Lavoisier (1743–1794), who saw oxygen as a great life force and carbon dioxide as a poison, are still widely accepted. His experiments with mice placed under glass domes along with a burning candle supported his view when the candle and mouse expired at roughly the same time as the oxygen supply was exhausted. Because only carbon dioxide remained, he concluded that it must be a poison.

In 1909, Professor Yandell Henderson at Yale University dared to disagree and said that "oxygen is in no sense a stimulant to living creatures" after he had observed that it was in fact a carbon dioxide deficiency that caused animals forced to breathe in experimental conditions to die. Few listened to him.

The toxicity of oxygen had been observed as early as 1899, but it was not until the 1960s that scientists, such as the young Professor Buteyko, began to understand it. Some premature babies who breathed in 100 percent oxygen during incubation developed a form of blindness known as retrolensil fibroplasia.

Even the most brilliant of scientists cannot change the composition of our atmosphere, which currently contains twice as much oxygen as we need to function well and 200 times less carbon dioxide. But many are now continuing Professor Buteyko's precepts and working with the adaptability and ingenuity of the human body to ensure that we control the elements of our air so that it suits us and our environment.

Overbreathing, or hyperventilation, was first identified in 1871 by the American physician da Costa, who observed the palpitations, coughing, and breathlessness, coupled with stress, from which many soldiers returning from the American Civil War suffered. His observations were studied later by the British doctor John Haldane, whose work on a large group of healthy soldiers set out the norms for breathing. We should breathe four to six liters of air into the lungs every minute. The norms are still in use today. Haldane recognized the importance of the balance between oxygen and carbon dioxide in the breathing process.

In 1905, the Russian physiologist, Verigo, and the Dutch physicist, Bohr, independently built on Haldane's work, demonstrating yet again the wonderful international chair of scientific and medical progress. They ascertained that without carbon dioxide in the body, oxygen cannot perform its regenerative function and, moreover, blood pressure will increase. Yet many hospitals still automatically pump asthma patients, admitted in crisis, with oxygen which they don't require and which can exacerbate their condition.

It was against this dawning of understanding that Professor Buteyko trained as a doctor in Russia and formed his interest in respiratory and related disorders. He came to realize that none of us needs to breathe in large amounts of air or compete with the stopwatch and breathe a set number of times each minute. He saw the dangers of hyperventilation, and he realized that taking in more than four to six liters of air per minute wrongly filled the lungs with an unnecessary amount of air. The central nervous system can be destabilized, and the digestive, hormonal, elimination, immune, and cardiovascular systems damaged. Fatigue and general weakness also occur. For Professor Buteyko, it became a matter of training patients to breathe deeply in order to witness the results. He then had to prove to other doctors that patients who were inhaling as much as 10 to 15 liters of air each minute were damaging their health.

He had noticed that patients' breathing often became deeper as the onset of death approached and he learned to judge very accurately how long someone had to live simply by monitoring his or her breathing. His passion for the study of respiratory disorder was awakened when he was a third-year medical student. He noticed that patients who were hyperventilating recovered if their breathing was encouraged to be more shallow. The first seedlings of today's knowledge about how correct breathing can affect many nonrespiratory illnesses were planted at this time, along with the early formation of Professor Buteyko's philosophy about diet and stress management. At first subjected to ridicule, Buteyko's ideas were eventually accepted by the Russian Ministry of Health, but it was to be years before his efforts were properly funded, recognized, and adopted throughout the Soviet Union.

Men—and women—of science who are ahead of their time, such as Joseph Lister, whose findings created the foundation for modern anesthetics, and Louis Pasteur, who taught the world about the importance of antiseptics, suffered the indignity of having much of their work ridiculed or unrecognized throughout their lifetimes. At least Professor Buteyko has lived to see his ideas widely accepted and adopted in Russia. A 95 percent success rate for his methods is recorded in Russia, and the remaining 5 percent of patients enjoy at least some relief if not a complete cure.

This book is about the importance of breath in our lives. It is so much more than a set of breathing exercises and a technique for hyperventilation. Nearly half a century of medical research and experience by Professor Buteyko has created a new medical system which addresses the relationship between oxygen and carbon dioxide in our bodies, thereby providing the key to our physical and mental health.

We at Breath Connection are very proud to be involved in the advancement of Professor Buteyko's life-saving message and hope that it will be a very short time before its obvious simplicity and effectiveness are regarded as the norm. Just as the achievements of Lister, Pasteur, and other scientific geniuses have formed the cornerstones of our modern concept of good health, Professor Buteyko and his revolutionary approach will form one of the vital foundations of our health in the future.

Appendix A: Recordkeeping Charts

BREATH CONNECTION WEEKLY PROGRAM FOR MILD ASTHMA: RECORDKEEPING CHART

Date	Time	Start Pulse	Control Pause	Shallow Breathe	Control Pause	Shallow Breathe	Control Pause + 5 seconds	Shallow Breathe	Control Pause + 10 seconds	Shallow Breathe	Control Pause	Final Pulse	Medication Intake and Physical Condition
	Morning												
	Afternoon												
	Evening												
	Morning												
	Afternoon												
	Evening												
	Morning												
	Afternoon												
	Evening												
	Morning												
	Afternoon												
	Evening												
	Morning												
	Afternoon												
	Evening												
	Morning												
	Afternoon												
	Evening												

243

BREATH CONNECTION WEEKLY PROGRAM FOR SEVERE ASTHMA: RECORDKEEPING CHART

Date	Time	Check Pulse	Control Pause	Decrease Breathing	Control Pause	Rest	Control Pause	Decrease Breathing	Control Pause	Rest	Control Pause
	Mor										
	Aft										
	Eve										
	Mor										
	Aft										
	Eve										
	Mor										
	Aft										
	Eve										
	Mor										
	Aft										
	Eve										
	Mor										
	Aft										
	Eve										
	Mor										
	Aft										
	Eve										

Do this exercise 3 times a day. For further instructions regarding continuation of practice, see chapter 6.

Decrease Breathing	Control Pause	Rest	Control Pause	Decrease Breathing	Control Pause	Rest	Control Pause	Decrease Breathing	Control Pause	Rest	Final Pulse	Medication Intake and Physical Condition

BREATH CONNECTION WEEKLY PROGRAM FOR MILD–SEVERE EMPHYSEMA: RECORDKEEPING CHART

Date	Time	Start Pulse	Control Pause	Shallow Breathe	Control Pause + 5 seconds	Final Pulse	Intake of Medication and Physical Condition
	Morning						
	Afternoon						
	Evening						
	Morning						
	Afternoon						
	Evening						
	Morning						
	Afternoon						
	Evening						
	Morning						
	Afternoon						
	Evening						
	Morning						
	Afternoon						
	Evening						
	Morning						
	Afternoon						
	Evening						
	Morning						
	Afternoon						
	Evening						

BREATH CONNECTION WEEKLY EXERCISE PROGRAM FOR SEVERE EMPHYSEMA: RECORDKEEPING CHART

Date	Time	Start Pulse	Control Pause	Exercises 1, 2, and 3	Control Pause	Final Pulse	Intake of Medication and Physical Condition
	Morning						
	Afternoon						
	Evening						
	Before Sleep						
	Morning						
	Afternoon						
	Evening						
	Before Sleep						
	Morning						
	Afternoon						
	Evening						
	Before Sleep						
	Morning						
	Afternoon						
	Evening						
	Before Sleep						
	Morning						
	Afternoon						
	Evening						
	Before Sleep						
	Morning						

247

BREATH CONNECTION WEEKLY PROGRAM FOR COLDS, FLU, AND HAYFEVER: RECORDKEEPING CHART

Date	Time	First Pulse	Control Pause	Shallow Breathe	Control Pause	Shallow Breathe	Control Pause	Shallow Breathe	Control Pause	Final Pulse	Intake of Medication and Physical Condition
	Morning										
	Afternoon										
	Evening										
	Morning										
	Afternoon										
	Evening										
	Morning										
	Afternoon										
	Evening										
	Morning										
	Afternoon										
	Evening										
	Morning										
	Afternoon										
	Evening										

248

BREATH CONNECTION WEEKLY SELF-CARE PROGRAM FOR STRESS AND BRONCHITIS: RECORDKEEPING CHART

Date	Time	Start Pulse	Control Pause	Shallow Breathe	Control Pause	Final Pulse	Intake of Medication and Physical Condition
	Morning						
	1 hour before sleep						
	Morning						
	1 hour before sleep						
	Morning						
	1 hour before sleep						
	Morning						
	1 hour before sleep						
	Morning						
	1 hour before sleep						
	Morning						
	1 hour before sleep						

249

BREATH CONNECTION WEEKLY BRONCHITIS PROGRAM: RECORDKEEPING CHART

Date	Time	Start Pulse	Control Pause	Shallow Breathe	Control Pause	Final Pulse	Intake of Medication and Physical Condition
	Morning						
	1 hour before sleep						
	Morning						
	1 hour before sleep						
	Morning						
	1 hour before sleep						
	Morning						
	1 hour before sleep						
	Morning						
	1 hour before sleep						
	Morning						
	1 hour before sleep						

BREATH CONNECTION WEEKLY PROGRAM FOR CHILDREN WITH ASTHMA AND BRONCHITIS: RECORDKEEPING CHART

Date	Time	Start Pulse	Control Pause	Number of Steps	Minutes of Shallow Breathing	Intake of Medication and Physical Condition
	Morning					
	Afternoon					
	Evening					
	Morning					
	Afternoon					
	Evening					
	Morning					
	Afternoon					
	Evening					
	Morning					
	Afternoon					
	Evening					
	Morning					
	Afternoon					
	Evening					
	Morning					
	Afternoon					
	Evening					
	Morning					
	Afternoon					
	Evening					

BREATH CONNECTION PROGRAM FOR SPORTS: RECORDKEEPING CHART

Date	Time	First Pulse	Control Pause	Shallow Breathe	Pulse	Control Pause	Shallow Breathe	Control Pause	Pulse	Intake of Medication and Physical Condition
	Before Sport									
	After Sport									
	Before Sport									
	After Sport									
	Before Sport									
	After Sport									
	Before Sport									
	After Sport									
	Before Sport									
	After Sport									
	Before Sport									
	After Sport									
	Before Sport									
	After Sport									

Appendix B: Most Common Health Problems and Symptoms That Can Be Treated by Breath Connection

Acidosis aklalosis

Agoraphobia

AIDS*

Allergies*

Anemia*

Anorexia nervosa*

Apathy

Arthritis (osteo and rheuma-
toid)*

Asthma attacks

Bed-wetting

Breathing without pause after
exhaling

Breathlessness

Bronchitis

Bulimia*

Cancer*

Cerebral palsy*

Chest pains (not in the heart
region)*

Chronic blocked nose

Chronic diarrhea

Chronic fatigue syndrome*

Chronic pneumonia*

Circulation problems*

Colds

Concentration problems

Constipation

Coughing

Cystic Fibrosis*

Depression*

Deterioration of vision

Diarrhea

Dizziness

Drug addiction*

Dry skin

Eczema

Edema

Epilepsy*

Far-sightedness

Fear without reason

Flatulence

Flu

Frigidity

Gulf War Syndrome*

Gynecological problems*

Hay Fever

Headaches

Heart attacks*

Heart conditions*

Heartburn

High blood pressure*

Hyperventilation

Impotence (male)

Infertility*

Insomnia*

Insulin-dependent diabetes*

Irritable bowel syndrome

Irritability

Itching

Kidney disease*

Lack of concentration

Loss of feeling in the limbs*

Loss of memory

Low blood pressure*

Memory loss

Menopause symptoms*

Mental fatigue

Migraine*

Multiple sclerosis (MS)*

Muscle pains

Nightmares

Pain in the heart region*

Painful and irregular periods*
   (female)

Palpitations*

Panic attacks

Parkinson's disease*

Post- and prenatal depression*

Posttrauma stress*

Premenstrual syndrom (PMS)*

Rhinitis

Scleroderma*

Short temper

Shortness of breath

Sinusitis

Skin problems*

Sleep apnea*

Snoring

Spasms of brain/heart/kidney/
   extremities/blood vessels*

Sterility*

Stomach sickness

Stress

Stroke*

Thyroid problems*

Tightness around chest

Trembling and tics*

Ulcers*

Varicose veins

Weight gain

Weight loss

The preceding list represents 90 of the 200 illnesses that Professor Buteyko discovered to be caused by hyperventilation. More than 90 percent of us suffer from these illnesses. When Professor Buteyko trained his patients to stop hyperventilating, their conditions either improved considerably or disappeared completely.

Anyone who suffers from asthma, emphysema, or bronchitis and one of the asterisked conditions (see above), is advised not to undertake the self-care programs in this book. You can still benefit from the Breath Connection program, but we strongly recommend that you do so under the guidance of a fully qualified and experienced Breath Connection practitioner. These illnesses are more difficult to treat and require a very individual approach for each patient. Although they will not be cured within a week, you should experience some improvement in your symptoms within a short period of time. You will, however, have to practice for some time, to remove the root cause of the condition.

Illnesses That Cannot Be Helped by Breath Connection

There are some illnesses that cannot be treated by Breath Connection. The most commonly known of these include the following:

Alzheimer's disease (although it can help in the early stages)	Manic depression
	Psoriasis
Autism	Psychosis
Back pain	Schizophrenia
Bad posture	Tonsillitis
Coma	Trauma/Accidents

Appendix C: Glossary

Acid/Alkaline balance: Otherwise known as the pH balance. This is the ratio of acids to alkalis measured in body fluids such as blood, gastric juices, and urine. Maintaining the correct pH value is essential for the normal, healthy functioning of every cell in the body. This balance, or homeostasis, can be detrimentally affected by a poor diet (including too much protein, sugar, or grains), stress, and hyperventilation.

Asthma: An inflammatory disease of the airways, resulting in bronchospasm attacks that induce coughing, wheezing, and gasping for air, among other symptoms.

Allergy: A defensive response by the body to a normally harmless trigger or allergen. Common allergens include foods, pollens, metals, household chemicals, dust mites, feathers, and animal fur. An allergy is an abnormal response, which indicates that the body is in a hypersensitive state.

Alveoli: Clusters of air sacs that are responsible for the exchange of gases between the lungs and the bloodstream.

Balanced breathing: Slow, shallow breathing that balances the delicate ratio of carbon dioxide to oxygen in the lungs and ensures optimum health.

Bronchitis: The inflammation of the mucous membranes of the respiratory system.

Bronchodilator: A drug taken by patients with respiratory conditions such as asthma. Bronchodilators artificially dilate the bronchial tubes in order to facilitate breathing. However, by forcing a greater intake of oxygen into the lungs, these drugs further exacerbate hyperventilation, leading to a greater deterioration of the patient's medical condition.

Carbon dioxide: A natural gas, and the body's own, natural bronchodilator. In its various chemical forms, carbon dioxide (also known as CO_2) is responsible for maintaining the correct pH balance of the blood and is a vital regulator of the body's systems.

Control Pause: A technique that allows you to measure the level of carbon dioxide in your lungs, and hence the state of your present (and future) health.

Emphysema: A severe respiratory condition in which the alveoli (air sacs) of the lungs fail to contract properly, thereby failing to expel sufficient air. This results in constant breathing difficulties, including serious shortness of breath.

Hyperventilation: Hyperventilation, or overbreathing, occurs when the intake of air is greater than the physiological norm of 5 liters per minute. This lowers the level of carbon dioxide in the bloodstream, which subsequently deprives the tissues of essential oxygen. According to Professor Buteyko, hyperventilation is a breathing disorder that causes a wide range of illnesses and is not merely a symptom of these illnesses.

Immune system: The body's overall defense system against internal and external attack. The immune system produces antibodies that help to protect the body against foreign substances and encourages the healing mechanism. A strong immune system deals with invaders, such as bacteria or viruses, quickly and efficiently.

Nebulizer: A method of administering bronchodilator drugs in very high doses.

Overbreathing: *See* Hyperventilation.

Oxygenation: The vital transportation of oxygen through the bloodstream, from the lungs to the body tissues.

Peak flow meter: An instrument used by the conventional medical profession to measure lung capacity.

pH: *See* Acid/Alkaline balance.

Respiration: The overall exchange of oxygen and carbon dioxide between the atmosphere, blood, lungs, and body cells.

Spasm: An uncontrollable contraction of one or more muscles. A spasm is one example of the body's natural defense mechanism against excessive loss of carbon dioxide.

Steroid: Natural steroids are chemicals such as cholesterol and hormones that are released by certain glands in the body. Steroids are also artificially manufactured, in order to mimic the actions of the body's own natural steroids. Artificial steroids are used preventatively for the treatment of asthma and other respiratory disorders, among other things.

Appendix D: Resources

Breath Connection U.S.	350 East 54 Street, New York, NY 10022-5049
Telephone:	Information on courses: Toll free: 1-800-259-4644
Fax:	212-415-9060
E-mail:	admin@breathconnection.com
Web site:	http://www.breathconnection.com
Telephone Advisory Service:	Contact email admin@breathconnection.com for further information
The Hale Clinic	7 Park Crescent, London W1N 3HE
Telephone	011 44 171 631 0156
Fax:	011 44 171 323 1693
Web site:	http://www.haleclinic.com
E-mail:	admin@haleclinic.com

Bibliography

Burne, Jerome. "Hyperventilation: The New Argument about Asthma," *Independent on Sunday*, 5 October 1997.

Carola, Robert, et al. *Human Anatomy and Physiology*, 2nd edition. New York: McGraw-Hill, 1992.

Chopra, Deepak. *Boundless Energy*. Rider, 1995.

Graham, Tess. "Self-Management of Asthma through Normalisation of Breathing: The Role of Breathing Therapy," *Australian Medical Journal*, December 1998.

Hale, Teresa. *The Hale Clinic Guide to Good Health*. Kyle Cathie Books, 1996.

Holford, Patrick. *The Optimum Nutrition Bible*. Piatkus, 1997.

Kenton, Leslie. *The New Ageless Ageing*. Vermilion, 1995.

McCance, Kathryn L., and Sue E. Heuther. *Pathophysiology: The Biologic Basis for Disease in Adults and Children*, 2nd edition. Mosby-Year Book Inc., 1994.

May-Ropers, Christine, and David Schweitzer. *Never Acidic Again*.

Perera, Judith. "The Hazards of Heavy Breathing," *New Scientist*, 3 December 1988.

Price, Sylvia, and Lorraine Wilson. *Clinical Concepts of Disease Processes,* 4th edition. Mosby-Year Book Inc., 1972.

Rowett, H. G. Q., *Basic Anatomy and Physiology,* 3rd edition. John Murray (Publishers) Ltd., 1988.

Shivapremananda, Swami. *Yoga for Stress Relief.* Gaia Books, 1997.

The Sivananda Yoga Centre. *The Book of Yoga: The Complete Step-by-Step Guide,* Ebury Press, 1983.

Stalmatski, Alexander. *Freedom from Asthma.* Kyle Cathie Books, 1997.

Weil, Andrew. *Spontaneous Healing.* Little Brown & Co., 1995.

Index

abdominal breathing exercises, for panic attacks, 123
accidents, 255
aches and pains, 126, 132, 254
  see also pain
acid/alkaline balance, see pH balance
acidosis alkalosis, 177, 253
acquired immune deficiency syndrome, see AIDS
acupuncture, 21, 26, 27
  for smoking cessation, 230
adrenal cortex, and steroid use, 68
adrenaline, treatment with, 61, 62, 66
  and asthma related deaths, 65
aging, premature, 179
agoraphobia, 186, 253
agrochemicals, 30, 128, 179
AIDS, 19, 184, 185, 253
air intake, ideal, 33, 47, 240
  see also inhalation
air travel, 74, 89, 201
alcohol use
  and elimination system, 128
  to handle stress, 125
  reducing, 164, 166, 193, 203, 229–30

allergens
  and asthma, 168
  inhaling, 171
allergies, 180, 182, 184, 253
  Breath Connection effect on, 22, 83
  as defense mechanism, 143
  to food, 30, 184
  and pH balance, 166
  suppression of, 62
  susceptibility to, 40, 171, 178, 184
alternative medicine, 6, 12, 236
  see also complementary medicine
alveoli, 36, 227, 239
  in emphysema, 103
  during hyperventilation, 167
Alzheimer's disease, 255
amino acids, 190
aminophylline, 65
anabolic steroids, 67
Andrews, Professor Gavin, 176
anemia, 253
anger, 186, 254
angina, 40, 162, 165, 175
animal hair, and asthma, 168
anorexia nervosa, 135, 166, 187, 253

rhinitis, 50, 254
rice, in diet, 192, 202, 231
Rimiterol, 64

Salbutamol, 64, 106, 220
Salmetorol (Serevent), 64, 77
  for emphysema, 106
  for severe asthma, 86, 89, 91
salt, dietary
  as asthma trigger, 42
  avoiding, 191, 202
schizophrenia, 255
schools
  asthmatic children in, 151, 158
  Breath Connection use in, 22
scleroderma, 254
scuba diving, 229
seasonings, for food, 192
self-care, 106, 119, 129–39, 212
  for children, 148, 153–6, 160
  daily technique for, 134
  improvement from, 225
  special techniques for, 135–7
self-help, in health care, 12, 26, 96
Severent, see Salmetorol
sex hormones, 182
shallow breathing, 50, 174, 213,
  214, 236
  and alcohol consumption, 203
  for asthmatics, 90, 91, 233
  for children, 146
  after exercise, 203
  and panic attacks, 123, 125
  for stress reduction, 126, 230
showering, and asthma attacks, 73
singing, 228
sinusitis, 50, 167, 171
  Breath Connection for, 21, 83,
  254
skin disorders, 184
  Breath Connection for, 254
  steroids to treat, 67

sleep
  Breath Connection effect on, 80,
  84, 98, 131, 233
  and children, 147, 159
  with plants/flowers in room, 231
  posture during, 39, 52–3, 74,
  139, 215, 225–6
  problems with, 126, 172–4
  taping mouth during, 39, 91,
  215
sleep apnea, 167, 172–4, 254
sleep disorders, 172–4
smoking
  as asthma trigger, 42
  and chronic bronchitis, 112, 113
  and emphysema, 100, 102, 104
  to handle stress, 128
  stopping, 164, 166, 230
snoring, 167, 172, 215, 254
  as defense mechanism, 134
  and hyperventilation, 220
  prevention of, 53, 142
  and sleep apnea, 173
sodium cromoglycate, 65
sore throat, 112
  Breath Connection for, 21
soy-based foods, 191
space travel, breathing methods
  for, 180
spasms
  of bronchi, 35, 57–9, 115, 118,
  178
  of muscles, 40
  treatment of, 254
Spence, Dr. Gerald, 22
spiritual beliefs, 18, 239
sports activities
  for asthmatics, 233
  during Breath Connection program, 203
  breathing during, 78, 138
  by children, 155

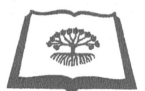

Getting Old Is
MURDER

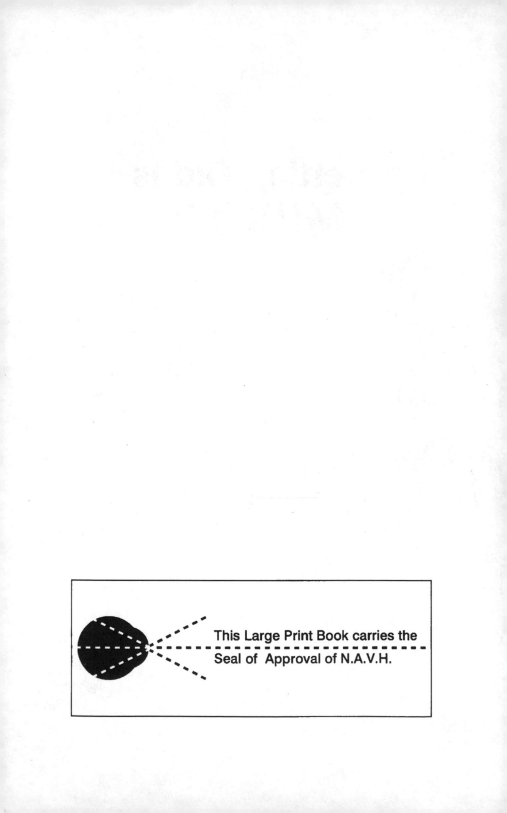
This Large Print Book carries the
Seal of Approval of N.A.V.H.

M

Getting Old Is
MURDER

Rita Lakin

Thorndike Press • Waterville, Maine

Published in 2006 by arrangement with The Bantam Dell Publishing Group, a division of Random House, Inc.

Thorndike Press® Large Print Mystery.

The tree indicium is a trademark of Thorndike Press.

The text of this Large Print edition is unabridged. Other aspects of the book may vary from the original edition.

Set in 16 pt. Plantin by Carleen Stearns.

Printed in the United States on permanent paper.

Library of Congress Cataloging-in-Publication Data

Lakin, Rita.
    Getting old is murder / by Rita Lakin. — Large print ed.
    p. cm. — (Thorndike Press large print mystery)
    ISBN 0-7862-8281-9 (lg. print : hc : alk. paper)
    1. Older people — Fiction.   2. Retirees — Fiction.
3. Fort Lauderdale (Fla.) — Fiction.   4. Florida —
Fiction.   5. Large type books.   I. Title.   II. Thorndike
Press large print mystery series.
    PS3612.A5424G48 2006
    813'.6—dc22   2005028291

For

My beloved mother, Gladys,
Who coulda, woulda, shoulda
been Gladdy Gold

and

My dearest Aunt Ann
Who inspired me all my life

National Association for Visually Handicapped
------------------------ serving the partially seeing

As the Founder/CEO of NAVH, the only national health agency solely devoted to those who, although not totally blind, have an eye disease which could lead to serious visual impairment, I am pleased to recognize Thorndike Press* as one of the leading publishers in the large print field.

Founded in 1954 in San Francisco to prepare large print textbooks for partially seeing children, NAVH became the pioneer and standard setting agency in the preparation of large type.

Today, those publishers who meet our standards carry the prestigious "Seal of Approval" indicating high quality large print. We are delighted that Thorndike Press is one of the publishers whose titles meet these standards. We are also pleased to recognize the significant contribution Thorndike Press is making in this important and growing field.

Lorraine H. Marchi, L.H.D.
Founder/CEO
NAVH

* Thorndike Press encompasses the following imprints: Thorndike, Wheeler, Walker and Large Print Press.

You know that old trees just grow stronger
And old rivers grow wilder every day
But old people just grow lonesome
Waiting for someone to say,
"Hello in there. Hello."

Hello in There
by John Prine

"Let's face it. We all have the same five relatives."

Billy Crystal

If one life matters
Then all life matters
A Christian meditation

"The golden years have come at last
Well, the golden years can kiss my ass."
Hy Binder,
taken from the Internet

Introduction to Our Characters

GLADDY & HER GLADIATORS

Gladys (Gladdy) Gold, 75 Our heroine, and her funny, adorable, sometimes impossible partners:

Evelyn (Evvie) Markowitz, 73 Gladdy's sister. Logical, a regular Sherlock Holmes

Ida Franz, 71 Stubborn, mean, great for in-your-face confrontation

Bella Fox, 83 "The shadow." She's so forgettable, she's perfect for surveillance, but smarter than you think

Sophie Meyerbeer, 80 Master of disguises, she lives for color-coordination

Francie Charles, 77 Always optimistic, Gladdy's best friend

YENTAS, KIBITZERS, SUFFERERS: THE INHABITANTS OF PHASE TWO

Hy Binder, 88 A man of a thousand jokes,

all of them tasteless

Lola Binder, 78 His wife, who hasn't a
thought in her head that he hasn't
put there

Denny Ryan, 42 The handyman. Sweet,
kind, mentally slow

Enya Slovak, 84 Survivor of "the camps"
but never survived

Harriet Feder, 44 "Poor Harriet," stuck
with caring for her mother

Esther Feder, 77 Harriet's mom in a
wheelchair. What a nag

Tessie Hoffman, 56 Chubby, in mourning
for her best friend

Millie Weiss, 80 Suffering with
Alzheimer's, and

Irving Weiss, 86 Suffering because she's
suffering

Mary Mueller, 60 and

John Mueller, 60 Nosy neighbors

ODDBALLS AND FRUITCAKES

The Canadians, 30ish Young, tan, and
clueless

Leo (Mr. Sleaze) Slezak, 50 Smarmy real
estate broker

Greta Kronk, 88 Crazy like a fox

Sol Spankowitz, 79 A lech after the ladies

THE COP AND THE COP'S POP

Morgan (Morrie) Langford, 35 Tall, lanky, sweet, and smart

Jack Langford, 75 Handsome and romantic

THE LIBRARY MAVENS

Conchetta Aguilar, 38 Her Cuban coffee could grow hair on your chest

Barney Schwartz, 27 Loves a good puzzle

AND

Yolanda Diaz, 22 Her English is bad, but her heart is good

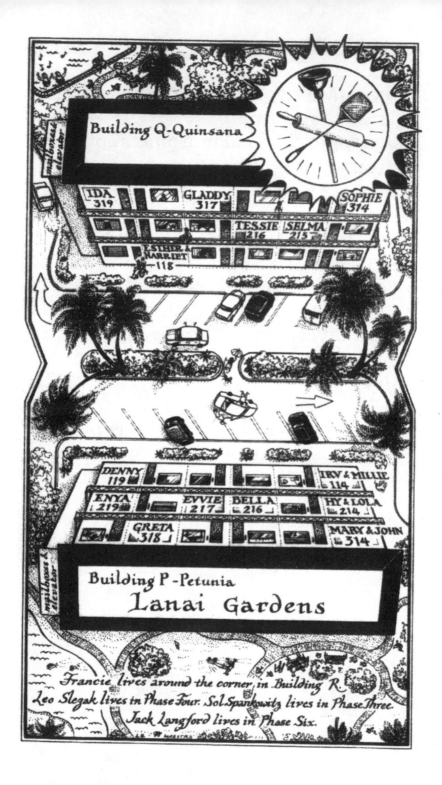

Gladdy's Glossary

Yiddish (meaning Jewish) came into being between the ninth and twelfth centuries in Germany as adaptation of German dialect to the special uses of Jewish religious life.

In the early twentieth century, Yiddish was spoken by eleven million Jews in Eastern Europe and the United States. Its use declined radically. However, lately there has been a renewed interest in embracing Yiddish once again as a connection to Jewish culture.

a choleria	a curse on you (get cholera)
a klog iz mi	woe is me
aleha ha-shalom	rest in peace
alter kuckers	lecherous old men
chozzerai	a lot of nonsense
dreck	dirt, filth
fahputzed	overly done
farbissener	embittered person
farblondjet	bewildered
gefilte fish	stuffed fish
geshrei	uproar
gonif	thief

Gott im Himmel	God in heaven
Kaddish	mourner's prayer
kasha	buckwheat groats
kasha varnishkas	groats & bowtie noodles
kibitz	someone offering unwanted advice
knish	meat or potato filled wonton
kreplach	like a wonton
kurveh	whore
kvetch	whining & complaining
maven	someone who knows everything
meeskite	ugly one
meshugeneh	crazy
mitzvah	a blessing
ongepatshket	overdone, cluttered
oy	an exclamation for emotions
oy gevalt	an anguished cry
pisher	a squirt, a nobody
putz	penis
rugallah	pastry with fillings
schlep	dragging a load
schmaltz	fat
schmear	to coat with butter or cream cheese
shayner boychik	darling boy

shayner kindlach	beautiful children
shikseh	non-Jewish girl
shmegegi	a fool
shnapps	whiskey
shpilkes	on pins and needles
vantz	bedbug
vay iz mir	woe is me
yenta	busybody

Death by Delivery

The poison was in the pot roast.

In a few hours Selma Beller would be dead. This was regrettable because tomorrow was her birthday and she was so looking forward to it. Her husband, Ernie, had keeled over at seventy-nine. Having beaten him at gin rummy and shuffle-board, she had gleefully intended to beat him yet again, this time to the big eight-oh. Alas, poor Selma.

While she was waiting to die, Selma was dusting.

Dust was her enemy. And she battled mightily. No fragile feather duster for her. And forget that sissy stuff like lemon Pledge. She used good old-fashioned Lysol, confident that neither dust nor germ escaped its lethal dose. Death to dust, she thought and then laughed, dust to dust.

Looking up, Selma glanced at the clock. Where had *the afternoon gone? It was nearly dinnertime. Too bad her best (and only) friend, Tessie, was busy tonight with out-of-town visitors. She should have gone shopping this morning. Oh, well, there was always cottage cheese, with a piece of cut-up peach and some sour cream. She wrinkled up her nose. What she really craved was red meat. Bloody and rare.*

There was a knock on the door.

Selma groped around for her glasses, misplaced, as usual. Giving up, she moved as quickly as she could manage toward the door, automatically straightening the doily on the arm of her emerald green recliner. Glancing toward the array of grandchildren's photos on her foyer table, she blew a kiss at the smiling faces.

"Who is it?" she trilled. She would never open the door to a stranger.

"Delivery. Meals on Wheels."

Squinting through the peephole, Selma, though her vision was blurred, identified the familiar shopping bags with the Meals on Wheels logo. A volunteer wearing jeans, a windbreaker, a baseball cap, and sunglasses stood there, arms full.

"Wrong apartment," she said wistfully.

"Mrs. Beller? Apartment two-fifteen?"

"Yes, but I didn't order —"

"Happy birthday to you from Meals on Wheels. A special introductory order."

"Really?" Selma was feeling the beginnings of hope. "Something smells wonderful. What's in the bags?"

The volunteer consulted a piece of paper. "Pot roast. Stuffed cabbage rolls. Mushroom and barley soup, potato pancakes with sour cream, and apple strudel for dessert."

Practically drooling, Selma unlocked the deadbolt her son, Heshy, had installed, then the other two safety locks.

She squinted again as the volunteer entered with the packages. "Don't I know you? You look familiar. . . ." But Selma was distracted as she sniffed the air in appreciation. "I can't wait," she said as she took the bags and carried them into her spotless kitchen. She quickly unwrapped the containers and began setting them out on her best Melmac dishes on her small white Formica dinette table.

"I just hope the soup isn't too salty. My blood pressure, you know."

A wrought-iron chair was pulled out for her. Smiling, she let herself be seated.

"At your service, Mrs. Beller."

"What a way to go." Selma giggled, tucking her napkin in.

* * *

Those were Selma Beller's final words.

The last thing she saw as she was starting to lose consciousness was the logo on the Meals on Wheels shopping bags as the killer calmly refolded them, and her last fading thought was that the pot roast had been a little stringy. . . .

1

Gladdy Gets Going

Hello. Let me introduce myself. I'm Gladdy Gold. Actually, Gladys. I'm a self-proclaimed P.I. That's right, a private eye. Operating out of Fort Lauderdale. When did I get into the P.I. biz? As we speak. My credentials? More than thirty years of reading mysteries. Miss Marple and Miss Silver are my heroines.

In case you were expecting someone like what's-her-name with her "A" is for this, "B" is for that — you know who I mean, working her way all the way to Z — well, that's not me. I'll be lucky if I make it to the end of this book. After all, I *am* seventy-five.

You think seventy-five is old? Maybe, if you're twenty, it's ancient, but if you're fifty, it doesn't seem as old as it used to. And if you're ninety, well, seventy-five seems like a kid. You ought to see those spry ninety-year-old *alter kuckers* trying to hit on me for a date. When I look in the mirror, I don't see that older, faded, wrinkled stranger who barely resembles some-one I once knew. I see a gangly, pretty, eager seventeen-year-old, marvelously alert and alive with glistening brown hair and hazel eyes.

Did you know that when you get older, and the brain cells start to turn on you, the nouns are the first to go?

For example, "what's-her-name" I just threw at you. I meant Sue Grafton, and this time it only took about two minutes for my brain synapses to make the connection and pull her name out of the cobwebs of my mind. Sometimes it takes days. All the while, it was on the tip of my tongue. My poor tongue must be exhausted from all the information I keep stored there.

Hey, you young ones — laugh. Wait 'til you get to be my age. Then the laugh will be on you. You'll ask the same questions we all ask: Where did the years go? How did they go by so fast? And even worse — where did all the money go?

Enough with all the philosophy. The question for now is how did I get into this private-eye racket? Before I retired, I was a librarian, so if you say this is a strange ca-reer move, I would certainly agree.

I was minding my own business in Lanai Gardens, Phase Two, building Q, apartment 317 on West Oakland Park Boulevard, Lauderdale Lakes, when a few of my neighbors died suddenly. Considering that the youngest of us is seventy-one and the oldest eighty-six, this is not something unexpected. I mean, *everybody* is on the checkout line. For example, we used to have five tables of canasta: now we're down to one. The Men's Sports Club used to fill four cars on Sunday for their trip out to Hialeah: now the only members left are Irving Weiss and his pal, Sol, from Phase Three. Even the nags that broke the guys' wallets have gone to thoroughbred heaven.

As I started to say — I was beginning to suspect foul play.

I am convinced that these deaths to which I am referring are not natural. There is a killer stalking Lanai Gardens. Nobody believes me, certainly not the police, but I intend to prove it. But first you need to meet the rest of the gang.

2

Walking

It's seven a.m. on a beautiful, very typical Friday morning in paradise. As usual I wake up a minute before the alarm goes off. I start my coffee perking — a vice I will not give up. I take out my one slice of whole wheat bread, pop it in the toaster. Get out my one teaspoon of sugar and my one-percent low-fat milk and I am ready to "seize the day."

I allow myself twenty minutes to work on the unfinished Sunday crossword that never leaves my kitchen table. I used to do the puzzle, in ink, on the morning it arrived. Now, it can take as long as a week to dredge up answers from my disobedient brain. Frustrating, but you do not give up *anything* that affords you pleasure at this time in life.

Lanai Gardens is situated in one of the many sprawling apartment complexes in this part of southeast Florida. A lot of people think of Fort Lauderdale as this ritzy community on the water, or the place made famous by all those college kids who take their clothes off on Spring Break — but that's not where we live.

Our condo isn't fancy, but it's pretty nice with its peach stucco buildings (just beginning to peel), swaying palm trees (look out for the falling coconuts), well-tended lawns (when the gardener shows up), pools and Jacuzzis, shuffleboard courts, duck ponds (watch your step!), and recreation rooms.

Now, into a pair of sweats, and I'm ready to begin the morning workout, such as it is. It's eight a.m. and my fellow residents are coming to life.

We used to go to the air-conditioned malls for our morning stroll, but not after reading those articles in the newspapers about older women being killed. Now we've decided to exercise at home. Exercise? Fast walking, slow walking, shuffling, barely moving at all; whatever the body will endure.

I'm the first one out on the third-floor walkway to warm up. And that's the signal for all the others to rush out.

My sister, Evvie Markowitz, is always the next one out. While I am in the Q building (Q for Quinsana), she lives across the way in apartment 215 in P building (P for Petunia. The builders were big on flowers).

She refers to herself as my kid sister. Seventy-three to my seventy-five. We don't look anything like each other. I am taller. She is heavier. (We're both shorter than we used to be.) Before we turned gray, she was a redhead; I, a brunette. I was the scholarly one; she the dynamic, dramatic one. I was the plain one; she was the beauty. This dictum came down from our well-meaning but unsophisticated immigrant mother who didn't understand what damage such labels could cause. It set the course for both our lives. We never really became friends until I moved down here.

Evvie starts her own warm-ups. She always says the same thing every morning, calling out to me over the tops of the cars parked between our buildings. "Glad, how did you sleep?"

"Pretty good," I call back.

"I only had to get up three times last night," she says.

"Don't complain. Five times for me!" This from Ida Franz, our whirling dervish, who pops out of apartment 319 in my building and fairly leaps into pace with me. Ida is seventy-one, with a body that's compact and wiry. Her salt-and-pepper hair is always in a tight bun which threatens to pull her face off her head. Her back is ramrod straight, which Evvie says is so she won't drop the chip on each shoulder. "And the last time was at three a.m. It didn't pay to go back to bed after that."

"So what did you do?" Evvie calls out from across the way, knowing full well what Ida will say.

"I called my son in L.A. He's still up at midnight."

Evvie makes a familiar disgusted gesture, flapping her arms. We are all used to Ida trying to make her children love her, a lost cause. She's the one who calls them; they never call her. And because her children make her crazy, Ida makes us crazy.

I hear what I hear every morning: Sophie, calling from her kitchen window. "Yoo-hoo, I'm coming. I'm coming. Wait for me!" Trust me. She'll be last one out.

Routine is very important to us. Ida, the perpetual wet blanket, says it's because we're all in our second childhood. Except for Sophie, who she insists never grew out of her first one.

Now the door to apartment 216 opens across the way in Evvie's building. Bella Fox, who is eighty-three, gingerly steps out.

"Good morning," she whispers.

The girls call Bella "the shadow" because she's forever trailing one step behind us. We are always afraid of losing her, because she is so forgettable. She's tiny, not even five feet, and she wears pale colors that add to her seeming invisibility. But I'm on to Bella. She may seem shy, but in her own timid little way she's not afraid to speak her piece. She says what she wants and she gets what she wants. "Hi, gang! Your personal trainer is here! Everybody ready?" This is from Francie Charles, calling up to us as she rounds the corner from her building.

Her arrival is the signal for all of us to go downstairs and meet on the ground floor. Then we walk together along a shady path that winds around the building.

Francie, who will be seventy-eight tomorrow, was a real beauty when she was young. Tall, elegant, and classy, a model in her younger New York days, she is still beautiful. She's our real athlete, the one who got us all started in this somewhat anemic form of exercise. "Something is better than nothing," she is always telling us. She is also our health nut, lecturing on the right way to eat, although no one really can, or wants to, change the bad habits of a lifetime. Francie's only weakness is advertised by her favorite sweatshirt, "Death by

Chocolate," given to her by her adoring grandchildren. She is wearing it today.

"How is everyone?" she chirps. "Isn't it a glorious day? Aren't we all glad to be alive!" As grumpy as Ida is, that's how cheerful Francie is. The perpetual optimist. She makes every day a gift. If it wasn't for Francie, I'd have left Florida years ago.

Bella begins taking slow, mincing steps — her version of exercise — along the path, apologizing every time anyone passes her.

"Stop apologizing for living," Evvie is constantly telling her. But Bella, who is fairly deaf, either doesn't hear or chooses not to. We all love her, but she doesn't believe it.

We walk and talk. With plenty to say, as if we don't see one another every single day and night. Not to mention phoning one another a dozen or more times a day.

Our half-hour workout is just about over when Sophie Meyerbeer, our roly-poly eighty-year-old, finally steps out of the elevator, bandbox-perfect in her pink, color-coordinated, extra-tight jogging ensemble. Pink sweats, pink sneakers with matching pom-poms, and a pink flowered sun hat. I might mention that this month's hairdo is also pink. Champagne Pink.

When she finally catches up to us, Ida mock-applauds her arrival. "So happy you could make it, Princess."

Clueless, Sophie takes her sarcasm as a compliment. Being incapable of sponta- neity, Sophie has to get all dressed up, in- cluding makeup (*fahputzed,* Evvie calls it), before she'll walk out her door. Her third husband, Stanley, who made a fortune in notions and novelties, spoiled her rotten. He babied her, never let her lift a finger. Insisted she dress like a Kewpie doll for him. (Boy, did we speculate on *their* sex life!) He left her well-off and impossible.

"We're just about finished," says Ida, cooling down by walking slower.

"Oh," Sophie says, pouting girlishly. "Well, I couldn't help it. I didn't sleep a wink last night. I had such a terrible night- mare."

Bella stops, glad for any excuse not to move. "Ooh, tell us." She sits down on a bench, fanning herself.

Sophie shudders. "I dreamed I had a heart attack!"

Bella gasps, fluttering her hands ner- vously. "Oy . . . just like Selma."

"Change the subject," Ida snaps. She is never comfortable talking about death.

"No, it's my dream," Sophie insists.

"Just because Selma had a heart attack doesn't mean you will," Francie says gently as she continues her stretches.

Evvie adds judgmentally, "Besides, she was overweight and never exercised."

"Yeah," Ida adds with a satisfied smirk, "she and her pal Tessie were both thrown out of Weight Watchers."

"Maybe something caused that heart attack," I say. "For example, you know how Selma waxed those floors?"

"Yeah," Sophie chirps, "you coulda gone ice skating on them."

"Maybe she slipped and fell. Or maybe something frightened her . . ." I continue.

"She was so scared of spiders," Bella chimes in, happy to be able to contribute. "Remember that time she fainted when a teensie one crawled on her chair . . . ?"

Ida puts her hands on her hips defiantly and glares at me. "So? Dead is dead. What difference does it make?"

"The point is nobody bothered to investigate," I say. "Nobody cared to find out what really happened. Maybe if she hadn't been alone, maybe if Tessie hadn't had company that weekend, maybe she wouldn't have died."

This gives everyone pause.

Ida's had enough, and starts for the elevator. "Well, I'm going to get my bathing suit on."

"Good idea," I say, sorry I even brought it up. What's the point in depressing them?

Francie puts a reassuring arm around me. "Hey, Ida called it." Mimicking her: "Dead is dead." She giggles and I join in.

The group disbands, each to her own building, to get ready for part two of the morning routine — the pool.

3

Swimming

Just as I'm ready to walk out the door and head for the pool, I look at the phone, count to three, and — it rings. I pick it up and say, "Yes, Sophie."

"Are we going to the pool?"

"Yes, dear."

"Can I walk down with you?"

"Only if you're ready."

"Well . . . I'll just be a minute."

Knowing Sophie's minute, I tell her as I always do, "I'll start down. You can catch up to me."

I hang up, but stay by the phone. I know my customers. It rings again. My daily double. "Yes, Bella," I say as I pick up.

"Are we going to Publix today?" she asks.

"We usually go shopping on Friday."

"Is it Friday?"

"Yes, dear. Now go knock on Evvie's door and she'll walk you down to the pool. Don't forget your towel."

"All right."

The phones. Umbilical cords. Lifelines. To keep connected. To counteract loneliness. God bless Bell South.

I walk down the three flights instead of taking the elevator, another small attempt to keep fit, and join the parade heading for the pool. Everyone's in bathing suits, sun hats, and thongs (not the kind worn by the young girls at Miami Beach, but the ones which adorn wrinkled feet) and carrying towels and small beach bags. Swimming time is also early in the morning — before it gets too hot to sit around the pool.

Francie is in the parking area chatting with Denny Ryan as he rakes up fallen palm fronds. He is a big six-footer, in his early forties, but you'd hardly know it. Perhaps being slightly slow-witted has kept him childlike. His mother, Maureen, died suddenly about seven years ago. Maybe it's cruel to say it, but he's better off. Even though she was his sole support and caretaker, she was a harridan. But there is a real sweetness to Denny, and we try to add to his small allowance from Social Security by giving him odd jobs around our apartments. He can and does fix everything.

It was poor Denny, just doing his job, who came up to Selma's apartment to fix a plumbing leak. He was the one who found her dead body, and he still hasn't gotten over it.

Francie and Denny have something in common: their love of gardening. Denny is very proud of the patch of ground the condo board gave him to raise flowers and vegetables. You should have seen the look of wonder on his face the first time a small shoot came up from a seed he planted.

"Good morning, Denny," I say.

"Hi, Mrs. Gold. Guess what Miss Francie gave me? A new plant." Denny will never address us by our first names. He feels it is impolite. Except for Francie, who is special to him. He squints down at the little identification tag, struggling with the Latin words. "Ge-nus of tu . . . tu . . . berous . . . herba . . ."

Francie and I exchange concerned glances. Her kind gesture is meant to help him get over his shock. "Forget the big words," she tells him. "Just call it dahlia."

"Dahlia," he says, smiling, committing it to memory. "Dahlia . . ."

"That's really pretty," I say.

Francie gets in step with me, and arm in arm we continue down the brick-tiled path toward the pool. In front of us, Ida is cursing our resident ducks as usual. They deposit their droppings right smack on our paths and it sends Ida into a tizzy.

The regulars are already at the pool. The seating arrangement is a tableau. Everyone has his or her designated place. And no one ever varies from it. Or there would be war.

At the farthest end of the pool, completely alone, sits Enya Slovak on a chaise longue. At eighty-four, she is a fragile remainder of a woman who was once very beautiful. She wears a big, floppy sun hat, but it's less to hide from the sun than from the rest of us. While her husband, Jacov, was still alive, he made her attend the various events we have in the clubhouse. The holidays were vitally important to him. Especially the group Passover dinner. Enya merely endured those celebrations. Now that he is gone, she has reverted to how she really wants to be. Alone. I say hello. She nods, then her head swivels back down to the book in her lap. Enya met her husband after they were released from Dachau at the end of the war. They had both lost their entire families. When I look into Enya's haunted eyes, I get the feeling she never fully left the camps.

Directly across the pool from Enya sits a small group who always congregate together. They are the snowbirds — the Canadians — renters and owners who fly in every winter to get away from the bitter weather up north. They're friendly but generally stick to themselves.

Moving clockwise from the snowbirds is another story and a half. Harriet Feder and her mother, Esther. Poor Harriet. Sometimes it sounds like it's already become part of her name: "Poor-Harriet." When Esther went into the wheelchair, Harriet gave up her Miami apartment and moved in with her. It's already four years. I swear that Esther, who looks like a sparrow and can out-eat anyone, is in better health than the whole bunch of us. But meanwhile, her daughter, Harriet, is stuck at age forty-four without much of a life. She's not bad looking, if she'd only use some makeup, maybe do a little something with her hair. . . . She's such a nice girl. Unfortunately for her, she grew up big-boned like her late father. And going to the gym every day . . . all those muscles . . . it doesn't help. Esther boasts that no one on her side of the family died before the age of ninety-five. And she is only seventy-seven. It's not that Esther is a bad person, she's just so demanding. Get me this, get me that. . . . Poor Harriet. See what I mean?

In the shallow end of the pool, by themselves, holding hands and bobbing up and down like two rosy apples in a barrel are "the Bobbsey twins" as we call them behind their backs, Hyman and Lola Binder — aka Hy and Lo, when we are playing cards, but more about that later. Lola would be all right away from Hy, but that's the point. She is never away from his side. They've been married for sixty-five years and she hasn't had a thought in her head that he hasn't put there. They are still in love if you call obsession love. Hy is short and chunky; Lola is taller and much thinner. We decided that the happiest day in Hy's life was when the children grew up and moved away. I once commented to Irving Weiss that he and Hy were the only men left in our phase. Irving, a man of very few words, shook his head and said, "Then I'm alone."

I glance toward dear Irving, sitting next to his Millie in the shade outside of the pool perimeter. His life is hell these days, but he never utters a complaint. Millie's Alzheimer's is getting worse, but do not mention putting her into a hospital to Irving. Not a chance. There she sits, totally unaware of all her friends around her. She stares down at her sundress, picking at a thread, muttering to herself. We all take turns helping Irving dress her and bathe her and do the shopping and it is breaking our hearts to see what has become of the funny, warm-hearted Millie we once knew.

Denny Ryan walks up the path carrying a rose from his garden. He reaches Millie and gives it to her. He whispers to her and she seems to answer him.

Francie and I walk over to give her a kiss on the cheek. She stares up at us, vacantly. "Good morning, Millie," we say.

"Do you see them?" she says shrilly. Irving stiffens. Here she goes again. "Do you see the children? There! There, sitting on the fence. No! No! Don't let them see you looking! Don't make them mad!"

Francie and I are distraught by her hallucinations, but Denny, God bless him, joins in her fantasies. "Yes," he says, "I see ghosts, too."

"Do they scare you, Denny?" She always knows him, although she hardly recognizes the rest of us.

"Oh, yes," he says, "they scare me, too."

Millie shudders. "They're out to get us."

Irving puts his arms around her. "I'll protect you." She pulls away angrily, shouting. "No, you can't, they're too strong!" Everyone's watching, responding in their own private ways. Some with sadness, compassion, fear, and even terror. All with the unstated *There, but for the grace of God* . . . Irving helps her up from the bench. "We better go back in," he says.

Irving leads Millie away, Denny following behind, as if to shield them. There is silence, but the mood lifts. We have been living with Millie's deterioration for a long time.

Swimming is a euphemism for what we do in the pool. Except for Francie who really swims, the rest of us walk. Back and forth across the width of the pool, walking and talking.

Now Hy Binder slogs through the water toward us. "Look out," my sister Evvie whispers. "He's got a new joke."

I groan.

"Hey, Gladdy." I try to move out of his path, but I'm not fast enough. He punches my arm. He always punches my arm. He makes me black and blue. "Didja hear this one? Didja? I got it off the Internet on my e-mail. Six old guys" — they're always about old guys — "are sitting around the old folks home, smoking stogies and drinking schnapps when Sexy Sadie comes by batting her eyelashes at them. She holds up her pocketbook and says, 'If you guess what's in the purse you get free sex to-night.' One old guy says, 'Ya gotta elephant in there?' She bats her eyes again. 'Close enough.' "

Hy screams with laughter at his joke. "Didja get it, didja?" It's in incredibly bad taste. But then, so is Hy. I paddle away and he heads back to Lola, delighted with himself.

Evvie shakes her head. "Meshuggener. That man is an idiot."

I sigh. "But he's our idiot."

Francie points. "And here comes the other one."

"Hell-o, here I am." In yet another of her hundred color-coordinated garments — lemon yellow this time with a matching parasol to ward off that nasty sun — wiggles our beloved Sophie. Just in time for the rest of us to get out of the pool and head for the showers. . . .

Years ago, when a group of us were sitting around and kvetching about our troubles, wise old Irving said, "Go ahead, everyone put your pains on the table and pick up somebody else's. Believe me, you'll take back what belongs to you." When I look around at the denizens of our phase — Enya from the concentration camps;

Millie with Alzheimer's, and Irving's anguish; Esther in a wheelchair; Harriet, lonely; and all the women, now widows, left to cope as best they can — Irving was right.

Little did we know the troubles soon to come would be shared by all of us.

4

The Designated Driver

I am in my apartment, showered and dressed and waiting for the others to get ready to go out for our typical late morning errands. And the phone rings.

"It's a matter of life and death. I have to get to Publix. I'm out of everything." This in a panicky whisper from Bella, she who has enough food in her pantry to feed all of Miami.

I reassure her, yet again that, yes, we will stop at Publix. I barely get the phone back on the hook when the next country is heard from.

Sophie, the fashion maven, sighs when I pick up. "Oy," she says, dropping one of her many philosophical malapropisms, "when did my wild oats turn to kasha?" I wait. She reveals that she has to drop off thirty or so garments at the cleaners. Of course I'm exaggerating. But only slightly.

Next. Evvie reminds me that she needs to deliver her latest review for the Lanai Gardens newspaper, which my sister started twenty years ago with a group of frustrated ex-New Yorkers who loved movies, plays, and all the arts. Everyone reads the *Free Press*, the pulse of Lanai Gardens, listing its Hadassah meetings, club activities, religious holidays, etc. The biggest draw is Evvie's famous movie reviews. We girls go to the movies every Saturday afternoon and afterwards Evvie goes home and dutifully comments on them. She has a big following.

Ida, cranky as usual, phones in, and in that imperious voice of hers, says she must go to the bank. Sometimes I think that tight bun of hers cuts off the air to her brain. She always goes to the bank on Fridays, and she knows I always make a stop there, but she will call to remind me — the Phone God must be served.

And *everyone* has to go to the drugstore for the usual assortment of prescriptions that have to be refilled. Not to mention vitamins and Dr. Scholl's foot pads and Ex-Lax. Francie has all of us on some herbs called Brain Pep. She swears that *Ginkgo biloba,* gotu kola, and Schizandra (I did not make this up) will save our memories. It obviously isn't working for me.

Gentle Irving now phones to ask that I please not forget the items on his shopping list. Things his Millie needs. As if I would forget.

"Everybody report in by now?" This is Francie calling to check up on whether everyone else checked in yet.

"All present and accounted for."

We both laugh at the daily absurdity of the phone calls. We know that before they even made these calls to me, they'd already talked to one another and gone through the exact same litany.

And why do they all call *me?* Because I'm the only one of the girls who can still drive and hasn't relinquished her car. Denny has his mother's old Ford Fairlane, which we use as a taxi occasionally. He also helps out by driving relatives to and from the airport — for a fee which we set for him, or he'd be too shy to ask. Hy Binder also drives, but no one in their right mind would get into a car with him, except Lola, who has no choice. God help her — he thinks he's racing the Daytona 500.

Harriet works; that lets her out. And Francie gave up her car when her car gave up on her.

"Well," Francie says, winding up, "enjoy your chores, Ms. Limo Driver."

"Sure you don't want to come along?" There actually is room for six in my old

Chevy wagon, but it's a tight fit. "You can always sit on Ida's lap."

"What, and get stabbed by her quills!?"

"Sophie?"

"And get stabbed by her parasol?"

"Coward."

"Glutton for punishment."

"What can I do? They *neeeeed* me." As if we haven't enjoyed this conversation a hundred times.

"Read my lips." And we recite it, sing-song, together. "Get a cab! Take a bus. Walk. Stay hoooome."

I smile as I hang up. I love that wonderful woman. She is my soul mate. What would I ever do without her?

5

Going into Town, Or Trying to

"Glad, can we please get going? I'm dying from the heat already." Evvie has a right to complain. We've been waiting forever, or so it seems, for everyone to get into my car. The pavement is burning our feet.

First, Bella, terrified of forgetting anything, left her shopping list on the kitchen table, so she went scampering back for it. Then Sophie, who would never let anyone break her record for lateness, went back for her sunblock even though we'd only be walking outside from the parking lot into the market.

"We can always leave them behind," I say.

"Then let's do it. Heckle and Jeckle are driving me up one wall and down the other," agrees Evvie, the impatient organizer.

"Bella! Sophie! Get down here already," screeches Ida, who has less patience than anyone.

Sophie waves gaily out her window. "I'm

47

almost ready. I got my head together, but the rest of me is falling apart."

Ida is in a bad mood anyway. As usual, her mailbox was empty this morning. She mailed an expensive birthday gift to one of her grandchildren. (She'd never admit it's bribery.) No one has bothered to thank her or even acknowledge receiving it.

I try not to open my mailbox when she is around. I feel guilty when I get so many wonderful letters from my grandchildren in New York. I'm truly blessed. And genuinely sorry for Ida.

Evvie is tapping her foot, a very bad sign. "I promised Meyer I'd get my copy over to the newspaper before noon. Now, he won't be there when I get there. I'm going to kill those two *shmegeggies!*"

She's furious; she's never late with her copy.

I've pulled the sunshade off the windshield, I've got all the windows and doors open, and I'll put the air on as soon as I see them coming. The car should be bearable enough to get in now. And we're still waiting.

Ida, trying to keep her temper in check, is now reading the notices on the bulletin board next to the elevator. "Did you see this, girls?" We turn.

"There's another flyer warning us about this guy who's killing older women. They say we should never go out alone at night, or go into bad neighborhoods."

"Well, we don't have to be concerned," Evvie says. "We're always asleep by nine o'clock and, anyway, we never leave our neighborhood."

"They're worried about us being followed home," I comment as I read over her shoulder. "This guy manages to get into women's apartments without breaking in."

"How can he do that?" Evvie asks. "You have to be pretty stupid to let in someone you don't know."

"Well, it happens all the time. My murder mysteries come up with tons of different ways. A guy carrying flowers poses as a delivery man. You'd open the door, wouldn't you? Or a telegram. Or someone in a cop's uniform? Or someone says your kids were in an accident and he's the good Samaritan they sent to get you. . . ."

Ida and Evvie are silent for a moment. "I see what you mean," Ida says. "Who'd ever question any of those?"

I suddenly feel my blood run cold. "Is it possible," I say, thinking about Selma yet again, "maybe it wasn't a heart attack or an accident — ?"

"Hey, dolls! Up here!"

Ida jumps, startled. We look up, to the second floor.

And guess who? It's our favorite pain-in-the-ass, Hy Binder, heading for the laundry room with a basket load of wash.

"We almost got away," Evvie moans.

"Didja hear this one?" he calls out to us. "What's the difference between a wife and a girlfriend?" Not bothering to wait for a response, he tells us. "Forty-five pounds."

"Get lost, Hy," Ida yells.

"What's it called when a woman is paralyzed from the waist down?" Pause, then a guffaw. "Marriage!"

There's no stopping him.

Evvie shrieks at him. "Why don't you go soak your head in the dryer?"

"Don't you mean washer?" Ida asks.

"Washer. Dryer. Who cares. Just get rid of him!"

Evvie starts to get into the car. "I'd rather melt than listen to his dreck!"

"Wait, but didja hear what happened real early this morning? No joke."

Lola comes out of their apartment with another basket of laundry. She continues it for Hy. "Guess who crazy Kronk got this time?"

"Who, now?" Evvie asks, changing her mind about the car in the face of a choice piece of gossip.

Greta and Armand Kronk lived here for many years. She was Spanish, he German. They hinted vaguely at being in "showbiz" and they would have nothing to do with any of us, although one year they did offer classes in flamenco. But they were so unpleasant, and their prices so expensive, very few people took their classes. Eventually Armand died and just about no one has seen Greta since. Food and liquor are delivered to her door. Especially liquor. A few years ago she started getting creepy, prowling the Dumpsters at night. First, she would smear garbage all over people's cars and front doors. Then she began scrawling juvenile kinds of poems on our front doors in greasepaint. Very short. To the point. And scary in their accuracy. No one can figure out how she knows so much about all of us. No one ever admits how close she comes to nailing us.

"The Muellers over us?" Hy comments. "I could hear them early this morning when John went out to pick up the newspaper. He woke us up with his yelling and Mary trying to quiet him. I looked out and he was pounding on Kronk's door, screaming, daring she should come out. So he can kill her!"

By now the two prima donnas have managed to come downstairs. And they want to know what's going on. Evvie shushes them.

"Wow!" says Ida. "What did she write this time?"

"Well, you wouldn't believe —" Lola begins.

Hy interrupts. "He got some soap and wiped it off the door real fast."

Sophie, the queen of pastels, tugs on Evvie, insists on knowing what she and Bella missed by being a teeny-weeny bit late. Evvie, annoyed, fills her in quickly.

"But before he finished wiping," Lola continues, "Mrs. Feder already read what Greta wrote."

"Wait just a minute," I say. "How did Esther Feder see from across the way on the first floor at the other end of the building to the Mueller's top floor at this end? What did she do, wheel her chair down the sidewalk?"

"She has binoculars," Hy announces, grinning. Hy is really getting a charge out of all this. "Well, old Feder told her darling Harriet. Harriet told Lola. Natch, Lola told me."

"I can't believe nobody blabbed about it by the pool this morning," Ida says, amazed.

"Not in front of the Canadians," says Lola.

We are always on our best behavior with our northern visitors.

Sophie, who reads the end of every novel first because she can't stand the suspense, pushes forward. "So, alright already, what did Kronk write?"

Hy beams from ear to ear, emoting dramatically. " 'Mary, Mary, quite contrary. Kick him out. Your John's a fairy.' "

Conversation comes to an immediate halt.

Bella is the first to recover. In her own inimitable way of thinking, she's gleefully made a connection. She delicately wiggles her hand to get our attention. "Is that why he always wears pink?"

Back to my car. I jump in and quickly crank up the air. Ida gets in, and I wait to hear what she will say. She never disappoints me. "Glad, turn down the air! You want me to freeze?"

"Get in already," Evvie says. "I'm melting out here."

"Now where are you beauties off to?" a

melodious voice wafts down the sidewalk towards us.

Oh, oh. From Hy's frying pan into Leo's fire. It's Mr. Leo Slezak, aka Mr. Sleaze, waving at us. That's mine and Evvie's name for this real-estate entrepreneur and slimeball. A not-too-bad-looking man, fifty-ish, if you like his type. Dapper in an oily sort of way. He favors creased white linen suits, Panama hats angled rakishly across his forehead. And a lot of gold chains.

He's standing with Tessie Hoffman, a hefty two-hundred-fifty-pounder, best friend of the deceased Selma Beller, and fellow Weight Watchers dropout. We all like Tessie because she can make fun of herself. If we ask what she's had for lunch, she'll say Shamu and fries. Like that. Selma's sudden death has devastated her.

Like a shot, the girls are out of the car again, ready to melt once more, but this time from Leo's baloney. Evvie and I cannot stand this man, but most of the other females in Phase Two think he is God's gift to women.

"Why are you here today, Leo?" Sophie gurgles.

"You, of course, know about Selma Beller. So sad. Well, her children gave me the listing and Tessie, here, is giving me the key to her apartment."

At the mention of Selma's name, Tessie's eyes tear up. She shakes her head and repeats her familiar litany. "She never even got to open her birthday present."

Smarmy Slezak pats her on the shoulder. "There, there," he says with his usual phony sentiment. He beams back at us. "I have a couple of hot prospects coming this afternoon."

I wonder how he gets those listings. Leo hasn't sold a condo in over a year. More than a dozen units just stand empty. He keeps moaning that business is bad. The snowbirds aren't buying much anymore. There are bigger and fancier condos going up all over the place, like the Wynmore or Hamilton House. If this keeps up, eventually we'll all have our choice of graveyards — Beth Israel, across town, or stay right here in our own apartments.

I swear if I didn't know better, I'd think he stands near the ambulance exit at the hospital and follows them when the sirens go off. One of us dies and that embossed card is out of his pocket and into the hands of a grieving relative faster than you can say "Escrow is closed."

"How do you ladies do it?" he says with that simpering lisp. "How do you keep so fresh and beautiful in all this heat?"

You don't want to hear their nauseatingly sweet answers. It would make your stomach turn.

Evvie leans over and honks the horn. "We have to go, girls."

Almost sighing, the three little twits begin backing away from Leo, the ladykiller. Like a magician, Leo whips a hand into his pocket and his cards instantly appear. His greatest fans take them lovingly. Evvie and I keep our hands folded. He reaches toward us.

"No, thanks. We already have a few dozen," Evvie says with ice in her voice. My sister does sarcasm very well.

Leo taps at the brim of his Panama and says what he always says: "Don't buy out the stores, ladies."

And we are off. Thank God. I have such a headache already. But as I drive through the wrought-iron gates out onto Oakland Park Boulevard, I think once more about Selma's death. It's the way she died that's beginning to nag at me. It reminds me of something. Someone I've seen before? But I can't drag it out of the cobwebs in my mind. Damn getting old and what it does to your memory!

6

Supermarket Shuffle

We have finally arrived at our local market. Picture a supermarket in any city in America. So, pardon me if I don't waste time describing where the cream cheese is.

But our Publix has one big difference: the customers. Shoppers under fifty-five are referred to as "the kids." The rest of us are seniors who live along Oakland Park Boulevard in the various condos, boarding-houses, apartment buildings, and retirement homes. The dress code? Canes. Walkers. Wheelchairs. The object? Shopping for food and surviving the experience. The secret agenda? Kill or maim everyone in your way. OK. Carts at the ready. Bracing ourselves, we take a deep breath, and start wheeling! Welcome to the Supermarket Shuffle!

Evvie and I watch as Ida, bun bobbing, teeth bared, relishing a chase, immediately dashes off on her own. Bella and Sophie, their four eager hands pushing one cart, meander their jolly way down the nearest aisle. And off Evvie and I go.

Aisle One. There goes Yetta Hoffman, ninety-seven, from our Phase Six, using her cane to dig into the back of eighty-eight-year-old Miltie Offenbach. He dares to block her view of the pickled herring specials. Move on. That cane is sharp.

Aisle Two. Look out for Moishe Maibaum, in fine fettle, using his walker like he used to fly his P51 Mustang fighter plane in World War II. "Oops, sorry, Mrs. Garcetti," he says, "just a flesh wound," as he knocks her against what was, only seconds ago, a tall pyramid of sugar peas.

Aisle Three. We are debating pineapple juice over prune.

Aisle Four. A store employee is giving out minuscule samples of lox on crackers the size of pinkie-nails and the line snakes around the perimeter of the entire store, punctuated by much pushing, shoving, and insulting.

"Putz!"

"Yenta!"

"Meeskite!"

"Lunatic!"

(Translation: Penis. Busybody. Ugly one and lunatic.)

A familiar announcement comes over on the loudspeaker. Cleanup on aisle seven.

No, not some careless child, only a senior with palsy. A jar of Korean kimchi has smashed. You know what kimchi smells like?

Look out! Eleven o'clock, wheelchair bearing down on us. Jump! Breathlessly we grab for a couple of the hanging salamis and hold on for dear life. (Well, actually we just step out of the way.)

In aisle eight, a drama is taking place. Two women. Photographs. A letter. Tears. We reach for our items and move past quickly and quietly.

Meat and Poultry. A tug-of-war. Two sets of spindly arms hold tight to two equally spindly chicken wings. A fight to the finish. Move on. Forget making chicken soup. Get lamb chops instead.

One long hour later, our shopping is finally done. Evvie, Ida, and I have checked out, but we have to wait for Bella and Sophie. And here they come, Tweedledum and Tweedledumber, basket filled to the brim. I sigh. This will take forever.

The checkout stand. One needs the patience of Job. Fifteen minutes for the first customer; one tiny change purse filled with coins and the slowest fingers in the world eking them out.

Then the next customer and an argument over two cans of sardines. "They were cheaper last week. So how come the price is higher this week?"

"No, they're exactly the same price as last week."

"Listen, you little *pisher,* don't tell *me!* I'm old enough to be your great-grand-mother."

Finally Bella and then Sophie.

Every item calls for a debate.

"How come the Bosc pears are so high?"

"How come the broccoli has no taste?"

"How come you don't carry the Del Monte peaches anymore? I mean the 'cling'?" Then there is the obligatory exchange of recipes. Complaints about the store. The attitude of the help. Local politics. World hunger.

Evvie taps her foot throughout, muttering obscenities, but that doesn't move them any faster.

When we're done, our clothes are rumpled and our faces are flushed and our pulses are beating just a little faster. All right. So I exaggerated. But, at our age, where else can we go to have this much fun?

7

No Rest for the Weary

Back home. At last. I'm beyond exhausted. Time to lie down and take our afternoon naps. I can't wait. We deliver Irving's groceries, then get our own packages out of the car and into the building's shopping carts. On the elevator, riding up, I hear this:

Bella: "Did we say we were eating in tonight or going out?"

Ida: "Out, we said OUT! Twenty times in the car."

Bella: "Oh, I didn't hear that."

Ida: "Well, if you wore your damned hearing aid —"

Sophie: "Not Chinese again. We ate that yesterday."

Evvie: "No, we didn't. That was *last* Friday."

Sophie: "So where did we eat last night?"

Evvie: "Home. We stayed home. It was canasta night."

Bella: "We played canasta?"

Sophie: (the light bulb goes on): "Oh,

61

that's right. I won."

Evvie: "No, I won. Didn't I, Glad?"

Me: "Who can remember?"

Sophie: "You won last week. I know I won."

Ida: "Who cares! When Sophie wins, it's by reason of insanity. She drives everybody nuts and we all give up!"

Evvie laughs. "Sore loser."

Ida: "Look who's talking. You almost filleted her with the cheese ball knife."

Evvie: "My finger slipped."

Bella: "I like Eleni's. Or Nona's. Can't we go there?"

"Next time. The birthday girl chose Continental. And," I remind them, "don't forget your presents."

We help Sophie in with her stuff from the cleaners, which took all of us to carry. We divide up the grocery bags from the shopping carts. Then Evvie starts to lead Bella back to the elevator, so they can take their things across the parking lot to their own building. Bella looks confused.

"Don't I live here?"

"No, dear, we live over there. We had to help Sophie."

"Oh." We once left Bella downstairs to wait while Evvie helped us carry, but she wandered away and it took us twenty minutes to find her, so now we just bring her up one building and down the other. Ida wants to put a bell around her neck.

Finally everyone is safely deposited in her own apartment. I turn up the air, start undressing. I head toward my bedroom, then remember. I rush to the phone. Too late. It rings. I wasn't fast enough to turn it off.

"Yes, Bella," I say.

"It's me, Sophie."

"Sorry. Yes, Sophie."

"So where did we say we were eating?"

"Continental," and I hang up before she can say another word. I quickly turn off the ringer.

Finally I am in my cool bed in my cool room looking forward to my nap with the utmost of pleasure. I might even get in a little reading later.

My eyes are closing and I feel myself letting go of consciousness when the doorbell rings. I try to ignore it, pulling my pillow over my head, but it doesn't stop. Finally, swearing and stumbling, I race to the door to find Sophie there.

"What!" I screech at her.

"There's something wrong with your phone. We got cut off, but when I rang again it didn't answer."

"No! *It* didn't answer, because *I* didn't answer! Go back to your apartment. *Now!*"

And Sophie scurries away wondering why I raised my voice at her. I want to bang my head against the door, but what did that door ever do to me?

8

Library and Liberation

Through the plate glass window, Conchetta Aguilar sees me staggering toward the entrance, carrying my usual load of returns. Grinning, she moves to the coffeemaker and pours me a cup full of her great Cuban coffee and hands it to me as soon as I put the stack of books down.

"Leaded? I hope."

"You betcha. I only needed one look at your face. Hard morning with the inmates?"

I nod, gulping the hot liquid down. "I left them in the clubhouse playing mahjongg. I feel like I escaped Alcatraz."

Conchetta is head librarian for the Lauderdale Lakes branch. She's in her thirties, about five feet tall and just as round, and a lot of fun. When she found out I used to be a librarian in my New York days, she reached out as one professional to another. When she realized that the library is my one escape from Lanai Gardens, we became even closer.

Not only am I designated driver, but I am designated book chooser. This is no mean feat, since I have to carry around each girl's list of what she's read before. Heaven help me if I bring home a repeat. Bella reads only romances in large print. Evvie wants biographies of the stars. Ida likes the best-sellers, Sophie prefers the *Reader's Digest* condensations, and Francie reads cookbooks. Happily, nobody else wants to make the trip, so coming here is like a vacation for me.

"Come on, *muchacha*. Tell *mamacita* everything."

"What a day. Those girls are wearing me out. Publix was bad enough. Going to the cleaners was maddening. It was the bank that did me in."

Conchetta leans her arms against the counter, ready to listen. "Good. A bank story."

"The bank is always mobbed on Friday. Everyone has checks to cash. Ida, who hates waiting for anything, gets this brilliant idea. She sneaks in a slice of her famous pecan coffee cake and slips it to a teller who knows Ida's cakes. The bribe gets her to the front of the line. Neither one of them being subtle. And what a *geshrie* from everyone on line!"

"*Geshrie,* I guess, means an uproar."

"You got it. Wait 'til you hear what happened next. Harriet Feder, who's near the front of the line with her mother, lifts Ida up and carries her bodily, feet dangling, and drops her back at the end of the line where she belongs. All the while, Ida is hitting her with her purse, thus emptying the contents all over the floor. Everyone's hysterical. Ida is mortified. Knowing Ida, she will never forgive Harriet."

"And . . . I can tell there's more. . . ."

"Greta Kronk struck again."

"Barney, quick. Another Kronk episode."

A tall, skinny, and proud-to-be-a-nerd young man strides over. "Fantabulous," Barney Schwartz says. "Our Lady of the Garbage."

"Our what?"

"We're having a contest to give Greta a title worthy of her accomplishments," says Conchetta.

Barney adds, "I want to publish her poems. I already have the title of the book: *From Under the Belly of the Alligator.*"

I burst out laughing. "You guys are so bad!"

"I especially love 'Hy and Lo put on a

show. They make me throw. Up.' Brilliant," says Barney.

Conchetta recites her favorites. " 'Tessie is fat. That's that.' And 'Esther's a pest and Harriet can't get no rest, yes.' "

"They've been benign up to now. Today took a different turn. She hit on a couple named John and Mary." I recite it for them and their eyes widen.

"Wow," says Conchetta. "I think her crazies are escalating."

"Is he?" asks Barney. "Gay?"

"I've always wondered, but how could Greta know?"

"That woman needs help."

"We've tried. But to no avail."

Conchetta is being beckoned. As she moves off to help a fellow book lover, she calls back, "Typical. The authorities are waiting for her to hurt somebody."

I head at last for the mystery section, perturbed by our exchange. But quickly my mood gentles. I am among my favorite things. Books.

A half hour later with a Virginia Lanier, a Barbara Neely, a Mary Willis Walker and a Ruth Rendell in hand (so many great women mystery writers these days), I have enough to keep me happy for a week. I pick out books for the girls. It's nearly dinnertime and I must gather up the lambs before they turn into lions.

Conchetta smiles at my customary stack as I check out. Then she picks up my Barbara Neely. "Like it so much you're gonna read it again after only two weeks?"

"What are you muttering about?" I pick up *Blanche Among the Talented Tenth.* "I didn't read this one. I read her first and third."

"Two weeks ago."

"Oh, yeah, smart stuff, what's this one about?"

"Blanche sends her kids to a snooty private school and they start getting attitude."

I smile sheepishly, and take it off my pile. "Well," I say, "if I ever get Alzheimer's, I'll only need one book from then on."

"And we'll be out of business."

I say my good-byes and *schlep* my books out to the car.

She knows I'll be back very soon. It's the way I stay sane. But all the way home I find myself thinking of Greta Kronk and what loneliness can do to people. But is Conchetta right? Is she dangerous? Would she do more than hurt someone? Would she kill?

9

Dinner at the Deli

The parking lot is already packed and the line outside the Continental deli winds clear around the perimeter of the minimall.

We're late, of course. Half past three is a shoo-in. Four o'clock is the right time. Four-thirty is pushing it and five is rush hour for the early-bird dinner ($6.50 for six courses plus coffee). It's now twenty-five minutes after five.

"I told you . . ." howls Evvie.

"Don't start," I caution my sister.

"The milk is spilled already," says Sophie, "so don't keep drinking."

Francie, the birthday girl, glances at Sophie and shakes her head. "I think she needs a translator."

"I think she needs a keeper," Ida snarls. "Why can't you say 'Don't cry over spilt milk' like everybody else?"

"That's what I said."

We get out of the car and head for the end of a very long line.

"Well, at least we can window-shop,"

70

Bella, our little ray of sunshine, says, eyeing the minimall with eagerness.

I keep time. Ten minutes stalled in front of Discount Linens. Fifteen in front of Klotz's Klassy Klothing. Sophie has disappeared into the deli to scope things out and now she returns with her report.

"The *kasha varnishkas* are already a dead duck. I told Dena to hide a plate of kreplach for us, there's only two left. If you were dreaming of the stuffed cabbage, wake up."

A few moans accompany the food report. Followed by a couple of I-told-you-so's.

Now a short wait in front of the prosthetics shop (a really cheerful window) and then the ninety-nine-cent store and finally we are in. It's ten after six and naturally everyone is starved.

The place is packed and we don't get our favorite waitress, Dena. Now you really hear groans. We get Lottie, she of the long, bushy black hair (a strand of which Ida swears gets in her soup every time we are stuck with her) and the very bad breath. She's so ugly and antagonistic, Francie swears she must be a relative. Who else would hire her?

As we sit down, she practically throws

the pickle and sauerkraut appetizer dish at us, then hurries away like Hurricane Hannah, whirling from table to table, hurling dishes and insults with equal fervor.

The deli customers consist of a smattering of families, some couples, but mostly women sixty and up. We're all of us regulars here.

We study the menu avidly, as if we didn't know it by heart. Before we even get past the soups, there's Lottie, order book in hand. "What'll ya have, gals?"

"I don't know yet," Bella says warily, bracing herself for trouble.

"I don't got all day, so lemme hear something before I die on my feet."

Intimidated, Bella blurts out her choices, stringing them together like Jewish worry beads: pineapplejuice-saladwithThousand-Island-matzoballsoup-broiledchicken-rice-spinach.

Ida, just to infuriate Lottie, goes into slow-motion mode. Every word takes forever to pass her lips. "Let . . . me . . . see. First . . . I might like the . . . tomato juice . . . with a piece of lemon . . . or maybe the grapefruit. . . ."

Francie interrupts, trying to avoid trouble. She places her order quickly. "Tomato juice. Pot roast. Baked potato. Salad.

French dressing." Evvie and I follow suit. We always get the same things, anyway.

"And . . . how . . . is . . . the kreplach soup this evening?" Ida's voice seems to get slower and sarcastically sweeter.

"It's the way it always is. In or out on the kreplach?"

"Well, I could say 'in.' "

"Say it!" we all shout.

"In. Alright already."

"And?!" Lottie is gritting her teeth.

"And . . . for my meat dish, I am simply torn between the sauerbraten and the sweetbreads."

"Don't be so torn, pick already!"

Ida looks her dead in the eye. "I do not like to be rushed. It is not good for my blood pressure."

"And I have six other tables to worry about. Think, dollink, I'll be back."

Lottie leaves and we all glare at Ida.

"Enough, already," I say.

"Why? I'm enjoying myself." She leans back, relaxed.

"Meanwhile, I'm starving," wails Sophie. She takes a bite of a sour pickle on the tray. "This is good."

"Then you should spit it out," says Bella, being bossy.

"Why?" Sophie asks mid-bite.

"My doctor says if it tastes good, then it's bad for you."

Evvie ignores this exchange and shakes a fist at Ida. "Why can't you behave? You are ruining Francie's birthday party."

"You certainly are," adds Francie, pretending annoyance.

Now that we've ordered, the bottles come out of the purses and the vitamins and the prescription drugs are lined up. Bella gasps. "I'm out of my Zantac. What should I do?"

"Tomorrow is another day," says our Sophie philosophically.

"I always take it before dinner."

Ida digs around in her purse. "I have some." She takes one out. As she hands it to Bella, "I'll take two dollars now, thank you."

Evvie swats her with her purse. "How can you! You would sell seltzer to a dying man in the desert!"

Ida is insulted. "My late husband, Murray, taught me that business is business. Supply and demand. Bella just demanded. I just supplied. I get paid. It's the American way."

Bella's eyes start to tear up. Francie takes a tissue from her purse and hands it to her. "Now you've done it."

"What did I say? I was talking about my Murray."

The tears flow harder, followed by pathetic little hiccups. Evvie rolls her eyes heavenward. "You said the *h* word. As in 'husband.' As in dead and not here anymore and we never go there! And furthermore, Zantac only costs a dollar seventy-five, you gonif!"

"Oh, if only my Abe, my angel, was here, things would be different." Bella was now going out on an old limb. Things would be different, all right, and not for the better. As the years pass, Abe's memory gets a whitewash. The mean-spirited, domineering Abe who often brought her to tears now brings her to tears because she's rewritten history. Now he's a saint!

Lottie is back. Ida sees five sets of steely eyes glaring at her. She shrugs. "I'm ready. Where were you? I'll have the noodle soup and it better be hot. Salad, oil and vinegar and no cucumbers. The steak rare and that doesn't mean well-done or medium or raw. Potatoes mashed and leave out your usual lumps. Oh, yes, and make sure we all have separate checks."

Lottie just stands there.

"What?" Ida asks, all innocence.

"Are you finished, Mrs. Have-it-your-way? I wouldn't want to miss something of vital importance."

Haughty now: "Yes, thank you. That will be all, my good woman."

"Oy," says Sophie, "I wish the food would get here so I can take home the leftovers."

And it goes downhill from there. Ida sends her soup back because it isn't hot enough. Bella chokes on a chicken bone. Ida pulls Bella's arms over her head and pounds on her back. Evvie makes her eat a piece of bread because that's supposed to prevent the bone from stabbing her. Francie makes her do special breathing. Sophie makes her blow her nose to free the passages. I am on standby in case we need the Heimlich, but finally, the bone is gone, and everyone takes credit for her method.

We give Francie her presents, apparently many minds with similar brainstorms. They all give her pretty soaps or bath salts. Francie good-naturedly wonders if we are trying to tell her something about her personal hygiene. I, of course, give her a book. A cookbook.

We all order dessert, but none of us eats it. We never do. There is always too much food to eat and dessert is taken home to be indulged in later. Naturally, Francie, the chocoholic, orders the chocolate cake with chocolate icing.

And finally the check comes. One check. Ida has a small fit, but there is nothing we can do but figure out who had what, which need I say takes another half an hour. Leaving the tip is one of the heavy decisions of eating out. Everyone is responsible for deciding her own. No one amount ever gets the same number of votes, with much debating on how fast the service was, how good, etc. But having Lottie makes it easy. Everyone tips the minimum. Except Ida, who tips nothing.

We drive home with Evvie leading us in a medley of musical comedy tunes.

10

A Waltons' Good Night

Wearily we each trudge to our apartments, bloated as usual with too much food, carrying our little doggie bags. We watch one another, making sure we each get inside safely.

"Don't forget to double lock," Francie calls.

"Don't forget, movies tomorrow afternoon." This from our social director, Evvie.

"Don't forget, I have an early dentist's appointment," Ida reminds me.

"Good night, Bella."

"Good night, Ida."

"Good night, Glad."

"Good night, Evvie."

"Good night, Sophie."

"Good night, Francie. Happy Birthday."

I am the last one in and I know at least one of the girls is watching out for me through her kitchen window.

We said good night, but we didn't know we were saying good-bye.

11

Death by Chocolate

All lights were off, but one. Everyone was asleep before ten except Francie.

She was too excited.

Francie Charles was at her favorite pastime. Surrounded by her cookbooks, she paged through Claddy's birthday present, a collection of the best desserts from Bon Appétit.

Naturally she was perusing the "fabulous cakes" section first. Her eyes glanced toward her doggie bag, still sitting on the kitchen counter. She was debating. Have it now or save it for tomorrow. She was practically drooling over the book's description of the double fudge cake with whipped cream. Or maybe she might try to make the triple mocha square first. It had been weeks since she'd baked anything. Maybe she'd surprise the girls tomorrow.

Happiness, she thought, is having a sweet tooth. She glanced up at the magnet on her fridge, last year's birthday present from her daughter-in-law, Ilene. She always giggled when she passed it. "Men think the greatest thing in life is sex; women know it's a Hershey bar."

There was a soft knock on the door.

Surprised, she called out, "Who is it?" She was even more surprised when no one answered. Now she wasn't sure there had been a knock. But she went to the door anyway. "Anybody there?" No answer. She looked through the peephole. Nobody. Slowly, she unlocked the door and as she did, the package leaning against it fell onto the threshold. Francie picked it up and looked outside onto the balcony. She looked both ways, but there was no one there.

The package was a square white box tied with a pretty red bow. Something inside smelled wonderful. She reached for the note taped to the ribbon and opened it. In an almost immature hand it read, "Sweets to the sweet. Happy birthday." No signature. Inside the box was a vision of beauty. A thick slice of chocolate almond mousse with fresh raspberries and chocolate chantilly whipped cream! Francie was astonished. Where did it come from? Who could have found something as elegant as this in Fort Lauderdale? Her meager cake from Continental went into the fridge. She grabbed a fork and very gently dug into her gift to have her first taste. Heaven! Absolute heaven.

Now I can die happy, she thought, smiling.

Francie heard the turn of a key in her lock. Thank God, she thought, someone will save me. She lay on the floor, clutching her stomach. She had been in pain for she didn't know how long, falling in and out of consciousness. She couldn't move. Her body was paralyzed and she knew she was dying. "Help me," she tried to cry out, but her tongue was also paralyzed.

At that moment Francie realized three things: 1) There was no help coming. 2) The killer had returned to finish the job. And 3) she had forgotten to double lock her door after bringing in the gift that would poison her.

Francie's eyes were the only things that could move. They watched the betrayal, as someone she thought she knew so well moved about her apartment, cleaning up. The plate and fork were washed and put away. The remains of the cake dropped into a plastic carry-away bag. The note crushed and put in a pocket. The crumbs wiped off the counter into the sink.

Her body was dragged along the floor until she was positioned lying near the phone. Her hand was placed as if she had been reaching for it and failed. Her eyes looked into the eyes of her killer and she realized begging was useless. What she saw reflected was a coldness beyond compassion.

Francie's last thought was that she would never see her children and grand-children again. And that was more un-bearable than the pain.

12

Getting Old Is Murder

It's Saturday morning. The day is beautiful. Nothing is wrong, so why am I depressed? Must have been a bad dream brought on by something I ate at the deli last night.

I'm down at the mailbox as are a lot of my neighbors. It's a favorite meeting place, located to the left of the parking lot on the side of our building facing the elevator. Get the mail, see what's new on the bulletin board, touch base with the people who are about to get into their cars and out to do errands. And of course, take a copy of our free newspaper from the newly arrived stacks.

Everyone reads Evvie's review first.

KNISHES OR KNOCKS
GOING TO THE MOVIES
WITH EVVIE
By
Evelyn Markowitz
Exclusive to:
THE LANAI GARDENS FREE PRESS

AFTER LIFE

OK, so it's a Japanese movie and who knows from Japanese? I love going to movies from other countries. You always see how the other half lives. Especially the French, ooh là là. My pet peeve against foreign movies is that they always put the subtitles on white backgrounds. So it isn't bad enough you miss most of what's going on in the movie while you're reading the long titles, but your head keeps jumping around trying to find them through all the white. Result: You haven't a clue what it was all about in the first place and end up needing an Alka-Seltzer.

When the video of this movie comes out, buy one — you'll be able to throw out your sleeping pills. Such a sleeper!

I liked the idea. When you die you come to this place and remember your favorite memory and you take it with you wherever it is you're going. But let me tell you, if where you're going is as dark and de-pressing as the place you're in in this movie, you shouldn't go anywhere with this crowd.

All that agonizing for two hours, and what memories do they come up with?

Flying in a cloud. Reciting a really nothing poem. Sitting on a bench. It's bad enough they have to eat all that raw fish, do they have to live such boring lives? They should make the director fall on a sword like they do in those other movies.

Now if my heroine, Barbra Streisand, was in this movie, she would have made them use the fluorescent lights like we have in the clubhouse so you wouldn't go blind trying to see what's on the screen. And she would have come up with a great memory, like finding this gorgeous hunk, James Brolin, for a husband after all those movies never getting the guy, and always being left alone, sad, but brave. And would that gorgeous Omar Sharif have been so bad? Too bad she couldn't keep both of them.

QUOTH THE MAVEN:

Enough already. I give it 1½ knishes. If this is all we have to look forward to after life, then as Hy Binder, in our phase, always says — I'm not going!

The End

Thank you, Evvie for another memorable movie interpretation. I shake my head. Just what I needed — an article about death in the mood I'm in.

Evvie's timing is always perfect. The celebrated editor-reporter-reviewer arrives downstairs for a round of kudos from everybody. And as always, she graciously takes the applause as her due.

"Loved it, just loved it," Mary Mueller gushes at her as she and her husband, John, get into their Buick on their way to the mall. John looks away, unable to face us these days because of what Kronk wrote on their door.

"Well, that's a movie we can miss, thanks for the warning," says Harriet Feder, as she installs her mother's wheelchair into the back of their van. "Off to another movie today?"

Evvie nods. "Every Saturday afternoon."

I chime in. "Harriet, why don't you join us?"

Harriet beams. "Why, I'd like that —"

"Allow me to say no, thanks, for my Harriet." Esther Feder's voice rings out from the passenger seat, where she is waiting. "We're already going to see a movie later."

"We are?" asks Harriet, puzzled.

"Yes, Harriet, darling, I just got this idea. After my doctor's appointment, we can pick up a tape from the video store and watch it when we get home. You know how we both love that sweet Fred Astaire. And maybe you'll make your mamma some microwave popcorn." Esther now directs herself at me. "That daughter of mine won't let me miss any pleasures just because the good Lord decided to make a cripple of me. Everyone should have such a good daughter."

"Poor Harriet," says Evvie as they drive off.

"I'm glad she didn't come with us," Ida says, still smarting from the way Harriet treated her at the bank.

Sophie giggles, remembering Ida's embarrassment. Ida pokes her in the ribs.

My eye is caught by the sight of Irving and his pal, Sol Spankowitz from Phase Three, sitting on a bench near his front door, foul smoke belching from their stogies. They are leaning over a newspaper, deep in concentration. The two friends are an odd couple, Irving being thin, almost frail and hunched over, quiet-spoken and polite, while Sol is chunky, pear-shaped, and bald, the only sign of hair his pencil-thin mustache. Sol is loud, brash, and as subtle as the butcher block he used when he was still working. I hurry over, Evvie on my heels, both of us thinking the same thing. Every Saturday morning we take turns sitting with Millie while Irving plays a little pinochle. And on Sunday afternoons in season, he and Sol go to Hialeah.

"I still like the six horse in the double," Sol says.

"Valenzuela's riding," cautions Irving.

"So, he's on a losing streak," Sol comments. "Maybe his winning streak will come back tomorrow."

"Who's with Millie?" I ask. "You didn't leave her alone?"

Irving's hands go up as if warding off any other words. His thumb motions toward the door. "Sleeping."

I smile. Irving, the ultimate cheapskate with words.

Many years ago, I once asked Irving why he didn't take a vacation in Europe. He could always go back to Poland and visit the place he was born. This was at a time all of us were still doing a lot of traveling. His answer to me was, "I been." And that was that. End of discussion. Short and sweet. Millie told us she thought the real reason Irving never went back is that he ran from the draft and was afraid the Poles were still looking for him.

"How are you, Evvie?" Sol asks, staring

at her bosom. Sol has the habit of never looking any woman in the eye. Somehow he never gets past their breasts.

"I'm up here, Sol," Evvie says, pointing to her face.

Sol, startled, drags his eyes away and looks up into Evvie's eyes. She barely hides her irritation. "We are what our minds are, Mr. Sol Spankowitz. Our bodies are merely the vessels that carry our heads."

Sol doesn't understand a word she says, but he manages a brief, "Uh-huh."

Irving taps his watch, then nods at Evvie and me. "By eleven?"

"Have a nice card game," Evvie says.

They walk away, heading toward the clubhouse, with Sol still scanning the sports page. "What should we do in the trifecta, Irv?"

"Wheel the three horse," answers the expert.

I poke Evvie in the shoulder. "You've got a potential suitor there, sister. He's hot to trot."

"Let him trot down at the track. I'm not interested."

"Well. He *is* available. Not too many of those left."

"Big deal. He was a lech even when Clara was alive."

I always tease Evvie about Sol, but somehow my heart isn't quite in it today. "Well, he's good for a nice dinner now and then."

"I can buy my own dinners, thank you. Besides, I still have dear old Joe hanging around, now that the broad from Miami dumped him. Besides, I like my freedom." She stops, seeing the amused expression on my face.

"Gotcha."

"And what about you? You are so busy fixing me up, how about your love life?"

"Let's change the subject."

Evvie smirks. She is about to open Irving's door when we hear another door open right above our heads and angry voices arguing.

From where we are hidden by a straggly ficus tree, we see Hy Binder hurrying down the second floor walkway, and Lola grabbing his arm trying to stop him. Evvie and I exchange glances. The Bobbsey twins fighting? This we gotta hear.

"But I got the lawyer hanging on the line." Lola sounds frantic.

"He can hang forever." Hy is really angry.

"You gotta talk to him sometime."

"When hell freezes over. Twice."

"But our kids will kill one another over the money."

"Let them."

"Please, Hy, the man wants to tell you about a living trust."

"The only trust I care about is the one I wear for my prostate."

"That's a truss. Not a trust. Stubborn man! Everybody has to make out a will."

Hy turns just as he starts down the stairs.

"I told you a hundred times. I don't need a will. I'm not going!"

With that he rushes past us, giving us dirty looks, gets into his car, and careens off. Lola, crying now, runs back into the apartment and slams the door after her.

Evvie erupts with laughter. She looks at me. "What?" she says. "Why aren't you laughing?"

I shrug. "I know it's funny, but it's also depressing, Hy being afraid to plan for death."

"Boy, are you grouchy today," Evvie says as she opens Irving's door. We walk in quietly, hearing nothing.

Millie is indeed sleeping, curled up on the couch in the sunroom. We also call it the Florida room, this screened-in porch. I remember when Millie decorated it with wild, brightly colored pillows and rattan furniture, how delighted she was with how it looked. She told me it made her think she was in a Bette Davis movie. "She looks so peaceful," I whisper.

"Like she's off in some other world," Evvie says.

We sit quietly for a few moments. What a day. My mood just keeps getting darker and I can't shake it. Millie's eyes open. She seems restless. Evvie reaches for the pitcher on the side table and pours her a glass of water. Millie grabs the glass and drinks the water down greedily. Then she flings the glass to the floor. Not a problem: We started using plastic dishes a long time ago. Evvie tries to take her hand. Millie shoves her away. Now, she tries to put a shawl around her shoulder, but Millie hurls that away, too.

"Ev, stop!" I say. It breaks my heart to see how hard my sister tries.

"I feel so helpless."

"I know dear, we all do."

I'm suddenly aware of shouting outside. "Glad! Evvie, are you in there!?" Then pounding on the door.

We both jump up. "That sounds like Sophie," Evvie says. "What's going on?"

I unlock the door. Sophie stands there.

And Denny. And Bella. All of them ashen-faced. Behind them I see other people standing around too, watching. For a moment everything is frozen. I am aware of half of Sophie's hair covered with curlers, the other half limp and wet. Denny has keys in his hands and his hands are shaking. Bella is moaning.

It must be bad. I shiver. "Who is it?"

Sophie sobs. "Francie . . ."

I shake my head violently as if to throw the word off. My mind refuses to accept this. Please, God, not Francie! I can hear Evvie gasp and I feel her grab my arm.

As much as I don't want to hear it, I need this to be over with. "Tell me . . ." My voice is a croak.

Sophie begins to hyperventilate and Bella's eyes lose focus. Denny tries. "I went up . . . the air-conditioning didn't work good . . . the air comes out warm it's supposed to be cold . . . I promised in the morning . . . She said come up, but not too early . . . She didn't answer, so I thought she went out . . . so I opened the door with my key. . . ."

He quits. This is all he can manage.

"Denny, tell me, how bad is she hurt?! Did you call nine-one-one?"

He looks at Sophie plaintively for help.

"I went to get you, but you weren't home. So, I went to Mrs. Meyerbeer. . . ."

I wait for the miracle I know won't come. Too late to plea-bargain with God . . . Too late . . .

Sophie can't stand it anymore. She screams. "She's dead! Francie's dead!"

Evvie gasps, starting to slide down. I clutch her arm and pull her back up.

"Bella." I try to get her attention. I touch her hand. She finally manages to focus and look at me. "Bella, please stay with Millie."

She doesn't answer. She goes inside. And I start running, pulling Evvie with me. Sophie and Denny follow right behind us. Denny and Sophie are both crying. Stupidly, I wonder where Ida is, and then I remember dropping her at the dentist this morning. I am dimly aware of people everywhere. Standing in the street, or on their balconies. Whispering. Crying. Shaking their heads in disbelief. Bad news travels fast.

Francie is dead. Francie is dead. . . . How can I go on without her?

13

Funerals on the Run

"Where are we now?" I ask for the hundredth time, or does it only seem that way?

"On four-forty-one and passing Twelfth Street," Evvie reports. As always she sits in the front seat next to me. The upper half of the opened map covers her side of the windshield, and the lower half is spread across both our laps. And she still doesn't have a clue as to where we are.

"It can't be," I tell her, once again pushing the map out of my line of sight. "We passed that corner five minutes ago."

"I told you we were lost!" wails Ida. "We already passed Fuddruckers twice!"

Bella is keening, "Oh, God . . . Oh, God . . . We shoulda been there half an hour ago."

"I knew we shoulda taken University. This traffic is killing us!" Ida's voice is sharp.

"Shoulda, coulda, woulda," singsongs Sophie for the third time in fifteen minutes.

All our voices are shrill. We are beyond our boiling points. Today, of all days, the air conditioner isn't working. Even Ida is hot, which should give you an idea of how bad it is. The windows are all open, and between the dirt flying in and the deafening noise of the trucks rumbling past us — I am not coping well. And naturally we are all dressed up in clothes that feel way too tight after living day after day in loose sundresses and bathing suits. We are sweating and miserable.

"We're so late, we're so late. . . ." Bella, who is in tears, sounds like a demented Alice, only this is no tea party we're going to.

Ida is now shouting. "Of course we're late. Because Sophie wasn't ready." She elbows her in her stomach. "How could you be late for Francie's funeral!"

"Stop already with the blame," Sophie says defensively. "You're a broken record, play another."

"I'll stop when you stop being impossible!" We have been driving around aimlessly for forty minutes and Ida has lost it by now. I think we all have.

"I knew we should have hired a car," Evvie says.

"Woulda, coulda, shoulda," says Sophie yet again.

"You say that once more, and I'll throw you out the door!" Ida's hand moves across Sophie's lap toward the door handle. Sophie shuts right up.

But Evvie is right. I should never have offered to drive to the cemetery. I am much too upset about Francie. I can't think straight, and I'm making mistakes.

Evvie grabs my arm, jerking the steering wheel.

"Don't ever do that!" I shout at her, trying to avoid a pedestrian crossing the street in front of me.

"Turn right! This is where we were supposed to turn right. On Davie Boulevard."

"No," I insist. "I did that last time and that's why we're right back where we started. Davie and Twelfth are the same street. It's left."

"No, right. You turned left last time."

"Gladdy's right, it's left, not right," says Ida, digging her fingers into the upholstery behind my back.

I know I'm driving erratically. Now I narrowly miss a Holsum's White Bread truck as I turn onto Stirling.

"Oh, no," Evvie gasps.

"What! What is it?" I ask, in a state of total panic.

"Look. Look where we are." She points

across the street and everyone stares out the window.

"No!" Ida says. "It can't be! We're at bingo!"

Sophie is so excited she is jumping up and down in her seat, her black wide-brimmed hat, with tiny red rosettes, bobbing. "Yes! And today's pick-a-pet day!"

And sure enough we've arrived at a spot that is very familiar to all of us: the Seminole tribe reservation where we go every week to play bingo.

I pull over to the curb and stop the car. I throw my arms across the steering wheel and lean my head on my hands. I am laughing and I am crying and I am laughing . . . I'm hysterical.

"What's so damn funny?" Ida asks.

"Pppick-a-ppppet day." I can't stop laughing.

"So? What's so funny about picking out a stuffed animal full of money when you win at Bingo?"

Evvie is beside herself. "You're babbling on about winning a stuffed animal and they're burying Francie!"

"I just realized," I say through hiccuping sobs. "We've been to so many funerals at Beth Israel Park Cemetery and we go to bingo every week and I never realized it before. The cemetery is on the same street as bingo."

Evvie starts to laugh, too. "If you go left you play, if you go right you die."

Ida and Sophie are stone-faced. "I don't see what's funny about that," Ida says, crossing her arms.

"You wouldn't," Evvie says.

By now my laughing has turned into sobbing. I bang my fists on the steering wheel. I just can't stop. "Francie is dead! Francie is dead and gone and we'll never see her again! And I can't find the damned cemetery!"

Good old Bella joins in with me. She hasn't stopped crying anyway, since she got in the car. Now her sobs escalate. A moment later, Evvie is crying, too, and leaning her head on my shoulder. And like falling dominos, Sophie and Ida grab onto one another as they erupt into tears.

If anyone driving by looked in our windows, what a sight they would see.

We all needed a cry. I finally compose myself. The others pull themselves together. I check the map one more time.

"OK, now I've got my bearings. We are directly east on Stirling Road. I know how to get there now. We're only about six blocks away."

"Thank God," Bella says.

I make an illegal U-turn, ignoring the honking horns and squealing brakes, and we are finally headed in the right direction.

We drive through the ornate cemetery gates, and I pull up to the main information office. Evvie jumps out to get directions as Ida yells for her to hurry. The rest of us climb out of the car and try to stretch our aching muscles, at the same time peeling our sticky clothes away from our bodies.

Evvie rushes out again waving at us a paper with a lot of small black-and-white boxes on it.

"Oh, no," says Ida, "not another map."

"Come on, we have to follow it. Look for row twelve."

"Aren't we taking the car?" Sophie wants to know.

"It'll be faster if we cut across," Evvie shouts.

We all race after her as best we can.

"Cut across what?" Bella asks with trepidation.

"Across the stones."

Bella stops in her tracks. "You mean walk over all those graves?" she says in horror, looking down at the seemingly endless rows of flat stone markers. "With all the people I know under there?"

Now everyone has stopped.

"All right!" Evvie says, exasperated. "So, walk on the grass around the stones."

"But they're still graves."

"Bella. Come on!" says Sophie.

"I can't. It's not right. I'll walk along the outside."

"Forget it," Ida says. "That'll take forever."

"Don't be ridiculous, Bella. You've been to plenty of other funerals here and you walked on the stones," Evvie says.

"I don't remember that."

Evvie is moving briskly along. "Here's aisle twelve, now we need to find plot two-eleven. . . ."

Ida grabs Bella by the hand and starts pulling her. Bella digs her heels into the ground. But with one good yank, Ida dislodges her. "One more word out of you and I'm throwing you into the next open grave!"

We follow Evvie, moving briskly along. Except for Bella who is trying to walk on her tiptoes and keeping up a litany of *Oh, Gods*.

Sophie keeps looking down at the grave markers. "Keep your eyes open for six forty-two."

I ask why.

"Because I changed my plot. I wanted one with a corner view and I wanna make sure I got it."

Bella utters a small screech.

"What is it now!?" Evvie calls without looking back.

"I've stepped on my cousin, Sarah! Oh, God . . ."

"Over there!" Sophie points. And sure enough, not thirty feet away, I can see our neighbors and friends from Lanai Gardens. And in an instant, I know this is not good news. They are not facing in the right direction. They're turned away from the graveside. In fact, they are all walking toward us.

We meet them halfway.

"Such a lovely service," says Mrs. Fein from Phase Three.

"How could you miss it?" asks Hy Binder.

"It was inspirational," says Lola.

"It's over?" Evvie says, totally dejected.

"By five minutes. Where were you girls?"

"Don't ask," says Ida.

I watch in misery as Francie's son, Jerry, and his wife, Ilene, and the grandchildren pass by, heads down, unable to see or talk to anyone. Denny is there, in a suit much too small for him, probably the last suit his mother ever picked out for him. He is sobbing uncontrollably. Harriet struggles as she pushes her mother's wheelchair over the uneven ground. Irving, with the help of his pal, Sol, is supporting Millie, who has no idea where she is or why. Tessie Hoffman passes us muttering something about another death so soon after her dear Selma. Enya, as always, walks alone. Even Conchetta and Barney have taken time off from the library to pay their respects. I recognize a few of our Canadians. And — no surprise — there's Leo Slezak with a few of his cohorts from the Sunrise-Sunset Real Estate office. The Sleaze, being what he is, is slowly sidling up to Francie's family, his hand in the pocket where he keeps his damned cards.

Evvie looks at me and I look at her. We are despondent.

We nod and watch mutely as everyone passes us on the path. We wait until every last person is gone and then the five of us walk up the knoll and over to where Francie's casket sits on an elevated hoist.

We stand there silent and bemused.

Bella looks to me for help. "Say goodbye," I tell her.

"How?" Without the rabbi, she doesn't know what to do.

"Any way you like, Bella, dear. She'll know."

And each of us in our own way quietly says our last words to Francie.

"Thank you for always being nice to me," Bella says.

"I'll miss you," Sophie says, "especially your baking." She stamps her formal black orthopedic sneakers, annoyed. "Oh, that's a stupid thing to say. I don't know what to say to a dead person."

Ida turns away. She chokes up, shakes her head. For once the words won't come. She picks up a stone and places it on the casket.

"Thank you for your friendship," Evvie says, sobbing. "There will never be anyone like you again."

I can't speak. I silently tell my beloved friend what is in my heart. What do I do now, Francie? You're the only reason I stayed down here. Because we shared the same interests and laughed at all the same things. Because we were intellectual snobs at heart and we knew we really didn't belong down here, but going back was too hard, so we made it work for both of us. Because we knew what the other was thinking before we ever said it. Because home is where the person you love resides.

And that person was you and I no longer have a home —

"Glad?" Evvie interrupts my reverie. "Remember how I first met Francie?"

I smile. None of us can remember what we ate for breakfast, but ask about the distant past, and it seems like only yesterday.

"I don't think I ever heard that story," says Ida.

"It was a couple of years before you got here."

"It was just after I arrived," I comment.

"I was here," Bella says, "but I forgot."

"So, tell us," says Sophie as she sits on the bench next to the plot. Bella immediately joins her. Ida and I sit on the bench opposite.

"Actually, we met Al first. It was twenty-five years ago, when the buildings were new and people were first starting to move down here. Millie and I are standing on the balcony with our laundry, gossiping, when we see this nice-looking man walking up and down in front of our building. He keeps walking, then he disappears around the corner and then here he is again. Then a few minutes later, we see this beautiful woman doing the same thing. We finally figure out they are looking for each other, but keep missing each other. Soon, I hear him calling 'Francie, where are you,' and then we hear, 'Al, where are you?' Millie and I start laughing. Finally Millie can't stand it and she calls down, 'Hey, Francie, if that's who you are, stand still!' She is so surprised she stops in her tracks. A minute later Al appears and they run to one another hugging and kissing. 'I thought I'd never see you again,' he says.

"Everybody used to get lost at first. This place seemed so big, and all the buildings looked exactly the same. But we all became good friends after that."

We sit quietly for a few minutes. Behind us a half dozen graceful flamingos meander by, unmindful of our presence. "That was a nice story," Bella says.

"Now what?" a very subdued Ida asks. All of us stare at this tiny piece of ground where Francie will stay forever. At least she is with her beloved Al once again.

"Now what, what?" Evvie asks in return.

"Are we going to the get-together? Everybody said they were going after the services," says Bella.

"Do we have to? I'm afraid to look anybody in the eye after missing it. We'll be the laughing-stocking of Lanai Gardens," says Sophie, Queen of Malapropisms.

"Well, I don't care. We'll get to talk to

Jerry and Ilene and the kids. It's the least we can do," says Ida.

"I agree," Evvie adds.

"All right," I say. "Where are they having it?" The incredible silence that follows says it all.

"Nobody took down the name of the restaurant? Or the address?" I say, gritting my teeth.

"I think it starts with an *M*," Sophie contributes.

"You mean like meshugeneh, like all of you?" I say to them. "I can't believe this is happening. Why do I have to be responsible for everything? I left one thing up to you to take care of . . ." I sigh. "Is it at any of the places we usually go? Everybody *think!*"

"No," Ida says. "I remember saying to someone I never heard of that restaurant before."

"It's someplace in Margate, or maybe Tamarac," says Sophie.

"It could even be Boca Raton," says Bella.

"Well, that's that," says Evvie.

Another long silence.

"I can't do it!" Bella cries.

"Do what?" I ask.

"Just go home and do nothing. I won't

be able to stand it."

"Me, too. I don't want to be alone," says Sophie. "I'll just keep crying."

"We can go somewhere for lunch by ourselves. I could eat." Ida says this with no conviction whatsoever. It gets the silence it deserves.

I walk over to Francie's coffin, sitting out here in the hot sun waiting for the groundskeepers to come and slowly lower it into that horrifying gaping hole.

I bend toward it, cupping my ear as if listening. "What? What's that you say?" The others turn and gawk. Finally I straighten up. "Well, it's peculiar, but if that's what you want, Francie."

I start walking away. The girls look at one another, befuddled. I call over my shoulder. "Francie told me what she wants us to do. Come on."

They just stand there. "Come *on*, girls."

They run after me, puzzled but obedient, as Bella says, "Oh, not again over those dead bodies!" And Ida calls back to the casket, "Rest in peace, Francie, you hear!"

Five minutes later I pull into the parking lot of the Seminole Indian Bingo Hall and Casino. They are staring at me incredulously, and I tell them as I park the car, "Francie said that we should win the

108

pick-a-pet for her!"

I open the trunk where all our bingo gear is always at the ready. Before they start grabbing for them, I raise my hand in warning. I tell them that they are never, never, under penalty of torture, to tell anybody where we went after Francie's funeral.

I had to think of something to save this god-awful day. And knowing Francie, if she could have whispered anything at all to me, she would have said, "*Carpe Diem*, babe — seize the day. What the hell — PLAY BINGO!"

14

Murder Will Out

The quiet is deafening, if that makes any sense. Since Francie's funeral last week, a pall has fallen over Lanai Gardens. Our friends and neighbors go about their day's activities very quietly. When people speak, they speak in whispers. There are none of the usual complaints about the weather. Francie made a difference in our lives and her loss is beyond measure. And maybe because it is Francie, we think about our own mortality. Especially we who live by ourselves. It brings an icy feeling to the back of the neck to think about dying all alone.

Francie's family went back to New Jersey after Evvie and I offered to take care of disposing of the rest of her things. Their instructions were: Take something to remember her by, and give everything else to charity.

Now Evvie and I are in Francie's apartment early in the morning. The first twenty minutes, we do nothing but just sit here and think of Francie in this place she loved. Her apartment reflects the bright and cheerful person she was. Her fabric colors are lemon, coral, and avocado green; her furniture style, light and airy wicker.

"Let's do the bedroom first," I say, to make a start. As we get up, Sophie flings open the front door and hurries in.

"Your coffee and bagels," she announces.

"Thanks, Soph," Evvie says. "Just leave them on the sink."

We start working on the closets, but are aware that Sophie hasn't left. We hear her clattering about.

"What are you doing, Soph?" I call out.

"You work, don't worry about me. I'll just kibitz."

Evvie and I exchange glances. Does that mean she plans to keep talking and drive us crazy?

We box Francie's clothes, and what a painful task it is. Remembering when she wore what. Remembering her laughter. And how she made everything fun.

Sophie's head pops into the doorway. "She did have aspirin," she says as if continuing some earlier discussion.

"Why?" asks Evvie. "Do you have a headache?"

"I read somewhere that if you're having a heart attack, someone should give you an aspirin. It could have saved Francie." She looks at us, eager to share her knowledge.

Exasperated, Evvie says, "But she was *alone*, Sophie."

"Well, maybe we should all carry aspirin all over our bodies from now on." She waits for a response.

"Thank you for sharing that. Don't you have someplace to go?"

"Not 'til two when we play cards." She disappears back into the kitchen-living room area.

Evvie holds up a beautiful peach organza cocktail gown. "Remember?" she asks.

"Jerry and Ilene's wedding."

Evvie nods and folds it away carefully. She opens the next drawer. "Oh," she cries out.

"What?" I pull my head out of the closet.

Evvie is holding up Francie's favorite sweatshirt, the one that says "Death by Chocolate." "She loved this crazy shirt." With that she starts to cry.

"We can't keep doing this. We'll never get done," I say as gently as I can.

"That's just it! I don't ever want to get done, because that will be the last we have of her."

We hear more noise from the kitchen.

Sophie calls out, "You know how neat and clean she was. If Francie could see the crumbs in her sink, she'd die!"

"I'm going to wring her neck," Evvie says through gritted teeth.

I laugh. Everyone should have some comic relief in their lives. "Just leave it, Soph, we'll get someone in to clean."

The doorbell rings. "I'll get it," Sophie calls. As she opens the door, we hear her voice turn all sugary. "Well, hello there. Please do come in."

"Bet you five dollars." Evvie smirks.

"No bet. It can only be —" I call out, "Is that you, Mr. Slezak?"

Evvie and I return to the living room and there he is — gold chains gleaming.

"Good morning, beautiful ladies," he says, saluting us with his dirty white Panama hat as he snoops around. "I see by your hard work you are earning stars in your crown."

Evvie snarls at him, "Jews don't get stars in crowns!"

"Well, so call it a mitzvah, this good deed."

"My Stanley used to say, 'One mitzvah could change the world, two could make you tired,' " Sophie adds.

"Why are you here, Mr. Slezak?" I ask.

"*Leo,* why do you fight calling me Leo?"

"So, *Mr. Slezak,*" Evvie says deliberately, "tell us what you want."

"I need a set of keys. The family, such nice people, gave me the listing."

Evvie groans. We forgot to warn Jerry.

"Grave robber," Evvie mutters.

"You'll leave the furniture for a while? A property always shows better with a little interior décor."

"What difference will that make," Evvie says, losing her patience. "You'll never sell it anyway."

"How can you show such cruelty?" He pleads, "Don't I live here, too, among you? Am I not one of us?"

Evvie smirks at his pathetic parody of *The Merchant of Venice.*

"I work my buns off for you ladies. And why haven't you taken advantage of my 'Save Your Family Grief' program? A little rider added to the will about disposal of assets —"

"*I* have," chirps Sophie.

"We've already saved our families from grief, thank you," I inform him. "We have it in our wills to give our apartments to the first homeless people they see, rather than let Sunrise-Sunset Real Estate get their paws on it."

Leo shrugs. He tried.

Evvie unclasps an extra key from her key ring and tosses it at him. "Don't slam the door on your way out."

"I'll walk you," Sophie says, almost drooling as she clutches at his arm and apologizes for our rudeness.

An hour goes swiftly by and we are making good progress. The refrigerator is almost emptied when a familiar doggie bag catches my eye. "Evvie, look. From dinner . . . our last dinner together. Remember, Francie took home the chocolate cake. She never ate it."

"That's not like her."

"Maybe she never got the chance." We look at each other considering what that means. For a moment I hesitate, and then I say what's been on my mind. "There's something I want to discuss with you. Something really serious."

Evvie looks at me, alarmed.

"Coincidences. I've been thinking there have been too many. Selma and Francie."

"What are you talking about?" Evvie asks, now more puzzled than alarmed.

"The birthdays for starters. Selma and Francie both died on the night before their birthday. Both were very healthy. Both died suddenly of heart attacks. With no history of heart attacks that we know of. They both died alone. Both were trying to reach for the phone. And there's something about that damn phone that's driving me up the wall and I can't remember what it is."

"But isn't it possible? Couldn't it have happened like that?"

"Yes. However, Miss Marple and I agree — we don't believe in coincidences."

"Oh, you and your mystery books —"

"I learn a lot from them. What it's beginning to sound like is an M.O."

"Again from the mysteries?"

"As in 'modus operandi,' the method used in a crime."

"A crime?" Now the worry lines appear on her face.

"As in murder —"

The doorbell rings and we both jump.

"Later," I say as I go to answer, hoping it isn't Sophie again.

Surprisingly, it is Harriet Feder, carrying a small basket.

"Come on in," Evvie calls out warmly.

"I hope I'm not interrupting. I took the day off, and I thought maybe I could help in some way." She indicates the basket. "A snack for the hard workers."

"Thanks, Harriet, that's really very thoughtful. You're not sick . . . ?"

"No. I just can't get over Francie. . . . I started to go to work and then I said the hell with it. The hospital can manage without me for a day or two. Considering how low the pay is, anyway. Then I sat around the apartment feeling depressed. I need to do *something*."

"We'll take all the help we can get," Evvie says.

"We're just about to start on the dishes," I tell her.

"I'll pass them down, you put them in the cartons," I say as I head towards the kitchen cabinets.

"OK. Keeping busy will help."

"How's your mother?" Evvie asks.

"She's fine. The usual aches and pains. I just wish I could find a way to make her accept being in that chair. She was always such an independent person."

Evvie and I exchange glances. To us, Esther Feder seems quite happy in that chair as long as she can boss everyone around. Especially Harriet.

We all work quietly for a while, then Harriet starts to clear the knickknacks off a corner shelf. She picks up one of many birthday cards that still linger there as a silent reminder. "This must be from Denny. He always sends such sweet, simple cards." She looks inside and smiles. "How does he always remember? I know the cards he sends me are always on time."

"That's easy," Evvie says. "About five years ago, we had a crafts class in the rec room and Denny attended. He made this birthday reminder calendar and it got him so excited, he went to each and every person in Phase Two and got them to mark down their dates."

"That's right. I remember when Mother and I moved in, he came and asked for ours. What a sweet boy." She smiles wryly. "Not a boy. He's actually about my age. The poor dear. He must be suffering terribly right now. Wasn't he the one who found both Selma and Francie's bodies?"

Evvie says, "Now that you mention it, you're right. Both times he was on his way up to fix something . . ." She turns to me as she says meaningfully, "What a coincidence."

"Thank God he has keys to all our apartments. Who knows how long poor Francie would have lain there, if he hadn't gone in." Harriet stops, aware of our tension.

Just then there is a knock at the open

kitchen window. It's Ida. "Harriet," she calls in a snippy voice, "your mom wants you." She still hasn't forgiven her for the bank.

"Oh," says Harriet, looking at her watch. "She must be waiting for her lunch. Call me later." She leaves.

"I forgot the board gave Denny those keys. Another coincidence?" Evvie asks.

"Speaking of lunch," says Ida through the window. "I have it ready and waiting in my apartment. Take a break."

"Maybe we should," Evvie says. "Right now, I need to get a breath of air. But somehow I lost my appetite."

Suddenly a comment Sophie made jogs at my memory. "Go on ahead. I'll be with you after I lock up."

Alone in the apartment now, I am in a turmoil of emotion. I hurry to the kitchen sink. Sophie, in her dithering, talked about it being dirty. Crumbs, she said. I see tiny bits of debris. I touch them. They are soft, like the texture of cake. Brown cake crumbs. I pick them up and smell them. It's chocolate. I know it is.

Two thoughts pop into my head. 1) Sophie's right. Francie would never leave a dirty sink. 2) If she didn't eat the chocolate cake from Continental, where did these crumbs come from? And now I keep hearing words repeating in my head. *Death by chocolate. Death by chocolate.*

15

Making a Decision

I am waiting for Evvie in her apartment. She's getting ready for swimming. We had dinner together last night and breakfast this morning because she wanted to talk about the bombshell I threw at her yesterday, and we are still talking. If you call going around in circles talking.

"I'm almost ready," she calls from the bedroom.

"No hurry," I call back. I am on her sun-porch skimming through one of her many movie magazines. While my apartment is a study in simplicity with a few nice antiques, a small collection of prints, and too many books, Evvie's place is a cluttered tribute to showbiz. If my sister "missed the boat," as she is fond of saying, she has certainly kept up with the ebbs and tides of her lost profession. Evvie wanted to be Doris Day. But Doris Day didn't have Joe Markowitz for a husband, who insisted she stay home and be a proper wife and cook and clean and care for the children. She had her one-week shot as a torch singer, performing in a small club in Jersey, and she was pretty good. (She swears Doris sang there, but I doubt that.) But then the war ended, and the guy she had met and married on a romantic weekend, before he shipped out for Korea, came home. That was the end of her career.

But the memories and dreams live on in her movie posters and recordings of Doris Day.

"I still don't think it was murder," she says as she comes out, rubbing on suntan lotion. She's only said that eleven times by my last count.

"But it is a possibility," I say, feeling like a broken record myself.

"It can't be anyone who lives here."

"I didn't say it was. I only said it might be."

We walk out her door and head down the stairs.

"I refuse to accept the possibility it could be Denny!"

"I never said it was."

"But he does have all the keys and he was the one who found them both."

"It could be a coincidence —"

"Which you don't believe in."

"But it could be."

We say our usual hellos to the usual gang and make our way down the path, passing our ducks in their pond, carefully avoiding the poop on the path.

"Look." Evvie grabs me. "There's Denny in his garden."

"So? He's usually in his garden at some time or other during the day." Denny sees us and waves.

"Does he look like he could kill anyone?"

"No, Ev, I don't think he could. But the truth is, anyone is capable of murder if provoked, or if they believe they have a strong enough motive."

"Or is crazy."

"He's retarded, Ev, not crazy."

"The Kronk is crazy."

"We don't know that she's crazy. Maybe she's just eccentric." Evvie has forced me into this role of devil's advocate and now she's driving *me* crazy.

"Is she dangerous? Is she capable of murder?"

"Who knows? Nobody has even seen her in years."

"But she might be. She could be a raving maniac by now."

We arrive at the pool. I shush her. "Quiet. Drop the subject now. I don't want anyone else to know what we're talking about."

We greet everyone, drop our towels and pool shoes, and wade into the pool. I'm glad I didn't tell Evvie about the chocolate crumbs. I'd never hear the end of that discussion. But I do feel I have to do something about my suspicions.

"Hey, girls, c'm'ere, I've got another great joke," calls Hy as he and Lola bounce up and down together at three feet deep.

Evvie whispers to me as she starts to get in. "Well, if the murderer has to be one of us, I hope it's Hy. I would love to see him in Alcatraz."

"Alcatraz is closed."

"Whatever."

Of course Hy has to "playfully" splash us before he begins his joke. "There's these three guys standing in a bar boasting of how great they are in the sack. The Eye-talian says he rubs olive oil on his wife before sex and she screams with pleasure for an hour. The Frenchie says he pats butter on his wife and she screams for two hours. The Jew says he schmears chicken schmaltz on his wife and she screams for *six* hours. The Eye-talian and the Frenchie are impressed. 'How did you get your wife to scream for six hours?' 'Easy,' he says, 'I wiped my hands on the drapes!' Didya get it, didja?"

A few of us actually laugh.

I glance over at Enya sitting in her usual place. When Hy is most vulgar I look at her, hoping she isn't listening to him. She seems oblivious.

Tessie swims by me. Chubby as she is, in water she's as buoyant as a sponge. She does her usual laps. I get an idea. I wait until she is through and I follow her out to where her chaise is parked between the Feders and the Canadians.

I speak very softly. "Listen," I say, "you cleaned out Selma's apartment after she died, didn't you?"

She responds to my seriousness. "Yes, I did. Why?"

"I'm just curious about something. Do you recall seeing anything at all that was odd or unusual in the apartment?"

"Not that I can remember." She pauses. "You think there's something wrong?"

"I'm not sure, but I do want you to give this some serious thought. We'll talk later."

As I pass Harriet, she gives me the smallest of nods and an OK sign as if she guessed what I said to Tessie and was giving me her approval. I start to walk toward her, then stop. Esther is tugging at Harriet's arm.

"Sweetheart," she says, "I think I need more lotion." Since she is covered up to the neck, this seems unnecessary, but Harriet gets out the cream and works it into her mother's face.

"No," she says, "on my shoulders. I feel the sun through my robe, pull it down."

"Mom," Harriet says with a patience beyond Job's, "you can't get a burn through clothes."

Esther looks toward me, slyly. "You don't want them to see the marks." Harriet throws me a weary look over her mother's head. Her glance says, *See what I put up with.* Mine says, *You have my deepest sympathy.* I change my mind about approaching. She has enough to deal with. "Talk to you later," I tell her and jump back into the pool.

Evvie paddles over to me. "What was that all about?"

"Later," I say to her, too. I am putting everyone on hold until I can figure out what to do.

Evvie says, "Irving didn't bring Millie down today. I think we better check."

"Good idea," and we both leave the pool.

"So, where are you going?" Ida calls after us.

"We're gonna look in on Millie."

"OK."

You may have noticed by now that everybody keeps tabs on everybody else. The Lanai Gardens FBI is always on the alert; God forbid somebody should miss something. Especially since our behavior is so predictable that any small deviation is cause for complete attention by a mob of people — especially the girls.

We arrive at Millie's. When we walk in we immediately see how frazzled Irving looks. He is sitting at the dining room table, the remains of breakfast still there, his head in his hands.

"What's wrong?" I ask.

"She had a bad night. I was up until maybe four a.m."

"What was she doing?"

Irving looks embarrassed. "She was yelling at the children."

Poor Irving. He's been living with Millie's hallucinations so long, he talks about them as if they were real. They're real to Millie, so he goes along.

"Why was she yelling?" Evvie asks.

Irving shakes his head, and turns red.

"They want to do disgusting things with him and I won't let them." Millie shambles into the living room, her hair disheveled, her robe a mess. Looking coy one moment and furious the next, she bends over her husband. "Don't they, lover boy?" She runs her fingers wildly through the few strands of his hair.

Irving has always been a very shy man. Millie used to tell us funny stories about how he would undress in the closet when they were first married. He's never used a curse word in his life and now his demented wife is talking unashamedly about sex in front of other people.

"The children like to fuck!"

Irving pulls away from her and hurries out to the kitchen, holding his hands over his ears. Millie laughs as she watches him go. It is more like a cackle. Alzheimer's is a horrible disease. The Millie we are looking at bears no resemblance to our old friend.

Then once again, that peculiar symptom — suddenly, the light goes out in her mind and the catatonia returns. She starts to fall down, but Evvie catches her. Balancing her between us, we walk her back to bed and tuck her in.

We join Irving in the kitchen. He is standing at the stove with a tepid cup of tea.

I start carefully. We've been down this road before and he always cuts us off at the pass. "Irving. Maybe it's time —"

"No."

"Maybe you need someone to come in during the days."

"You all help . . . ."

"You need more. You have to be able to sleep. You can't watch her twenty-four hours."

He says what he always says. "I'll think on it."

We start for the door. "We'll get one of the girls to come and spell you, so you can take a nap," I say.

He nods and we leave.

"I can do it," Evvie volunteers.

"No," I tell her. "I have other plans for us."

16

Keystone Kops and Nosy Neighbors

"Do you think we can make our getaway without anybody noticing?" Evvie is whispering, as if that would help.

We are walking very quietly down the stairs from my apartment on the third floor. "Ha ha," I say, "fat chance."

Ida's door flings open and she steps out onto the walkway. She sees us round the second floor stairwell and calls down to us over the banister. "Where are the Siamese twins off to now? First it was dinner, then breakfast. Now out to lunch I suppose?"

"Here we go," I say. "Send in the clowns!"

Evvie sighs. "If three-nineteen is out, can three-fourteen be far behind?"

And sure enough, Sophie's head pops out of her kitchen window. "So where is everybody off to?" she calls out.

"Maybe if we don't answer . . ." Evvie says softly.

"Dream on," I say.

From across the parking area, Bella's third-floor door opens and she peers out. "Am I missing something?" she calls out in her whispery little voice.

Evvie and I are now on the ground floor tiptoeing to the car. God bless them — they may be half deaf and half blind and well on their way to senility, but they don't miss a trick.

Now we pass the Feder apartment, 119, which is two doors away from my parking spot. Esther Feder is at her usual post, sitting in the doorway behind the screen, so the bugs won't get her. Which is actually a bizarre sight if you think about how she looks with her head pressed against the dark mesh partition. She raps at the screen to get our attention. "Where are you girls going in all this heat?"

Ida, the acrobat, now hangs over the balcony. "So, what's the big hurry?"

Sophie trills, "If you're stopping at Publix, maybe you'll bring me a pint of sour cream? I'll pay you back later." Which is a joke. Sophie borrows money from all of us, and we've yet to get a penny back. Ida calls that the lifestyle of the rich and disgusting.

The three-ring chorus is getting louder.

"We can't just ignore them. We have to

tell them something," Evvie says.

"You're the writer. Make something up."
I open the door and turn on the air so I
can cool off the car.

"We're going out on blind dates," she
calls out.

"That's the best you can come up with?"
I say.

"Oh, yeah? They'd have to be desperate
to want *you* old ladies." And now dear Hy,
the snake charmer, comes out of his apartment carrying the garbage, adding his two
bits.

All the clowns are laughing. The idea of
us having dates is just too funny.

Ida especially loves this. "Who's your
matchmaker, Yentl Frankenstein?"

Esther, excited, now pushes her screen
door open so she can see better. "You got
dates? Maybe you can fix my Harriet
up?"

There is a loud clatter from inside the
kitchen and Harriet appears quickly, wiping her hands on her apron. "Oh, Mom,"
she says, embarrassed. "Please!"

"Well, you told me to sit in the door and
spy on them."

Harriet turns red in the face. "That's not
funny!" She spins her mother's wheelchair
around sharply. "Go inside now! Eat your

lunch. You know I have no time for this. I have to get back to the hospital!"

"I didn't mean anything. Don't hit me." Esther wheels herself in quickly.

Harriet looks at us. "I'm sorry," she says. "Sometimes Mom can be so difficult." Then she smiles and leans in toward us and whispers. "You really have dates?"

Evvie whispers back. "Of course not. We're going to the police station and we don't want anybody to know. You know what yentas they all are."

"Evvie!" I say sharply. "My sister, queen of the yentas."

Harriet joins in the conspiracy. "I knew it! You do think there's a connection between their deaths. Don't worry, I won't say a word. Good luck. Let me know how it goes."

We get into the car and make our escape, leaving a lot of disappointed faces peering after us.

"I'm sorry," Evvie says. "I didn't think it mattered if I told Harriet."

"I just didn't want anyone to know until we were sure there was a crime. You know how rumors spread."

"Yeah, like cream cheese on bagels," she says with a sigh.

We leave Lanai Gardens and I make our

turn onto Oakland Park Boulevard, and I can finally breathe a sigh of relief.

"Come to think of it," Evvie says, "when was the last time you and I had some time alone away from the gang?"

"When you had to cover that speech by that Israeli fund-raiser. No one else wanted to go. If I hadn't had to drive you, neither would I."

"Oh, yeah. He lectured on 'Is Israel In Trouble?' "

"Which YOU slept through. Though I did love your review."

Evvie bristles, ready to be insulted. "Why, what was wrong with it?"

"Nothing, because it was so . . ." I stop. "A senior moment. What's the word that means 'short and sweet'?"

"I don't know. What's wrong with 'short and sweet'?"

"Because I can't stand it when I can't think of the word that won't come out of my mouth when I want it."

"Good? Was the word good? My review was good?"

"That's not the word. Never mind."

"My review wasn't good?"

"That's not the point. I am talking about my loss of memory."

"Now you've got me not remembering. I

don't remember what I wrote in that review."

"You said, 'Yes. Israel is always in trouble.'"

"That was it?"

"Yes. It was pithy." Now I get excited. "That was the word — pithy!"

Evvie points. "There it is. The police station."

As I make the right turn from Oakland Park Boulevard into the parking area, I say as sternly as I can, "Evvie, promise me you'll let me do all the talking."

"Mum's the word."

We are finally shown into the office of Detective Morgan Langford, and I'm already exhausted. The waiting seems endless. The paperwork, too. The sergeant at the front desk would not let us go any further until we first explained to him what we wanted. I held my ground. I would only speak to someone in Homicide. Why should I waste my time going through it twice? Finally, I used the "age card" and pretended senility. He was glad to be rid of me. But, I think, as punishment, he sent me to Detective Langford.

It's amazing that in all my seventy-five years, I have never really seen or been in a police station. In movies, in books, but not in reality. I have to admit to a little shiver of excitement. I want to yell out, "Hey, Agatha, look at me!"

Evvie is also all a-twitter in her first police station appearance, but she is off in another art form. She is preparing to become the actress she should have been. Suddenly she has an attitude. She is trying to look sophisticated and worldly. I just hope she doesn't decide to sing.

Detective Langford is busy reading the very little information I grudgingly filled in while waiting. This gives me a chance to study him. He's in his thirties, very, very tall, and skinny. His clothes hang on him. He seems to favor loud checks and plaids. He is very relaxed. Maybe too relaxed.

"So," he says, "you insisted on talking to Homicide. Are you planning one, reporting one, or looking for one?"

And cynical.

Before I can stop her, Sarah Bernhardt begins to emote. "We are here to report two murders. They are Selma Beller, who kept a very clean house, and Francie Charles, who was the best pastry maker in Fort Lauderdale."

"When did these murders occur?" asks long and lanky, trying to keep a straight face.

"Evvie . . ." I growl, but she ignores me.

"One month ago and one week ago."

"How come they haven't been reported?"

"Because nobody knows they were murdered. Everybody says they had heart attacks, but we know better. Only my sister, who is an expert in murder mysteries, and myself, a writer for the Lanai Gardens *Free Press*, know the truth."

"Are you finished yet?" I hiss at her. I notice she doesn't mention that the "*Press*" is a throwaway.

"Would you like to add to this, Mrs. Markowitz?"

"I'm Gold, she's Markowitz, my blabbermouth sister. I know this may sound far-fetched to you, but two women did die in our buildings. But their deaths . . ."

Evvie obviously can't stand my slow, logical pace. "Too many coincidences. Agatha Christie doesn't believe in them and neither do we!" Pleased with her pronouncement, she folds her hands, waiting for the detective to take over the case.

"And what are these coincidences?"

Evvie blabs, "Tell him about the cake Francie never ate and that the girls both died on the night before their birthdays and that Denny had keys to their apartments and they both died reaching for the phone."

Hearing the way my sister lays out our case, I could just about imagine Langford's opinion of us. He is drumming those long bony fingers impatiently on the desk.

"And these are the devastating facts that make you suspect murder?"

Evvie, totally missing his sarcasm, blathers on. She gets a brainstorm. "What about the serial killer? He kills old women. What's his M.O.? That means his method," she explains to the Homicide detective.

If his tongue was any farther back in his cheek, he'd choke. He asks dramatically, "Interested in the M.O.'s, are we? Well, our killer sneaks into apartments of women who live alone. Late at night, he creeps up on them when they are sleeping and strangles his victims. Were your victims strangled?"

"They didn't look strangled. But then, we're no experts," Evvie grandly admits.

I've had it. I reach over and smack my hand over Evvie's mouth. Evvie, eyes widening, looks at me, horrified. She tries to speak, but I keep my hand firmly pressed on her mouth. I turn to Langford. "Listen. I know none of this sounds incriminating — but there is something wrong with their deaths. Can't you give it a little time and investigate?"

Langford gets up — rather, it's more like unfurling himself — and he is an awesome six foot six or so. Evvie gasps in pleasure amidst her pain. He is moving toward the door, which is his way of moving us to the door — and out.

"I really would like an autopsy," I say in desperation.

"You wouldn't like it. It hurts like hell," he says and roars with laughter.

As firmly as I can, I make my last-ditch stand. "I think they were poisoned. I am a reasonable, rational woman, unlike my sister here." With that I let go of her, and glaring at her, I dare her to make a sound. "Please do not condescend to me with bad jokes. I do not make such statements lightly. These women were murdered. In my heart I know I'm right."

He opens the door. "Well, thanks for dropping in." And we are dismissed.

As we head for the door, Evvie, oblivious, punches my arm, delighted with her premiere. "How'd we do, sis?" she asks.

I tell her she deserves an Academy Award. And I deserve what I got for taking her along.

All the way home, I simmer. The detective wouldn't take me seriously because I'm old in his eyes. Well, I'll show him, that snotty string bean.

I wake up suddenly, look at the clock. It's nearly eleven. I must have fallen asleep reading. The light is still on. Suddenly I am jumping out of bed, throwing my robe and slippers on. Scrambling through my junk drawer for my flashlight. I grab my keys and I'm out the door. I don't want to do this. I don't want to walk around alone at night, but this can't wait until morning.

Maybe I should wake Evvie. No. Coward. It's not the middle of the night. What am I afraid of?

I know what I'm afraid of.

I truly believe there is a killer loose around here.

It's a beautiful night with a wild, full moon. The kind of moon that once upon a time meant romance, not terror. I walk down the stairs. I tell myself, *See, there are a few people still up.* I can see the flickering of TV sets. Then I giggle. Maybe I'll run into Greta Kronk. Maybe she'll tell me what's so great about digging around in Dumpsters in the middle of the night.

So far so good. Now I have to walk around the corner. It seems darker as I make the turn, but that's silly. Between the moon and the streetlights, I can see what's ahead. But then again, I can also be seen.

I curse the memory lapses that come with getting old. Two wasted days to remember what should have clicked the instant I saw it. And now I'm walking around in the dark.

I jump, startled, then realize it's a stupid palm tree swaying and what I saw was its shadow. But, finally, I'm at Francie's apartment. I curse the key. I curse my hands that won't stop shaking. When the lock finally gives, I go straight for the kitchen. I don't even turn the lights on, the flashlight will be good enough.

The proof is in the pudding, I think, giggling with relief that I got here safely. The poison will be in the chocolate. I will bring it to Detective Langford and say, "Here's your proof." He'll have to listen to me!

I flash the light over the sink. Even as I see it, my mind refuses to accept it. No!!! Damn it, no! The chocolate crumbs are gone! Someone has scrubbed the sink clean.

I crumple into Francie's favorite armchair and start to cry. In my mind the heroes and heroines of every murder mystery I have ever read are wagging their fingers at me, shaking their heads ruefully. *We taught you so much and you learned nothing. Failure. You had it and you lost it. You old woman, you old failure.*

Whatever courage got me here is gone now. I sit in the armchair all night, just an old lady waiting, trusting in the safety of daylight.

17

Canasta

It's Sophie's turn to host the weekly canasta game. Not my favorite place to play cards. First of all, Sophie's apartment is enough to give me a headache even before we play. Her decor is what Ida calls Early *Onge-patshket*. This is almost untranslatable, but the closest meaning would be overdone to the max. If there is an empty space, something must be put in it. And something is never enough. Too much is never enough. Why one doily on a couch, when five would be better? If you get my drift.

In everyone else's apartment, we get served some nuts and raisins, tea and maybe sponge cake. Not in the home of Sophie, the bountiful. A huge bowl of fruit. Boxes of candy. Later on, coffee and three kinds of pie. Bella calls her generous. Ida calls her a show-off.

Ida is not here yet. But when she arrives, the battle of the air conditioner will begin. Sophie will want subarctic temperatures. Ida will want the tropics. Speak of the devil. Here she is.

"Turn down the goddamn air," she announces before even getting through the door.

Sophie folds her arms. "No. My house, my rules. In your house we sweat like pigs!"

Bella, the pacifist, says meekly, "Put on your sweater, Ida dear."

The card game begins.

"So how much do we need to open?" Bella asks.

"It's one-twenty. It's always one-twenty!" Ida snaps at her.

"I forget."

Evvie asks Bella, "Did you bring your hearing aid?"

"What?" she asks.

"Never mind."

"So, partner, are you ready to open?" Ida asks Evvie.

"Already, they're starting. This is a card game, not a discussion group." Sophie glares at them.

"I'm close," Evvie says, ignoring Sophie.

It is my turn to sit out the game. We play a round robin, alternating who gets to play. Bella would prefer never to touch a card since there are already four of us, but the two sadists insist she can't just sit and watch. She hates to play as much as they hate playing with her. What can I tell you? This is the way it is. I'm glad I'm sitting out. I don't think I could concentrate.

It's Ida's turn. She looks at Evvie. Evvie comments ever so lightly, "Have you seen *Hy* lately?"

"Yes, indeed I have," says Ida, putting down a jack. Evvie blows her a kiss.

Sophie glares. She knows what they're up to. "Cheater," she mutters. "As if you give a hoot about Hy Binder!"

Ida stands up. "How dare you!"

Sophie says, getting surly, "Next time it'll be 'and how is dear old *Lo*' and you'll give her a *low* card —"

Evvie throws her cards down on the table. "That's it! You have some nerve!"

Bella looks from one to the other thoroughly confused.

War is about to begin.

"Girls," I say, "we need to talk. Girls!"

They take one look at my face and know something is up. Reluctantly, they throw their cards into the middle of the table, still simmering, except for Bella, who is relieved.

It takes a few minutes for them to calm down and plump up pillows and generally get comfortable. Finally I have their attention.

"You all wondered where Evvie and I went the other afternoon, I'm sure."

Ida answers huffily. "We certainly did."

I drop my bombshell. "We went to the police station. To report the murders of Francie and Selma."

For maybe three seconds there is a stunned silence. Then they are all talking at once in a barrage of words. *Murder? Francie? Selma? Not possible. Oy gevalt! What are you talking about? You're kidding, right? Police, really the police? What did you say? What did they say?*

Finally Evvie bangs on the table. "Shah! Be quiet and you might learn something!"

Slowly they settle down, all eyes glued on me in horror and excitement.

Bella looks confused. "You mean you didn't have dates?"

I say, "No, Bella, no dates."

Evvie, of course, jumps in. "Gladdy thinks they were both murdered but that cop wouldn't believe her!"

"After he just dismissed us as crackpots, I tried to forget about it, but Francie won't let me. I keep hearing her in my head: *Find out who did it. You have to.* It was the crumbs that convinced me."

A chorus of "What crumbs?" follows.

Evvie looks at me suspiciously. "You

146

never mentioned crumbs."

"I know," I say guiltily. "It was the crumbs that Sophie found in Francie's sink. Chocolate cake crumbs. If Francie didn't eat the cake she brought home from Continental, where did they come from?"

Evvie is hurt. "You didn't tell me."

"I'm sorry."

"I told you Francie wouldn't leave a dirty sink! I knew it!" Sophie is delighted with herself.

"Maybe she didn't like the cake from Continental," says Bella. "Maybe she baked a new one." Then gleefully, "From her new cookbook." Bella is pleased with her theory.

"And ate an entire cake herself? Puleeze," says Evvie disdainfully. "Our health nut who eats tiny portions?" Evvie realizes what she just said. "Who *used* to eat . . ." She stops, on the verge of tears.

"I don't understand," Ida says. "Who would want to kill them? They didn't have enemies."

"And why? Why would anyone hurt them? They never hurt a fleabag," Sophie insists.

"It was the coincidences," my sidekick informs them. Evvie proceeds to list my suspicions.

"If it wasn't heart attacks," Sophie asks me, "what made them dead?"

"I think poison."

There is a group gasp at this as each of the girls tries to absorb this momentous information.

"I went back to Francie's apartment. I went to get those chocolate crumbs. It could have been the proof we needed. . . ."

Evvie gets it first. "Oh, no. The cleaning girl was there after we left."

"Gone," I say. But was it the cleaning girl? Or did the killer get there first?

"Why are you telling us this?" Ida asks softly.

"I want you all to help me find the killer."

There is a long moment as they digest the earth-shattering things I have been saying. Bella and Sophie reach out and hold hands. Ida jumps up, needing to move around.

Bella sighs. "How can we? A killer could be anywhere."

"Yeah," says Ida, "maybe he's the serial killer."

"The serial killer is a strangler, the cops told us," Evvie informs them.

"You're not saying . . ." Sophie begins.

"I am saying. I think the killer lives here

or comes here, somebody we probably know or have seen hanging around."

"*A choleria!* A plague on him! I can't believe such a thing," Sophie cries out.

"I'm never going out of my apartment again," wails Bella.

"They were both killed *in* their apartments," Ida says with evil relish.

"*Vay iz mir,* I'm dying!" Bella is in tears.

Sophie screeches, "Whose birthday is next?"

"Does anybody know when it's my birthday? I can't remember," asks Bella plaintively.

"We don't know for sure if that means anything," I say, trying to calm them.

Evvie takes a stronger tack. "Snap out of it!" she says, the movie critic paying homage to *Moonstruck.*

"I really do need help," I say. "I want us to go around and talk to everybody. Find out if they saw anything unusual the nights of the murders."

Again, silence as this is absorbed. Finally Sophie sighs. "*Oy,* I wish I were only seventy-eight again!"

Ida pats her on the back. "Don't worry, Princess, you'll find the strength. We all will, for Francie's sake."

"I don't know," Sophie says. "Maybe

we're opening up a can of snakes."

Bella whimpers. "Maybe you'll make the killer mad and he'll come after us."

"God forbid," Evvie says.

"I'm more worried we'll scare a lot of people, but it has to be done," I reply. More silence.

"Everybody in?" I ask.

I get a chorus of "in's."

"Then, hopefully, we'll get real information, so the cops will believe us and take over."

The girls get up and start clearing the cards off the table. We always help the hostess clean up.

"You should have told me about the crumbs," Evvie says accusingly.

"I know," I tell her. "I know."

"*I* would have remembered!"

"I know! Don't keep rubbing it in!"

Suddenly we hear sirens very close. Ida runs and flings open the door. "Police cars! Coming in here!"

"Murder! Another murder!" Sophie screams.

And Bella faints.

I feel very guilty. What have I unleashed?

18

Old-Timer's Disease

We don't even wait for the elevator. In spite of our age, and the possible damage we can do to our bodies, we are running down the three flights of stairs and across the parking area to where two policemen, and a small group of our neighbors in a varied assortment of sleepwear, are gathering. The flashing lights from the police car zigzag across the watchers like strobe lights at a "happening." Something is happening all right and we are terrified.

All the activity is centered at Millie and Irving's apartment. The police are pounding at their door. Thoughts crowd my head. Making assessments. It's after nine p.m. They must be asleep. It's not an ambulance, thank God, so Irving didn't call the paramedics. So, why are the police here? Please, God, don't let anyone be hurt. The officers keep hammering. No one is answering.

We arrive at the door, hearts throbbing with fear and overexertion. Throwing questions at them, although we are so out of breath we can barely speak.

"What is it?"

"Why are you here?"

"What's wrong?"

"Please talk to us. We're their friends."

The taller policeman with an orange mustache tells us they got a 911 call.

The short, stubby one says, "The woman was screaming that she was being raped and someone was trying to kill her."

The girls breathe a collective sigh of relief. "Boy, have you got the wrong address," Evvie informs them.

By now the group is beginning to look like a crowd. Hy and Lola, in matching robes, peer over the balcony right above our heads. Peripherally, I am aware of Harriet, tying her robe, as she hurries across the parking area. Tessie is not far behind her.

On this side of the building, Denny pokes his head out of his apartment. He looks disheveled, wild-eyed. . . . When he sees me looking at him, he turns and scurries back in. The expression on his face is pure fright. Poor thing. After having discovered both Selma's and Francie's bodies, I don't blame him for not wanting to be witness to yet another fearful situation.

All eyes turn as the door squeaks open to just the barest sliver. "Who is it?" Irving whispers.

"Open up. Police." Orange mustache is very forceful.

The door opens slightly farther. Irving is in his pajamas, his eyes sleep-encrusted and barely open, still not really awake. I sigh in relief. He looks at his visiting assemblage with alarm. "What is it? What's wrong?"

"We're here on a nine-one-one. Did you phone the police?"

"No," he says, still befuddled.

"I did," says a raspy voice behind him. The door is flung wide open.

How can I describe what Millie looks like? We all stare in awe. She can hardly move because she is wearing so many layers of clothes. I would guess she tried to put on everything in her closet and finally stopped when no more would fit. After the eye has absorbed that, the real horror seeps in. Millie has a huge pair of scissors in her hand which then makes you notice that most of her clothes have been mutilated. I hear someone moaning behind me.

Then there is the makeup. Millie's face is layered with cosmetics. And her hair! There are ribbons wildly tied to every possible strand. As I wonder where she got ribbons from, I realize they are the cut portions of her clothes.

Millie hits Irving on the back with her fist. "Rapist!" she shrieks. "Sodomist!" Where did she ever learn that word? "Assassin!" Irving freezes, mortified, standing there letting the blows fall on his bent shoulders.

I am vaguely aware of someone quite tall pushing his way forward through the growing crowd. But I can't take my eyes off Millie and Irving.

"She's ill," I finally say to the two policemen. "She doesn't know what she's doing."

"Irving wouldn't hurt a hair on her head," I hear Sophie say behind me.

"This is all a terrible mistake," Evvie says.

The short one speaks kindly to us. "Can you handle it from here, or do you need our help?"

"We'll manage," Ida says.

Millie's fit is already lessening. She now leans her head on Irving's shoulders, dropping the scissors as she does. He reaches behind and holds onto her. Taking charge, Ida hurries in to help him.

As Ida closes the door, the crowd begins

to disperse. The patrolmen walk to their cars, but stop to greet someone. "Detective," I hear one say, and I wheel about. And there's Morgan Langford.

I hurry over to him, Evvie following right after me, with Sophie clutching her arm.

"What are you doing here?" I ask.

He bends as if in greeting and smiles. "Mrs. Gold. Mrs. Markowitz."

"Such a good memory," Evvie marvels.

"Just call *me* Sophie," Sophie says, pushing her way in front of Evvie.

By now Harriet has joined us and she introduces herself as well. Evvie pointedly explains to Sophie and Harriet, "This is the cop we talked to, the one who wouldn't believe us when we told him about our murders."

"Enough, Ev," I say. "He's here now."

"I heard the police call," Detective Langford says. "I thought I'd check it out."

"Then you did believe me!" I am feeling vindicated.

"I didn't say that," he answers mildly, bursting my balloon.

"Morrie!" I hear an excited voice coming up behind me.

To my astonishment, there's Bella, obviously recovered from where we left her resting, hurrying over as fast as she is able.

And then, standing as high as she can on her toes (all four foot eleven of her), which still only brings her up to his belt buckle, she reaches up (as Langford leans way down to accommodate her) and gives Detective Morgan Langford a big, gushy kiss. Good thing he didn't pick Bella up, she could have gotten a nosebleed.

Morrie?

"You know him?" Evvie asks, beating me to it.

Bella grins. "This is Jack Langford's son from Phase Six. You remember, I was in Hadassah with his mother, Faye, until she passed, aleha ha-shalom, may she rest in peace."

Langford smiles way down at her. "So, you're one of these troublemakers, are you?" Bella looks confused.

Ida rushes up to join us, worried she is missing something. "Millie's back in bed," she reports. "And who is this tall, handsome stranger?" she gushes. Next she'll start to bat her eyes.

Evvie fills her in. Ida, being Ida, immediately leaps in where fools would fear to. "How dare you not believe Gladdy!"

"Hey, whoa. Easy, ladies."

"Lay off," I growl at Ida. Making an enemy of Detective Langford is not smart.

"Look," he says to me, "just find me a shred of something to go on, then I promise to get involved."

"Fair enough," I say, thinking guiltily of the cake crumbs I let get away.

"But, Mrs. Gold, be very careful. If there really is a killer, he's smart. He hasn't made any mistakes. That makes him very dangerous. Do not, I repeat, do anything foolish. If anything comes up, call me!"

Langford leaves and everyone voices an opinion.

"Gorgeous," breathes Ida.

"Ooh, so tall," says Sophie.

"Wow!" says Harriet. "Next time take *me* to the police station.

"I'm reserving judgment," says Evvie.

"Such a *shayner boychick,*" says Bella. "I know him since he was this tall." Her hand moves up and down trying to measure the man as boy. If we believe Bella, Lanky was six feet tall at two years old.

I smile. So, he's Jewish? Well, what do you know!

You've heard of the immovable object and the irresistible force. . . . Well, that's stubborn us seated in a row in the Weiss living room, facing even more stubborn Irving. After all the excitement, we went

157

back to check on Millie and found Irving in tears.

"Enough, Irving," I say. "No more discussion. Things have to change."

"I never heard her get up."

"It could have been worse," Evvie says, shuddering. I know she is thinking about the scissors.

"All right. I'll unplug the phone. I'll hide it before I go to sleep."

"She'll think of something else," Ida says. "Remember how she got out of the apartment that night and wandered down to Oakland Park."

"I put double locks on the doors. I hide the keys. She doesn't get out any more."

"No, she calls the cops in," says Bella.

"No more putting off, Irving," says Sophie. "If you're in a hole, you better start digging."

"It's time to get real help. Full-time help," I say.

"Around the clock," adds Evvie.

"No," Irving says. "I have no room for a stranger to sleep."

"You can't stay up all night and watch her."

"I'll nap during the day if someone is here."

"Irving," Ida says carefully. "You know

158

she'd be better off in managed care."

Irving puts his hands over his ears. "No! I won't hear this."

I get up. I feel so weary and so helpless. Through the bedroom door, I can hear Millie softly snoring. "All right, dear. We'll try hiring someone. But if that doesn't work . . ."

Irving turns his back on us.

We all tiptoe into the bedroom and take a look in at Millie. She is curled up with her thumb in her mouth. She looks almost young lying there, as though the Alzheimer's has made her face soften as she gives up her worldly cares. Her eyes open and she smiles slyly at us. Almost like she knows what havoc she causes and it tickles her.

We take turns kissing her good night. Suddenly Millie says pleadingly, "Where's Francie? Why doesn't she visit me anymore?"

My precocious granddaughter, Lindsay, when she was younger, mispronounced Millie's illness as old-timer's disease. As we watch Millie's suffering and try to remember happier days to offset our reality, maybe that's a gentler way to put it.

19

Gladdy's Gladiators

It is Sunday afternoon and we are sitting in the clubhouse, our chosen headquarters, strategizing. Now we are six. Since Harriet met that cute Morrie Langford the other night, she has begged to be allowed to join our merry band of private eyes. Ida, naturally, is not thrilled. She still hasn't forgiven Harriet, even though Harriet apologized for the bank incident.

We have a chalkboard and chairs. What more do we need? Except that the PA system keeps spewing out songs of the thirties and forties so loud we have to shout to be heard. The stereo music is supposed to play outside around the pool. Manuel, our groundskeeper, turns it on and up every morning before he heads out to do his landscaping chores. However, he didn't do it today. The music is inside and blaring at us instead. None of us knows how to figure out the complicated panel, so Evvie is on her hands and knees (not easy with arthritis) searching every wall,

160

looking for the plug to shut the whole thing off. With no success. Hopefully, Manuel will be back soon, or those of us who aren't deaf will be.

The first half hour is spent wasting time with general nonsense, all at the top of our lungs. Sophie suggests we give ourselves a name.

Ida informs her this isn't bingo, this is not a club, it's very serious business.

Bella, not hearing her, suggests "Gladdy's Girls."

Ida says, "No names, dammit!"

Sophie, always happy to spite Ida, says, "How about 'Gladdy *and* her Girls'?"

Bella says, "I like 'Gladdy's Gladiators' better."

"Where did you come up with that?" Evvie says from somewhere under one of those industrial-type tables.

"Gladiator is like Gladdy, and Florida has alligators."

"That has a certain logic, I think," says Harriet.

She's even beginning to make sense to me and that's scary. "Thanks for all the credit," I say. "But maybe we should get down to business."

"It'll look good on T-shirts," says Sophie.

"No T-shirts!" screeches Ida.

"With our names maybe on the pockets," says Bella.

"No, I don't like pockets," Sophie adds.

Ida picks up her copy of the Broward *Jewish Journal* and swats them both. "I'll give you a T-shirt, you meshugenehs! What has seventy-five balls and kills idiots like you!"

"I give up," Evvie says, getting up from the floor and brushing off her clothes. "I can't find the switch and somebody should really sweep better in here."

"Is it time to take our coffee break?" Bella asks.

"We haven't started yet," Ida says with disgust, "and she wants a break."

"I brought rugallah. Raspberry." She offers up a handful sweetly. This activates the bringing out of other plastic Baggies.

Another fifteen minutes are spent dividing up our coffee and tea and Danish and cinnamon rolls and all the other various goodies everyone brought, "so no one should go hungry until lunch in two hours."

As everyone eats and chats, I look at the dozens of group photos lining the walls. I can feel the spirits of twenty-five years surrounding me. This building could tell some stories!

Ida sees me glancing around.

"Ghosts," I say.

Ida nods. "So many people gone. But what good times."

"Tell me," Harriet says.

"Such parties," Ida says. "We'd use anything as an excuse to celebrate. Besides having all the real holidays and the Jewish holidays, there were birthdays and anniversaries and welcoming new arrivals and the births of grandchildren. . . ."

Evvie laughs. "Harriet, you should have seen us in the beginning, fresh from New York. The men had all retired and we came here planning to do nothing but have a good time."

Ida says, "Correction. Murray retired, I never got to retire. I still had to cook and clean and shop. . . ."

Evvie cuts her off. "At first, in winter, everybody wore their fur stoles and wool dresses. Until we wised up and dumped them for shorts and sundresses and muumuus."

"You shoulda seen the pool in those days, not like the ghost town it is today," Ida says. "Standing room only. Every lounge chair was spoken for. You would put a towel down to reserve your seat, turn your back, your lounge was gone. We had to bring chairs down from the apartments. All the kids came visiting at the beginning. With all the grandchildren. So much giggling and laughing . . ."

"Don't forget the weekends in Miami Beach," says Evvie.

"The New Year's Eve parties were the best," says Sophie. "Everybody got snockered and a little *farblondjet.*"

"Evvie jumped into the pool naked one year!" says Bella, giggling.

"I told you a thousand times, I was wearing a body stocking!"

"You couldn't tell from where I was standing, dearie," says Ida. "You shoulda seen the men's eyes bugging out."

"I got drunk. That was when I knew Joe was going to dump me for that blonde. He dumps me the week before New Year's Eve, that bastard."

"Everybody was alive and healthy then. . . ." says Bella. "My Abe looked like Valentino in a tux." The tears start to well up.

"Remember, Evvie, how your choir used to sing for us?" This from Sophie.

Evvie shakes her head. "Gone. All of them gone."

"Now the pool is always empty. None of the kids come down anymore," says Ida bitterly. "We're lucky if we even get a letter."

"We only got each other," Bella says.

Uh-oh, I think, this trip down memory lane is taking us up the garden path. I pick up a piece of chalk and tap it sharply on the board. "OK, my gladiators, enough with the food and gabbing. Time to get down to business. For Francie's and Selma's sakes." With the rustling of the cleaning up of packages and such, and a few last sniffles, they pull themselves back into the present.

I draw a diagram on the chalkboard dividing up the six buildings in our phase. Each building has thirty-six apartments, so that's a lot of ground to cover. I suggest we each pick a building and go by ourselves, but Bella says she's too scared to go alone, so she insists on going with Sophie and that's OK.

We agree on what to ask. We are looking for any suspicious behavior. Or any people seen hanging around who don't belong here. Especially anyone seen near Francie's or Selma's apartment on the days they died. A discussion evolves about what to tell people as to why we are asking.

I say we should tell the truth.

Sophie is afraid of scaring everybody.

And she has a point.

Ida believes in being devious. "Let's tell them we're thinking of hiring a security guard and we want to find out if we need one. Like if we've seen any weird characters around."

Harriet is afraid that will backfire and I think she is right.

Bella is nervous. "We can't just out-and-out say we think Selma and Francie were offed."

We all stare at her. She giggles. "I heard that on the TV last night."

Evvie, who loves lawyer shows, says it should be on a "need to know" basis. "We'll say we're doing a survey, but if they ask, we tell them more. If they don't, we don't."

Harriet agrees, but is dubious. "Evvie has a point, but suppose someone should want to get into it? What do we say is the motive? Who would kill them and why? And how? You think poison. How can we be sure? We have no proof. We have nothing. We don't want to make fools of ourselves."

Evvie speaks. "Listen, my sister Glad has intuition. I remember when we were kids, once she was out shopping with our mother and she insisted they rush home.

And there I was lying on the floor sick as a dog. Glad just knew!"

"That sounds more like ESP," says Ida.

"Whatever," says Evvie. "I trust it. And we have to start somewhere." Evvie puts her arm around me to show her support.

I thank her. "I'm hoping we'll get lucky and someone will have seen or heard something. For now, let's agree to try what we've been talking about and see how that works."

Evvie and I volunteer to start with the P building, her building.

Harriet volunteers to take Q, the building where we live.

Ida volunteers the R (for Rose) building around the corner where Francie lived. Since Selma lived in Q, these two are the key buildings, and we want to tackle them first.

Sophie and Bella will tackle S (Sweet William) across from where Francie lived. That way, we are dealing with all the apartments closest to the murder scenes.

"Do you think anybody will talk to us?" Bella worries.

"Everyone but crazy Kronk," says Ida. "She never opens the door to anyone."

"Probably Enya won't talk to us, either," says Harriet.

"Well, do the best you can," I say. "But I have to impress upon you very strongly what Detective Langford said. We have to be very careful. We are playing with matches here. Stay cool and calm and don't do anything foolish."

There is a knock on the door. I quickly turn the chalkboard around. It has a lot of our ideas written on it. Evvie goes to unlock the door. Hy is standing there in a bathing suit and a towel around his neck. Like some fierce bantam cock, he struts aggressively into the room.

"So, what's with the locked doors and secret meeting? You girls planning a revolution?"

"Yeah," says Ida, "we're planning to get rid of the few men who are left. Especially those who tell stupid jokes."

"Geez," he shouts, "it's loud in here. Why don't you turn down the hi-fi?"

"Because we don't know how to work the PA, Mr. Know-it-all," says Evvie.

Hy looks around the room briefly, then walks over to the panel, selects a switch, and turns it to Off. There is silence. Glorious silence. He shrugs and starts singing, "Oh, it's nice to have a man around the house. . . ." wiggling his butt as he does.

168

"Didja hear the news this morning?" Hy asks.

"No," we chorus. "And not interested."

"CNN announced that senior citizens are the leading carriers of aids."

"What!" Ida hollers. "You nutcase!"

"Yup. Carriers of hearing aids, Band-Aids, Rolaids, walking aids, medical aids, government aids, and especially monetary aids to their children!"

Evvie picks up a volleyball and throws it at him. "Get out, you *vantz* . . . you bed-bug, you!"

He grins, covering his head with his arms. "I'm going, I'm going." He runs out the door. A moment later he's back. "I forgot. I came to deliver a message. Glad and Evvie are wanted at Irving's. He's interviewing and needs your help. Hey, so don't kill the messenger!"

Hy starts out the door again.

"Hey, Hy," Evvie calls, "you make out your will yet?"

He gives her a dirty look. "None of your business, yenta."

"Yeah, right, we know — you're not going."

"I'd be glad to help you go," says Ida maliciously, lifting up a heavy ashtray.

Sophie joins in. "You're so ugly now, I

hate to think what you'll look like when you're a hundred and fifty."

"Yeah, you and Mel Brooks, the thousand-year-old man," says Evvie nastily.

Hy gives us all the finger and walks out again. Everybody laughs.

I quickly erase the board. "Meeting adjourned," I say as Evvie and I hurry to the door.

20

Job Descriptions

We can see them as far away as the path to the pool. A sizeable group of women milling about the Weiss apartment. The ad we wrote must have been better than I thought, or a lot of people need work. Even from where we are, I can see they are quite an assortment of ages. Different heights. Different skin tones. The few seats on the bench are taken; the others either stand or lean against the wall. Most of them carry worn purses, shopping bags, or lunch sacks.

We hear shouting from inside the apartment and we quicken our pace.

In the living room, three people sit rigidly, not looking at one another. Irving is sitting ramrod-straight on a dining room chair, staring into space, his face red from anxiety. A thin woman who looks fortyish also sits on a dining room chair. She is speaking very gently to Millie, who is on the couch, her fingers tearing away at a bit of thread on the hem of her sundress and her head turned toward the window. Millie is shouting, "No, no, go away. I hate you."

The woman must be from Haiti. She speaks in that wonderful lilting way, trying to calm Millie.

"But I don't hate you, hon. Not at all. You and me, we could be friends."

"Never," screams Millie. "You make the children angry."

The woman smiles at us when we come in. "I must have said something to anger her, but I don't know what."

"It's just her sickness," Evvie says.

"Maybe she'll get used to me?"

"No. No — get out." Millie, with little strength, manages to pick up a pillow and weakly throws it at the woman. The woman gets up.

"I think maybe she won't," she says, and starts out. "Good luck to you, Mr. Weiss."

Irving can't speak so we say his good-byes for him.

"What's going on out there?" I ask. "Didn't you set different appointment times when they called?"

Irving shrugs. "I just said come."

Millie tosses another pillow to protest this conversation.

"I thought maybe she'd watch TV in the sunroom . . ." Again he shrugs helplessly.

Millie cackles. "Trying to put one over

me, heh, old man? Millie is too fast for the old man."

"This won't work," he says. "Tell them to go home."

We attempt to get Millie to go into the bedroom to take a nap, but she sits as if glued to the couch. She knows what's going on and no one is going to get any job without her approval. My heart sinks. She isn't going to approve of anyone.

The afternoon drags on with painful slowness. One after another the women come in, give their resumes, and try to enchant the little princess who behaves more like the wicked queen. Haughtily the petitioners are each and every one rejected. The "children" whisper in Millie's ear, goading her into shamefully cruel comments.

Evvie and I exchange glances. We are getting nowhere, fast. Irving left us six women ago to take a nap. "You pick," he said, turning the thankless job over to us.

Finally, the last woman is gone. Millie has defeated us. She seems to be dozing on the couch by now.

Evvie whispers to me. "Next time we do this upstairs."

I start gathering up the paper cups from the many coffee and water offerings and bring them into the kitchen. Evvie goes off to the bathroom.

I think back on that god-awful day when we all faced Millie's doctor together and heard for the first time what we suspected anyway. Millie started to tell the doctor how terrified she was of the possibility of having Alzheimer's. This doctor, who, I suspect, along with too many others, came down to Florida to suck the money out of the elderly, didn't even bother to look at her. "What are you worried about, lady? It takes about ten years for Alzheimer's to kill you. You'll be dead long before that, anyway."

We were all too shocked to say anything.

Later, I cursed him and hoped *he'd* die horribly and soon.

I'm pulled out of my reverie. "Come in, come in," says a high, pleasant voice. "Don't be a stranger." I turn, startled to see Millie through the kitchen pass-through window, beckoning to someone at the front door. I turn again and there is a very young Hispanic woman standing uncertainly on the threshold.

Millie walks to her with ease and graciously reaches out to shake hands. The princess has returned. The young woman smiles a wide, gold-toothed, lopsided grin.

Millie pulls her into the living room and whirls her around. Then she proceeds to do a right-on-target parody of husband and two closest friends. Evvie returns to my side and we both watch this bizarre scene. Millie has our voices down pat.

"And my dear, do you have experience? No, never mind, I don't care about that. The important thing is can you dance?"

The woman, by now introduced as Yolanda Diaz, is enchanted by Millie and says, pretending insult, *"Qué mujer de Guadalajara no puede bailer?"*

"*La rumba?* Cha-cha? Lambada? Tango?" asks this expert of the salsa scene.

"Naturalmente," says Yolanda.

"Perfecto," says Millie, who has never before uttered a word in Spanish. With that, she drags Yolanda by the hand over to the ancient hi-fi, which hasn't been used since Millie took sick years ago. She tosses records every which way until she comes up with an old Pérez Prado album. Millie pulls it out of its sleeve, dusts it off by blowing on it and unerringly manages to get it onto the record player.

Evvie and I are beyond dumbfounded.

And then, there they are, the usually catatonic eighty-year-old woman doing a mean rumba with this very young, puzzled, yet willing applicant, to "Cherry Pink and Apple Blossom White."

Irving comes out of the bedroom in his stocking feet, rubbing the sleep from his eyes. "What's this racket?" he asks.

"Irv, come meet Yolanda," Evvie says, smiling. "We just hired her." With that, Millie collapses to the floor and falls asleep.

21

Kronk Strikes Again

Yolanda — the Spanish dancer, as Irving refers to her — seems to be working out. Sort of. Millie is thrilled with her. Irving is less than thrilled. He is finding all kinds of things to nitpick about. Too many taco-and-refried-bean dinners instead of his favorite cholesterol killers, steak and potatoes. Too much hot salsa in everything. Suddenly Millie, who never ate Hispanic food in her life, is scarfing down any food whose name has an *a* or *o* at the end of it. Irving now lives on Tums. I try to calm him, promising I will give Yolanda a weekly menu to follow. "But, isn't it worth it? Millie is better than she's been in a long time."

"Ulcers, I'm getting," Irving whines.

He grudgingly agrees, but he doesn't understand why he is upset. Suddenly Yolanda is telling him to go outside and get some air and smoke his cigars, or go play cards, she'll watch Millie. So used to being tense every moment of every day, how can he let down his guard?

We all like Yolanda. She smiles a lot and hums when she works. And takes time to talk to Millie. She doesn't speak much English, so her communication skills are part Spanish, part English, part pointing, and part miming. Millie thinks this is all being done to entertain her. Yolanda makes her laugh. We haven't heard Millie laugh in a long time. Millie was right to make her own choice.

The Gladiators are hard at work. Carrying their newly bought clipboards with attached pens, they are canvassing the buildings. Dutifully making notes when people aren't home, so they'll remember to call back. In protest, because we wouldn't let them have T-shirts, Sophie and Bella are wearing their bingo shirts.

So much for the lecture on keeping cool. Pandemonium has struck. Everyone wants to know everything. The suggestion of two murders churns up all the neighbors, either with fear or excitement, and everyone is comparing birthdays, wondering who will be next — even though we try to assure them that probably no one will be next. I think we are spreading hysteria more than gathering information. Eileen O'Connor in the R building is having a birthday next week. She has suddenly decided to leave tomorrow for a visit to her sister in Boca Raton. She has not made any plans for returning.

Esther Feder's birthday is in two weeks. She has been quoted as saying, "I have only one word to say to that killer — he better not mess with me!"

More and more, I feel guilt-ridden about having opened this Pandora's box. We haven't seen this much excitement since the uproarious Florida election of 2000.

"Who could forget?" Ida comments. "It took thirty-seven days! We got a president, and by then, who cared?"

Sophie scowls. "They didn't have to insult us in the newspapers." She mimics: "If you think we can't vote, wait 'til you see us *drive!*"

"I never did get what 'electile dysfunction' means." Bella says, mutilating the pronunciation.

Evvie puts an arm around her. "Don't even ask!"

I am sitting in the kitchen doing my least favorite chore — the monthly bills — before going outside for our morning workout. It already feels like another scorcher. Suddenly I hear a piercing shriek and my heart starts pounding. I remember Detective Langford's warning. Has our snooping forced the killer to strike again? Running out onto the walkway I see Ida, first one out, leaning over the rail and pointing, her hand shaking. Following its direction, I see my car. Its windows are covered in soap.

. As Ida and I hurry downstairs, the other girls are not far behind us.

"That damned crazy Kronk!" swears Evvie.

I sigh. I guess it was finally my turn.

We stare at the words that are soaped on the windshield. *You know. I know two.*

"I'll get water and a rag," Sophie volunteers, hurrying back to the elevator.

"That miserable pain in the neck. When will we ever get rid of her?!" Evvie asks angrily. "I'm taking it up at the next board meeting again. Enough is enough!"

"Oh, hell." The others react to the tone of my voice. I am looking down at my front right tire. It's been slashed. Too late, I remember needing to replace the faulty spare.

"What does she mean?" Ida says, trying to decipher this latest Kronk poetry-in-code. " 'You know'? Know what?"

Sophie adds, "Maybe crazy Kronk's really the killer and she's confessing. Like 'I killed two.' "

"How come no one ever sees her!" Bella cries, stamping her feet in frustration.

When the tow truck arrives, I convince the girls that since there is only room for one person alongside the driver, I'll go alone. I decide that since I'm taking the car in, besides buying a new tire, I might as well get it lubed and attend to all the other things I've neglected to fix. Maybe I'll even splurge and detail it.

"Who did that to your windows?" the driver asks after practically ripping my arms out of their sockets as he pulls me up into the seat next to him.

"It's a very long story," I tell him.

The girls wave as we head out.

In all the excitement I didn't give any thought to the meaning of Greta's scribblings on my car. I would be very sorry later.

22

Ye Olde Curiosity Shoppe

The repair department said give them a couple of hours. Usually I have a book in the trunk. All I need is a coffee shop and the time will fly by. Hmm. No book. I guess I forgot to leave one.

So, I decide to walk. Even though this is an industrial area, maybe I'll find something of interest. I find myself relaxing. A few hours to myself. What a luxury. To my surprise, I see a bookstore sign up ahead and that gets my attention.

A huge red banner announces the Grand Opening Today: J. Marley's For Mysteries. The proclamation under it defiantly states "Who's afraid of Barnes & Noble?" I move closer to read all the captivating information splashed across the window in Day-Glo paints. Party! Free! Exciting Panel Discussion! Special Famous Mystery Guests! Come as your favorite sleuth! And indeed, cheerful participants are crowding in wearing a wide array of costumes. Apparently I'm just in time and I join the throng.

A jovial and diminutive gent, dressed in a costume right out of a Dickens novel and wearing a name tag — J. Marley, Proprietor — stands at the doorway waving us in.

Once inside, I admire this charming little shop, done up as a classic Victorian English gentleman's library with wonderfully uncomfortable horsehair sofas and high-backed wing chairs slipcovered with hunting scenes. A drop-leaf oak side table set up in front of the small gaslit fireplace holds the makings of a proper English tea — crumpets, cucumber sandwiches, scones, trifle — all of it looking delicious. I look closer. Alas, not real.

Seats are being set up for the panel discussion in a large adjoining conference room and I am lucky to get one of the last chairs. There is much friendly banter as strangers get acquainted by guessing one another's identities. I sigh happily. How lucky to have accidentally found this place. I am prepared to have a very good time.

J. Marley moves up to the front podium. He makes a delightful welcoming speech which not only lauds his own bravery for opening up an independent shop, but also the courage of those who come here willing to pay retail! "Those megawarehouses that call themselves bookstores don't scare me. True book lovers will gather where others of their ilk assemble, and you here today are proof of that." This gets a round of applause. He grins mischievously. "I do hope you're not only here for the free punch and entertainment. You *will* buy something."

Marley now turns to the group seated onstage. "Today's guest speakers, the world's greatest detectives, will address the intriguing subject of 'How To Solve A Murder.' And allow me to admit what trouble it was getting them here, since they all exist only in the febrile imaginations of some of the greatest mystery writers of all time."

There is a nice round of applause.

"How fortunate I was to find this amazing group of players who swear they are being channeled by their literary originals."

Marley indicates a delicate elderly lady in a modest print dress and very sensible black laced shoes, who all the while has been attending to her knitting. With a flourish he introduces, "Miss Jane Marple!"

Miss Marple smiles primly. "I bring you a message of regards from St. Mary Mead."

"And now, Monsieur Hercule Poirot," says Marley with vivacity.

Poirot stands up, tips his bowler and bows stiffly. "*Bonjour.* I, too, wish to extend salutations. From Hastings and, of course, Miss Lemon."

Miss Lucy Pym is next and she is all atwitter. "Oh, I do appreciate the applause. It's because of my new book, isn't it? You readers do want some new thing, don't you?" With that she quickly sits back down, blushing.

"Mr. Sherlock Holmes."

"Yes, yes," hc says intolerantly, "if we must exchange these tiresome greetings, then I shall, of coursc, mention Dr. Watson, who even as we speak is chasing my deerstalker hat which the winds blew from my head." This brings much laughter and Holmes sneers nicely at it.

"Last, but not least, Lord Peter Wimsey."

Lord Peter wipes his monocle, then smiles. "Regards, of course, from her ladyship, the former Harriet Vane. And Bunter would be sorely tried if I neglected to mention him. A pleasure to be here in the Colonies again."

The discussion begins with amusing questions from the floor, answered wittily by the sleuths. But I hear nothing because of the roaring in my ears as I listen to person after person chat about murder.

A pathetically weak voice calls out, "I have a question."

To my astonishment, I am rising, and although I don't recall doing it, I am the one who spoke. I stand transfixed. What am I doing? All eyes are on me. I can hear my own breathing, and suddenly, I blurt out: "I'm investigating a *real* murder! Two murders, actually. And I desperately need help!"

The audience holds its silence for a moment before bursting into appreciative applause. Marley, chortling, says, "And what a clever opening gambit from the lady sitting next to Charlie Chan."

It's as if everything that has been troubling me has surfaced without my permission. To my horror, I am the center of attention.

Miss Pym pipes up. "Well, best left to the police, dear, I always say."

"But they don't believe me. And I think the murderer lives among us."

"Madam. Don't let's shilly-shally here. Where is your proof?" Holmes says with disdain.

"That's just it. I don't have any."

"Dastardly clever, the killer, eh, what?" comments Lord Peter.

"Yes. He hasn't made any mistakes yet."

"He will eventually. They all do," says Miss Marple sagely, not even missing a stitch.

"You must use the little gray cells, Madame, and all will be revealed." Hercule Poirot plays with his thin, waxed mustache.

"Suspects. Who are the suspects? Do not waste our time with frivolity!" Holmes bullies me.

"Well, there's Denny, our handyman . . ." I say hesitantly.

There is a burst of rude laughter from both audience and panel.

"Yeah, and he lives in the Bates Motel!" screams someone from the audience.

"And his dead mother done it," howls another.

"You better not take a shower, lady," shouts another.

"Order. Order," says Marley, clapping his hands to calm the waves of laughter.

Holmes tamps down the tobacco in his pipe, chortling. "He's as much a cliché as the 'butler who done it.' "

I try to keep my voice steady. "There's also the real-estate man who goes after the property of the deceased."

Miss Marple tut-tuts. "Quite nearly as bad as the janitor person."

"Is there a redheaded man on a bicycle?" asks Holmes snidely.

"No."

"Perhaps a vicar who's had a bit too much port?" asks Miss Marple.

"Of course not."

"A headmaster who has absconded with school funds?" asks Miss Pym.

"No. No. No."

"I say — surely the bloke left a weapon? A croquet mallet? A spade? A lead cosh?" Lord Peter winks at me.

Now everybody is hooting with appreciation for what they think is my impassioned playacting.

I stand up, furious. "Stop it. This is real!"

"But *they* aren't," snickers someone in the audience.

"But did the dog bark?" adds another wag in the crowd.

I can't believe it; I'm actually starting to cry.

Marley wipes his tears, too — of laughter. However, he decides that I have taken up enough of the panel's time. He interrupts, making an assumption. "Well, good luck with your novel, lady. Any other questions?"

I am briefly applauded and then forgotten. The panel continues on.

I look around befuddled. I run out of the conference room and back into the quiet library section and throw myself down into one of the armchairs.

Shaking and crying, I just sit there unable to move. Whatever got into me to do that!

I am handed a handkerchief. I look up to see a tall man peering down at me. He's in his seventies, with a full head of hair, the colors of iron and steel, and a lovely smile.

"I believed you," he says.

"Why? No one else did!"

I use his handkerchief gratefully.

"May I?" he asks indicating the chair next to me.

He has a gentle, deep voice with just the faintest touch of an English accent. Still snuffling, I nod.

"I'm sorry they upset you," he says. "But I don't think they were making fun of you."

"I know. It was all a game and I was spoiling it." I look up into his eyes. Such twinkling blue eyes. "What am I going to do about my murders? Someone has to find the killer."

He takes my hands and holds them gently. "If I were a mystery writer, I'd suggest that you look for someone who is behaving out of character. Who is behaving in a way that is alien to his or her personality?"

The man smiles at me, and for a moment I think I know him. "Thank you," I whisper gratefully.

"And don't forget," he says, now grinning, "the killer is always the one least suspected. As Holmes would say, 'It's elementary.' "

I get up, and return his handkerchief, then head for the door.

"Gladdy?" the velvety voice calls after me.

I turn, startled. How does he know my name?

"It is Gladdy Gold, I presume? May I buy you a cup of coffee?"

23

Lust in the Heat

"Don't you just love the name Fudd-ruckers?" I say.

"Works for me," says my mystery man.

We have just been seated in this overly bright popular hamburger hangout and the stranger has promised he'll tell all once we get our coffee. We drove around in his spiffy 1985 Cadillac 'til we found this place, and all the while he remained stoically quiet. I can hardly wait.

He smiles benignly at me as I study him while pretending to read the menu.

Dignified comes to mind. Built like a teddy bear, the way I like them. What *am* I thinking? Who *is* he and why am I blathering on like this? I feel rattled, and skittish.

The coffee is served by someone who looks young enough to be my great-granddaughter. Good, I think, now we can get started.

"Do I know you?" I decide to get the old ball rolling. And he does look familiar.

He takes a sip of his coffee. "We met briefly fourteen years ago. At a New Year's Eve party at Lanai Gardens. We were all standing around the pool in Phase Five drinking the obligatory inexpensive champagne in paper cups."

"Fourteen years ago and not since?"

"Unfortunately, no. But under the circumstances . . ."

Unfortunately? Interesting, that. Now I'm beginning to realize I am unconsciously mimicking his British accent. "Should I apologize for not remembering you?"

"Nonsense. I was just one in a dreadfully large group of people, but you — you were unique. You wore this lovely pink flowery dress and a matching hat with ribbons. Roses, I believe. I remember thinking you looked simply fetching."

"Did your wife mind that you thought me fetching?" I might have been fetching then, but I am fishing now.

He smiles. "I belong to the Jimmy Carter school of adultery. I lust only in my heart. And rarely. You were one of those rare occasions. You were sitting alone on a bench, sipping your bubbly and looking rather pensive. There was an aura about you. . . ."

With a sharp pain, I remember now. It wasn't me being pensive it was me responding to bone-chilling sadness. It was the anniversary of my husband, Jack's, death. No matter how many years had gone by, that date would always remain devastating for me. I would never get over it. How could I? Now here I was, uprooted, trying to get through my first New Year's Eve in a place far from home. I felt totally lost and adrift.

I had been at loose ends when Evvie had called me from Florida, begging me to fly down from New York and stay with her. Joe had left her and she was threatening suicide. I forced myself to stop thinking about myself and focus on her. Came down for a visit and never left. But that night was hell.

"Jack," I murmur aloud. Moaning in memory of my beloved. It's been so long since I've allowed myself to think of him.

"So, you do remember," he says, delighted.

"What?" I am having trouble pulling myself back into the present. "What did you say?"

"I never thought you'd remember my name. It was long ago and our meeting so brief. I'm awfully flattered. Funny we should meet like this. Just the other day, my son Morrie happened to mention your name. You know, the police officer?"

I quickly put it together. "Your name is Jack," I say, looking closer at this tall, tall man. "Of course. Jack Langford." The recently widowed Jack Langford, or so I'd heard. But where? And from whom? The final click. Bella. Who knew his wife in Hadassah.

He almost blushes. He's that pleased.

He reaches his hand out across the table and we shake formally.

"It's hard to believe, isn't it," Jack Langford says, "that we've lived in the same place fourteen or so years and have never occasioned upon each other."

"Well . . . Phase Two and Phase Six . . . We *are* separated by Three, Four, and Five." I sound positively idiotic.

"And speaking of Phase Two, that which you implied in the bookstore — your friends were murdered?"

We were on safer ground than talking about early lust. If safer is the right word when dealing with murder. "I'm afraid so."

"And Morrie doesn't believe you?"

I quickly come to his son's defense. "I have no way to prove my suspicions. It sounded far-fetched to him."

"He always was stubborn. Takes after his father."

"Well, you gave me good advice. I'm going to look at everybody and see who's behaving differently."

Jack senses that he is upsetting me and changes the subject. He begins to ask me all sorts of lovely questions about myself, and I have a lot to ask him, too.

We have all these years of catching up to do and we talk and talk until I finally realize just how long I've been away. The girls must be worried.

Even my car feels better after a day away from — dare I admit it? — the girls. The new tire makes me feel like I'm driving on air. C'mon, who's kidding whom?

And just because Jack Langford said hello. No, he didn't *just* say hello; he said he lusted after me. Had been attracted to me. Intimating that if he hadn't had a wife, he would have made a pass. Never mind it was fourteen years ago. Very flattering. Alas, wasted, since I never even knew it. And I was a mere sixty-one then. Truth? When's the last time *any* man looked at me? As a woman. At what age did I become invisible? I think this is one of the hardest things to deal with when getting old. Men no longer look. Not in that same way. That sly I-can't-wait-to-get-into-your-pants look. Gone forever. I'll never again feel that extraordinary wild passion of reckless youth. That's the true unfairness of age. No matter how old, you still remember it, but you can't have it anymore. Youth belongs to the young. And what a waste. They don't appreciate how tenuous is this gift, and how carelessly they abuse it.

So, I'm attracted to someone! I thought I packed that emotion away in mothballs with my winter coats.

I think about what Jack said to me when he dropped me off at the garage. "After all, I might have been sprightly back then, but now I'm just an elderly gentleman. Surely you couldn't be interested?"

"And what am I — a spring chicken?" That was the pathetic retort I was able to come up with to hide my absolute amazement. I wanted to jump up and down and say you bet I'm interested, you cuddly darling, you. But sanity prevailed. Good breeding prevailed.

"Call me!" I shouted after him as he drove away. I could see him grinning as he *vroomed* off like a teenager in a hot rod.

"You'd be proud of me and Harriet. We

partnered and together we came up with our first clue." Evvie is jabbering at me even before I get out of my car.

"Really? Sounds like you girls were busy."

"We talked to Tessie and she remembered something she found in Selma's apartment when she cleaned up."

"This could be important!"

"She said she found a little piece of wrapper stuck to the bottom of the dining room chair. She recognized it as a piece of bag the Meals on Wheels people use to deliver. She didn't think anything of it at the time. But, now she wondered. She couldn't remember Selma ever being a customer of Meals."

This was something real. At last. "Then we've got to call them! They'd have a record of the food going out on that date and who delivered it to her."

"Way ahead of you, sis. Harriet called. Nobody remembered anything."

I'm disappointed. But it would explain why Selma would open her door. The murderer must have knocked and offered her a delicious meal. I was beginning to see a pattern. Someone offered Selma food. Selma, who dearly loved to eat. Someone offered Francie chocolate cake. Someone

197

who knew she loved chocolate. This someone knows us very well. I shiver as if he just walked over my grave.

And what did Greta's soaped message on my car mean, if anything at all? Or were they just the ravings of a poor lost soul?

At dinner I tell the girls about the unusual party at the bookstore. But I do not say one word about Jack Langford.

24

Death by Dumpster

The first blazing rays of Florida sun were about to light up the sky. But in those few moments while Dawn played coy, a hand scribbled erratically in a whitewash paint: I SAW YOU KILL 2 — YOU DEVIL YOU.

Anxiously, Greta Kronk skittered away from the door, the small paint can wobbling from her bony wrist. Her heart was pounding because she knew what a terrible chance she had taken. She pushed her wild black hair back into the fiercely colored magenta scarf that encircled her face, and pulled her voluminous lavender dancing skirts and petticoats around her knees. Were it not for her deceptive clothes, Greta would look like the emaciated wraith she was. She glanced up at the sky and feared she had waited too long, that the light would betray her.

Holding her breath, she moved as quickly as the clumsy skirts allowed her, around the corner to the far end of Q building. Again she looked around. It was all right. This was a wall without windows. She could breathe. Quickly she hid the paint can deep in the first Dumpster. Now she would attend to her regular early morning business — searching all the Dumpsters for treasures. She opened her gunny sack, eager to plunder the riches this morning's trash would provide. The first thing she found was a twisted soup strainer. Good, she thought, this I can use.

The killer opened the door of the apartment. With a few quick strokes of a rag, the damning words were washed away. The killer also looked around, not really concerned. It was still much too early for anyone to be up.

Greta was so pleased with her take — a slightly bent set of plastic dinnerware and a wonderful black wig — that she wasn't aware she was no longer alone.

She gasped as the killer loomed over her.

"What you want?" she said, trying not to show her fear. "This my stuff, get your own fluff." Talking was hard for her. It had been so long since she had spoken to anyone.

"I don't want your stuff, you fool —"

"Then go 'way. Don't want play."

"It's not nice to paint on people's doors."

Greta stared, worried, because the killer's hands were hidden.

"I ain't got paint. . . ." But her eyes betrayed her as she instinctively looked toward the Dumpster where she had hidden the can.

"Wanna see what's behind my back?" The hands came out with nothing in them. Greta looked confused. Her eyesight was not good. She didn't notice the thin, colorless latex gloves.

"What did you see, Greta? Tell me!"

Greta moved backwards, but the killer kept pace. Her eyes looked into eyes that showed no sympathy. She knew she was doomed.

"You know what you're gonna see now?" The killer pulled her by her hair and dragged her back to the Dumpster. Greta tried to run, but her feet were pedaling in air.

"I don't tell . . . I not told. I not be so bold. . . ." she said, gasping.

"Bad news, Greta. No pot roast for you. No chocolate cake. You love garbage, now eat your last meal!"

The killer pulled a rancid onion from the trash can and forced it down her throat. "You like your salad? Sorry, no dressing."

Greta gagged, and the food was retched out, but the killer pushed it in again and held her mouth shut until it went down. "Ready for your main course?" Her eyes widened and teared as horrible remnants of foul-smelling food were shoved into her mouth. In her terror, she was not aware of the powdery substance that was forced in along with a slimy strand of what had once been spinach.

For a few more minutes she coughed and dry-heaved. Finally, she stopped struggling — paralysis began to set in. Her body sank to the ground, as the voluminous skirts cushioned her.

The killer took a moment to retrieve the paint can from where Greta had hidden it. At the corner of the building the killer turned and smiled.

"Too bad, Greta, you're about to miss your greatest literary masterpiece."

Greta's last thought before she lost consciousness was of a doll she had had as a child in the old country. A gypsy dancer she could gently fold up into its beautiful gown. Its eyes would close and the doll would go to sleep. She, too, would now go to sleep at last. She hoped Armand would be waiting for her and would forgive her for taking so long.

25

Sing Gypsy, Cry Gypsy, Die Gypsy

I come home from my early dentist appointment and I know immediately something is wrong. Too many people are hovering about outside, most still in robes, moving every which way. An ambulance and a police car are parked near the side of my building. Oh, God, I think hysterically, who is it now?

I don't stop to ask. I head where the flashing red lights beckon.

The girls are there. Quickly I count them off. Bella. Sophie. Ida. Where's Evvie? Oh, no, where — ? There she is, thank God. Standing with Harriet and Esther, who is seated in her wheelchair. Hy and Lola stand next to them, clutching one another for support.

The girls see me as I approach and they all grab at me, crying, all talking at once.

From Ida: "Hy went out to the Dumpster —"

Then Bella: "He was schlepping this big carton from a new TV, though I don't know what was wrong with the old one —"

And Sophie interrupting her. "He saw a nightmare in the daytime and then he ran around the corner yelling —"

I am trying to see who the paramedics are bending over, but I can't tell who it is.

"This all happened a couple of minutes ago," Evvie tells me.

"We only just came downstairs," Sophie adds.

"Tell me already!" I can't stand it. "Who is it?"

"The Kronk!" they say in unison.

"Greta?" I ask incredulously. I turn to Hy. "Tell me what you saw!"

He shrugs. Clears his throat. Hitches up his inevitably loud-patterned shorts. Clearly he's told his tale a few times already. "First I don't see nothing. The TV box is bulky and I can hardly see my way around it. I'm just about to lay it down and start to stomp on it so it'll fit in the Dumpster and I see a bunch of what looks like colored rags. Then I go closer and it's a body laying inside of them rags. I don't even recognize her. It's maybe five years since I even laid eyes on her."

Hy, always loving the spotlight, is determined to squeeze out every ounce of drama. And Lola, truly in shock, for once is not interrupting him. "At first I think it's a stranger, but, no, she looks familiar. I know it's nobody else, because everybody else I would recognize, so logic tells me it's Greta Kronk. All I know for sure, she doesn't look sick. She looks dead. So I run for somebody to call the nine-one-one."

His audience is rapt. Hy always did know how to tell a story. But this one was no joke.

"Could you tell what killed her?" I ask.

"I don't see no blood, so I figure she died of old age, or from eating that putrid garbage. Her mouth was full of that crap."

Everyone responds with horror, making gagging and gasping noises. Bella, turning pale, leans against the wall that separates us from Phase Three, for support.

A policeman comes toward us, his notebook at the ready. It's orange mustache again. I remember him from the infamous night Millie called 911. "Does Mrs. Kronk have any relatives?"

"Nobody," we all chorus.

"Do *you* know what killed her, Officer?" I have to ask.

He shakes his head. "Maybe her heart gave out. Looks like she just keeled over."

I move closer and watch as the ambulance attendants lift her onto the gurney. It's the first time any of us have seen Greta in years. She looks so thin. She must have been starving herself. I remember the dress she's wearing. It was the gypsy costume she wore when she gave dancing lessons that one year and very few people showed up. In those days, she was buxom and she filled out that dress pretty good. This body lying here is like a skeleton. Now I can see Greta's face clearly, and I jump back, startled. Her face! My God, her face! She looks terrified. As if something frightened her to death.

Sol Spankowitz ambles over. "Did you see what she wrote?"

I stare at him, puzzled.

"That crazy broad wrote another poem. On her own door. Like she wrote it to put on her gravestone. Weird. Come take a look."

The girls and I follow Sol around the corner, and now I realize what people were staring at when I arrived: Greta's front door on the third floor of P building.

"What does it say?" Bella asks tugging at me.

"I don't know. It's hard to read from down here."

Mary and John Mueller, her neighbors, are up there with a few other people from the building. They hear me and they all look down from the balcony. John calls to us. "It says, 'Get fed. Get dead.'" His voice is bitter. "Well, that's the last nasty poem *she'll* ever write."

His wife, Mary, turns away, embarrassed. Who can forget the cheap shot Greta took at John's masculinity?

We finally end up in Evvie's apartment, drinking tea. Needless to say, this is accompanied by a plate full of cheese Danish. As is typical, we are seated at the dining table in our usual card-playing seats. Harriet has pulled up an extra chair to join us.

I sigh. "Now I'll never get a chance to ask her why she wrote what she did on my car."

"Poor, sad lady," Harriet says as she reaches for another pastry. "What a way to die. All alone like that."

"And we were trying to get her thrown out." Bella sighs. "I feel so guilty."

Sophie giggles behind her hand. "Look at you," she says pointing at Harriet. "You're eating all the Danish."

Harriet laughs nervously. "Just neurotic

eating," she explains. "From all the excitement. I better start working out at the gym more often. By the way, did I tell you I'm starting my vacation? Maybe I better spend it exercising."

Considering what good condition her body is in, she doesn't have to worry about working it off. We should be in such good shape.

"How many heart attacks are we gonna have around here?" Sophie demands to know.

"*Another* heart attack?" I ask pointedly.

Evvie looks at me. "*Another* coincidence?" We exchange glances. She knows what I am thinking.

"That was only a guess the officer made. He couldn't know for sure," says Ida. "Maybe she's been sick for who knows how long and she just happened to die right then and there."

"What are you saying, Glad?" Harriet asks.

"Now a third woman dies suddenly for no apparent reason? All having just eaten food that came to them oddly?"

"Garbage is eating?" sniffs Sophie.

Bella jumps up, spilling her tea on her lap. "You think she was poisoned, too!"

"You are turning into a one-track train," says Sophie.

"How could that be?" Ida asks me. "How could the killer know she was going to eat garbage?"

"You mean he had to put poison in all the garbage cans?" Bella surmises.

"Every day until she picks the right can to eat out of? Nonsense!" Ida shakes her head vehemently.

"No," I say, grossing myself out even as I suggest it, "but what if he forces the poisoned food down her throat?"

"How could he make her eat it?" Sophie says. "I, personally, would clamp my mouth shut."

"I wish you would," says Ida, glaring at her.

"A gun. He had a gun! Oy, a gun in Lanai Gardens. That I should live to see the day!" Bella is getting hysterical.

"Bella, dear. He didn't need a gun. She was undernourished and very weak. It wouldn't take much to overwhelm her," I say quietly.

"Why would anyone want to kill that poor pathetic creature?" Harriet asks.

Bella asks shrilly, "Was it her birthday? Does anybody know?"

"I don't think so," Evvie says, musing. "April comes to mind."

Sophie gets up and starts pacing,

wringing her hands as she does. "You wanna know why!!! I'll tell you why! Because he's a serial killer, that's why. He's gonna kill us all before he's through! Eating us to death with our favorite food!"

Bella fans herself furiously with a paper napkin. "Garbage was her favorite food?"

"Please, everybody calm down," I say.

"Yeah," says Evvie, "before we all really get heart attacks."

Bella is shaking her head agitatedly.

"What?!" Ida demands.

"I'll never eat gefilte fish again," Bella says wistfully of her favorite food.

"Fool!" Ida mutters under her breath.

26

Death of a Poet

It's mid-afternoon and Lanai Gardens is at rest. Nap time. *La siesta.*

I'm too overwrought to sleep. I sneak out of the apartment building under cover of silence.

Now that Kronk is gone, Marion Martini, who has been hiding her car around the corner from U building, has driven it back. She's been secreting it there since the night the Kronk smeared raspberry juice all over her new upholstery. And all the other car owners who've had to wipe garbage off their windshields won't miss her, either. How sad. No one cares that she's gone.

I drive to my place of refuge, the library.

"So," says Barney with mock seriousness, "what's been going on at Lanai Gardens? This last week, the library has been recipient of a thousand rumors. Everybody has a different story."

"Ten people have died, we've been told," says Conchetta, hardly able to keep a straight face, "but maybe it's four, or maybe two. They've been strangled, poisoned, knifed, and put under Haitian voodoo spells."

I laugh in spite of my sorrow.

"And you," says Barney, "are the inciter of said rumors. You are now a private eye?"

Conchetta grins. "That's what you get from reading too many murder mysteries. So, give us the real enchilada."

And I fill them in on what has happened up until today.

My friends silently absorb what I'm saying. For a few moments the only sound in the room is the minute hand ticking its way around the big old maple library clock.

Barney whistles. "Whew. That's heavy. No wonder you haven't been around."

"Too many coincidences," says Conchetta.

"My point exactly."

Barney asks, "Did you really go to the police? I love that the rumors escalated to the FBI and the CIA. Someone even mentioned that you might go into the witness protection program. That's my favorite."

"Oh, boy," I say, "there's Pandora's box and then there is a Jewish Pandora's box. . . . Yes, I did go to the police, but they didn't believe me. And now there's been another death. This morning."

"No!" Conchetta stifles a cry.

"Who?" asks Barney.

"Greta Kronk," I say. The two of them stare at me, dumbfounded.

It's quiet today in the library. Few people choose to battle the midday heat, and wisely stay home. In almost complete privacy, we three move over to one of the reading tables and sit down with the inevitable cups of Conchetta's Cuban coffee.

"How?" they both ask.

"She died next to the Dumpster behind my building. Her mouth was stuffed with rotten food —"

Madre mia!" Conchetta says, "How awful! And I thought she would be the one who would hurt somebody."

"Now, I'll never get a chance to meet her," says Barney wistfully. "I'll miss her rhymes."

"There was one left on her door," I tell them.

"What did it say?" asks Barney, barely able to contain his excitement.

I recite. " 'Get fed. Get dead.' " That quote will be engraved forever in my mind.

For a moment neither of my friends speaks.

"Wow. . . ." Barney finally whispers in awe. "But how could she have written 'get dead' after she died? She certainly wouldn't have done it before."

"Exactly. I finally figured out that was the killer's idea of a sick joke. Trying to make it look like Greta wrote the poem."

A lone straggler comes out from behind the stacks and brings his books to the checkout counter. We wait until Conchetta returns.

We tip our cups in memoriam for the poet who gave us such memorable rhymes as "Tessie is fat and that's that."

Conchetta says, "I especially loved 'Sophie shop til she drop.' "

Barney adds his favorite: " 'Leo buys. Leo sells. Leo tells. Lies.' "

"It's the recklessness of the killer this time that puzzles me," I say. "Considering that the other two murders were conceived and carried out with icy meticulousness, this time he had to have forced the food down her throat. And to attack in daylight. What a chance he took."

"Was it her birthday, too?" asks Conchetta. She pours us some more of her coffee, but I can't drink it. My stomach feels like acid is eating my insides.

I am suddenly sick to my stomach.

"No!" I say, as realization kicks in. "Damn it!" I am so angry at myself, so angry that once again my slow memory synapses have failed me.

I am shaking with the frustration I feel. "Greta wasn't on the murderer's list! She knew that he had killed. Twice! She knew that and tried to tell me by soaping the words on my car, and I just didn't make the connection! If I had only realized she was probably a witness to the crimes, I could have saved her life! And found out who the killer was."

Conchetta comes to my side and puts her arm around my shoulder.

I am distraught. "What am I going to do?"

"Go see that detective again, and this time you'll be able to convince him," Conchetta says.

As I drive home I think that maybe the killer finally made a mistake. Please, God, let it be true.

27

Digging up the Dirt?

I'm practically living by my phone. Maybe one of these days I'll give in to progress and get an answering machine. But who knows. One thing could lead to another. I might get tempted to buy a car phone, then a beeper or cable TV or, God forbid, a computer. I've managed to live this long keeping life simple. . . . Ignore me, I'm rambling. This waiting is driving me crazy. I've been trying to get an appointment with Detective Langford but he's been away for two days at some cop conference in Miami. I know he's back today. I've already left three messages.

Speaking of the phone, it hasn't been ringing off the hook as is usual. Where are the girls? I'm grateful, because I would have to get them off the line pronto. And they'd insist on knowing why. And if I tell them, Evvie especially would demand to go with me, and there is no way I'll put myself through *that* again. But what are they up to? I wonder. Mah-jongg is over by now. Curious.

The phone rings. It's Langford at last. I beg to see him as quickly as possible. Can't I tell him over the phone? No, I insist. It's too important. I can hear the weariness in his lethargic voice. Too many mai tais on the beach? Too many blond shiksas around the piano bar? Miami Beach can be a dangerous place. Reluctantly, he tells me if I can get over there in five minutes, he'll fit me in. Beggars can't be you-know-what. I'm out the door as fast as I can grab my car keys.

As I start to pull out of my parking space, I catch a glimpse of movement across the way in P building. Bella is tiptoeing into Greta Kronk's apartment behind Sophie. Can the others be far in front? Now I recall hearing something about Evvie, as a member of our condominium board, giving herself the authority to look through Greta's papers. Since there aren't any relatives that we know of, maybe there's a will, or something. Evvie tells me this has never happened before, that there isn't some person to contact. So yes, we do need to do something. About her remains, for one, poor thing. And the apartment and her possessions. Having just seen what she looked like, I shudder to think what her apartment looks like.

Naturally, the gang isn't about to be left out of that juicy adventure, so I see she's taken them along and I can imagine them drooling over the prospect of uncovering Greta's secrets. Four yentas in search of dirt. What a concept! Or five. I think Harriet has started her vacation today. Now I know why they didn't call. They don't want me spoiling their fun by being the voice of their consciences.

Morrie (I can't think of him as Morgan anymore) Langford is a man of his word. He doesn't keep me waiting, but the fact that he stands in the middle of his office tells me he intends to make this short. And I intend to be there as long as it takes to convince him. So I sit down.

I go through it all, Selma to Francie to Greta, step by step. I am proud of my logical presentation. Finally, *he* sits down.

"Wait a minute." He stops me. He rifles through the papers on his desk. "I have the officers' report on Mrs. Kronk."

"Save your eyesight," I tell him. "It will say probably natural causes." Now I'm behind him, reading over his shoulder. "But note where he says there was food in her mouth —"

Langford moves away from my prying

eyes. "Do you mind?"

"Sorry."

"The police do not make assumptions on how a person died. They merely report what they see. If violence has obviously occurred, it becomes a crime scene and they call it in. If nothing looks suspicious, their job is over after the body is picked up by the coroner's office." He sees my frustration. "Look. She could have been hungry."

"Nobody's that hungry. She had money for food."

"You know that for a fact?"

"She had money for rent, for condo fees, for gas, electric. . . . Those things I know for a fact. And besides, she had delivery people bringing her bags of groceries."

"What is it you want?"

"Once you speak to the coroner, you'll see that I'm right. I want to know what the autopsy said. I tried calling them but they wouldn't give out that information. I need you to call up for me."

"What makes you think they did an autopsy?"

"Don't they always?"

"Not if the death seems natural." He looks at the report again. "The woman is what — in her eighties? Seemingly emaciated?"

"The woman was found near a Dumpster, for God's sake. Isn't that suspicious enough? Please call."

"Being found near a Dumpster, rather than in it, may not necessarily seem suspicious."

He looks at me for a long moment.

"In your board members' many earlier complaints to the police department about Mrs. Kronk harassing people, they refer to her as a possible mental case."

Boy, is he thorough. The man has done his homework. Over the last five years, as Greta's behavior escalated, we complained plenty. But, funny, he doesn't mention how many times we were ignored. Bring proof, they demanded of a spirit that moved invisibly in the night. Call us if she hurts somebody. Yeah. Right. When it will be too late. Well, now somebody hurt *her.* Permanently. I pull myself out of my dark thoughts.

"Crazy people might eat garbage," he insists.

"Then again, they might not."

"Her death might be considered bizarre, but there's nothing —"

I don't let him finish. "The poem on the door — wasn't that bizarre?"

"It doesn't prove that whoever wrote the

poem killed her. You say she alienated just about everybody in your buildings with her nasty poems. Somebody could have seen her dead body and then written the poem as a mean prank."

"Puleeze. It would mean reacting to the fact she was dead, getting this cruel idea very quickly, and then finding her paint can and rushing up to her third floor apartment and composing the poem in her style and painting the poem, returning the paint can to the Dumpster, and then getting away without being seen. Two things come to mind. Do you know how many people live right there in those two buildings? Who are forever snooping out their windows? Besides, eighty percent of them are way too old to be able to move that fast. For a prank? Not likely."

"But possible."

"Not probable. C'mon, Morrie. Excuse me. Detective Langford. The only person vicious, devious, and fast enough to do all that has to be the killer. Please call. They must have finished the autopsy by now."

Langford picks up the phone and dials a number. I hold my breath. He gives them the relevant information and waits. I can hardly sit still. I feel like I'm jumping out of my skin. He thanks them and looks at me.

"Well? Well!" I shout. "What's with the suspense? Tell me what they found."

He takes a deep breath. "Do you have any idea how many dead bodies show up at the morgue every day?"

I'm beginning to get a bad feeling about this. "I don't know and I don't care. I only want to hear about Greta."

"They signed her death certificate and she's been released to a mortuary. Natural causes, Mrs. Gold."

Befuddled, I ask, "You mean the autopsy didn't find any poison?"

"I mean they didn't see any need for an autopsy."

I cannot believe this. I cannot! "Detective Langford. Hasn't anything I've said to you today given you cause to believe there is at least the possibility of foul play? Come on!"

"Let me give this some thought."

"Think fast. Please. Before she's plowed under and you'll have to dig up the dirt again."

I start out the door.

"Mrs. Gold?" This is a softer tone of voice.

I turn.

"My father mentioned he met you recently. . . ." Obviously he's trying to lighten my black mood. I see the beginnings of a smile on his face as he watches mine looking for a reaction.

He's caught me off guard. I think I am blushing. I hope I'm not. "Nice man," I mumble. And I rush out.

I have murder on my mind. How can I think of men? Especially a sexy, good-looking older gent with a twinkle in his eyes. Then again, I must be a fool not to. I need all this aggravation like I need the heartbreak of psoriasis.

28

Where Did Everybody Go?

I am so wound up from my visit with Langford that it takes me three tries 'til I can get my car parked properly.

I am beyond depressed. I was so sure there'd be an autopsy. How could they look at that poor body and not know something was very wrong? Just to look into those dead, tortured eyes. The terror, the knowledge that she was about to be killed. Couldn't they see that?! We were so close to finding out the truth. . . .

I decide to stop at the mailbox. I never did get my mail while waiting for the phone to ring.

"Gladdy, hold up."

I reluctantly turn, knowing the owner of the voice. Sure enough Leo, the Sleaze, is rapidly bearing down at me.

"Do you know where Evvie is?"

My answer is snotty. "Am I my sister's keeper?" Truthfully, I am, but I'm not about to tell that to Slezak. "Anyway, isn't she in her apartment?"

"No, I just came down. No answer. Then I figured she was in with one of the other girls, but no soap."

It annoys me Leo Slezak is so informed about our lives, who we pal around with, our whereabouts. Another yenta living in our midst.

"She wasn't at Bella's?" Bella being her next-door neighbor made it a fair guess. The two of them were forever visiting back and forth.

"Not Bella. Not Sophie. Not Ida. I didn't see your car so I guessed you drove them somewhere, but here you are and where are they?"

I hide my own surprise. This is atypical. "What's the big rush to talk to my sister anyway?"

He at least has the decency to blush. "Well, since it don't look like Greta Kronk has relatives, I thought Evvie, being on the condo committee, would know who has the right to sell her apartment. . . ."

Why did I bother to ask? As Sophie might say, vultures don't change their feathers. "While we are on the subject of real estate, Mr. Slezak —"

"Leo, please," he interrupts.

"Leo. What's the news on Francie's place? I haven't seen any action around there."

"Well, business is slow. . . ."

"And Selma?"

"Equally slow."

"The Canadians are here. I don't see you hustling."

"The Canadians are not buying. I thought I explained to you about that."

"Something's rotten and it's not in Canada, Slezak."

Slezak makes a gesture with his hand to say he is through with this discussion and walks away from me. Without turning, he calls back. "Tell her to call me. I'll make it worth her while." He gets into his car and drives off. I stick my tongue out after him, knowing how childish I'm being and glad of it.

Tessie Hoffman passes me. I have to ask. "Tessie, have you seen the girls?"

She starts toward the elevator. "No, but there's some function in the clubhouse. Maybe they're there."

"What is it, a lecture?"

"You know — that klezmer group from Israel. It started forty minutes ago. Me, I personally hate klezmer." With that she disappears into the elevator. Tessie doesn't like much of anything. Except food.

What have I got to lose? I might as well check it out. I walk down the brick path. It is starting to get dark, but the overhead lights illuminate my way. The ducks, as usual, have dirtied the path, so I have to watch my step. Out of the corner of my eye, I sense movement. Sure enough, there's Denny in his garden. I can tell by his posture that he is digging hard at something. I wonder how he is able to see in the failing light. Walking over to him I call out, so as not to startle him.

"Denny. Hello."

His back springs up and he turns toward my voice. I am close enough to see his face now. He's sweating and he looks angry. "Who's there?"

"It's only me. Gladdy."

"Waddya want?"

So unlike Denny, my mind is telling me. I don't want to hear this. Where is our gentle giant? Who is this angry man?

"I'm just on my way to the clubhouse and I saw you digging. Just came to say hello."

He stands very still, waiting. I want to ask what's wrong, but I don't dare.

"Have you seen my sister, Denny?"

"No." Abrupt. Cold.

The garden glitters in the near darkness. There is a profusion of a beautiful white flower I do not recognize, not that I know much about plants anyway. I suddenly re-alize I have not seen this garden in a very long time.

When Denny started out, he began with a very few little beginner shoots. We en-couraged him by buying him a variety of different kinds of seedlings, and his confi-dence grew. He planted simple little rows of pretty colored foliage and shared this beauty with all of us. Now the garden is overgrown. And no longer orderly. It's wild, almost haphazard, and out of control. *Like Denny himself?* I wonder. Is he going through some kind of personality change and his garden reflects this?

"It's getting pretty dark," I comment mildly, trying to hint that perhaps he should go home.

"I don't care! I don't want to go inside."

I am startled. Is this why he stays out-doors most of the time? He no longer feels comfortable in his apartment? Something is wrong with him and I must stop pre-tending there isn't.

"Why not?" I ask carefully.

"They wanna get me. If I stay out they won't get me."

"Who, Denny? Who wants to get you?"

But he is shoveling again, ferociously, his thick hair falling over his face, covering the rage and fear. I walk away quietly, wondering what to do about this.

The klezmer concert is ending and the residents are exiting, many humming the catchy tunes. But there is no Evvie. Or Bella. Or Ida. Or Sophie.

Just as I reach our building, Harriet's van pulls up and all the lost ladies pile out. I see from their shining, excited faces, they've had a big adventure and they are dying to tell me. Believe me, I'm dying to hear it.

Everyone starts talking at once.

29

My Worst Nightmare

Since they are all chattering at once I have to extricate their words as I would unravel a tangled line of knitting.

Ida: "You wouldn't believe the day we had!"

Sophie: "Oy, I'm starving. We haven't had a bite."

Harriet: "I have to leave you girls. I must get Mom her dinner. Fill Gladdy in." With that she gaily waves and leaves us.

Evvie: "Where *were* you? You should have gone with us! You missed such a day!"

Sophie and Bella slap high fives.

Bella: "Are we good or are we good?"

Evvie: "You wouldn't believe what we found."

Ida: "Or what we got done. What a team!"

"Stop!" I say. "Start at the beginning."

Evvie grabs my arm. "Right. We got to do this in order. First come up with us to the Kronk's apartment."

"You're not going to believe," says Bella, eyes glittering, as she pulls on my other arm.

"I got to eat or I'll perish," cries Sophie.

"So go eat," says Bella. "We'll go without you."

Sophie considers this for a moment, but hell would freeze over before she'd miss anything. "I'll eat a cookie at Greta's. She wouldn't mind."

I must admit I am curious about the condition in which they found Greta's apartment. Ten or more years of all of us speculating on the mystery of Greta's existence, never able to get into her apartment, never invited, blinds always shut, no way to snoop. Ten or more years of Greta never speaking to anyone except on the phone to order in supplies. Undoubtedly going to her mailbox in the middle of the night to get her Social Security checks.

I remember how many times we wondered if we should call the Board of Health. God knows what was crawling around in there. Even when we sicced the police on her, she never let them in. She stood inside her doorway to talk to them.

When we got the social worker to visit, she did get in, but afterwards told us Greta's file was confidential. Then turned down our request to remove her from the premises to some kind of health care facility, without saying why. Am I dying of curiosity? You bet!

Evvie unlocks the door, reaching in to turn on the lights. And wonder of wonders — I walk around inside taking it all in — the place is immaculate.

Evvie looks at me and grins. "Surprise!"

So, Greta prowled all night and scrubbed all day. Wow! The furniture was as I remembered it; she'd bought nothing new. But it was polished to a shine. Every surface gleaming. The windows spotless. A condition worthy of *House & Garden.*

Again the girls are grabbing and pushing me.

"The best is yet to come," says Ida. And I am pulled into the sunporch where a small table lamp is lit.

Here it is: testimony and only witness to the result of Greta's late night wanderings. Newspapers are carefully spread all over the floor and covered end to end with an astonishing collection of . . . things. In awe, I examine what Greta Kronk was able to create out of garbage. There must be nearly a hundred of these objects, these remarkable sculptures. Every size and shape imaginable. Everything we threw out as useless, Greta reinvented. Dancing costumes made from paper doilies, tissue, and wrapping paper. Dolls from wire, wooden sticks, and bits of metal like silverware and such. Damaged lamps, chairs, torn books, pots, and pans all recreated into other forms. Broken dishes and tiles had been reglued into vases of her own design. There was some craziness in the designs, but mostly they were unique and highly imaginative. And touching. How lonely she must have been.

Sophie is jumping up and down from excitement. "Look at the walls!" She turns on the overhead fixture and the entire room lights up. Bella and Ida join Sophie in crowding me to watch the expression on my face. "You coulda knocked us down with a feather bed when we saw!"

I stare incredulously at the collection of picnic paper plates lining the walls. Sketches in pastel, crayon, and acrylics of the residents of Lanai Gardens. Primitive as they are, they are each pretty good likenesses of us. If there was any doubt who they were, you only needed to read the poems she wrote beneath them. The same poems she matched to the doors. And there they are, all twenty-seven of them! I have to call Barney and Conchetta at the library tomorrow. They must see this.

The women are babbling behind me. "How about this!" "Look at that!" But I tune them out. I have to think.

Suddenly I am getting excited. Did she . . . did she paint one of the murderer? A picture to identify, a poem to accuse? I race my eyes up and down the rows, reading and recalling each and every one. No such luck. Except . . . except . . . the very last row. There's a nail hole. I glance down. The nail is lying on the floor behind a chair. I pick it up and hold it up to the light. I can see the tiniest trace of white cardboard still stuck to it. Again! Damn it! The killer is always one step ahead of us.

"What are you looking for, Glad?"

"The killer was here before us. He took his poem."

Bella looks around fearfully. "*Oy gevalt!* Maybe he's still here!"

"I doubt it," I say. Bella calms down.

Amazing. All of it amazing.

We go back into the dining area and the girls press me into sitting down. Sophie is hovering. I can tell she wants to raid the pantry and find something to eat, but she is having second thoughts about touching what belonged to the dead.

"Wait 'til you hear the rest," Evvie says.

"You have my undivided attention," I say.

"You have to admit, it was my duty to come up here. After all, with no relatives, we had to find out if she left a will."

"Absolutely," I tell her.

"And sure enough she had papers —"

Sophie interrupts, cutting to the chase. "Boy, were we surprised. She made Evvie her executor!"

Evvie beams and nods. "She had a paper she wrote by hand saying if anything happened to her, I should be in charge."

Sophie pouts. "I still don't see why she picked you."

Evvie puts her hands on her hips. "Why not me? I was always nice to her and besides, I'm on the board."

"No heirs?" I ask.

"Nobody. All her stuff goes to any charity we pick. Her bankbook has a few hundred dollars in it. That goes to some starving actors' fund. And she left a letter authorizing me to dispose of her remains as she asked."

Bella pipes up. "So that's what we were doing today."

Ida continues. "We called the coroner and they wanted to know what mortuary to send the body to, but first we had to prove Evvie had the right to say so."

"We needed you, but we looked everywhere for you, and you were gone," Sophie adds.

"Thank God we had Harriet. She did the driving."

"Lucky for you," I mutter. What turncoats.

"She knew just what to do about everything," Ida says. "We were already over the twenty-four-hour period for burial, so were we ever rushing."

Sophie continues. "We had to go to the bank and get it notarized who Evvie was, and make copies of Kronk's final instructions, then we had to run it over to the morgue and then we had to arrange it with the mortuary."

Bella grins, fanning herself. "I don't know how we ever got it all done in one day, but we did it!"

"Thank God for Feinberg's," continues Sophie. "Since everyone we know goes to Feinberg's when they die and they know us there, when we rushed them a copy of the death certificate they ran to pick up the body."

"And the cremation is," Evvie looks at her watch, "just about over now."

Everyone looks up at me, smiling, waiting for my words of congratulation for an impossible job well done. Instead, I scream, *What cremation?!*

"That's what the Kronk wanted."

I am hyperventilating now. I sputter. "Jews don't get cremated. It's against Jewish law."

Evvie grins. "Guess what. That's the joke. We did all that running around just to get everything done today because we thought the Kronk was Jewish."

Ida laughs. "We always think everyone is Jewish."

"Feinberg, of course, won't have anything to do with a cremation," Evvie continues. "He insists there must be some mistake. So we reread the papers again, and there it is. Turns out, after all that, that the Kronk was Catholic, so Feinstein ships her to O'Brien's right down the street on Sunrise."

I get up. My face must be purple. If I had high blood pressure I'd be having a stroke right now. I smash my fist down on the kitchen table so hard they all jump. *Do you idiots know what you've done!!*

I see the bright eyes dim and the smiles

turn to frowns of resentment.

"Do you know why you couldn't find me?" I shriek. "Because I was at the police station demanding an autopsy on Greta so we could find poison in her body! You cannot find poison in a charred hamburger! You cannot find poison in a jar full of ashes! You knew the only way we'd ever prove Francie and Selma were murdered was if we could find poison in a body!!! And we had Greta's body! *What the hell were you thinking!*"

It slowly sinks in, and one by one they realize what I am saying. And what they have done. They cringe.

"Whose idea was it to do all this today! Who!"

"Well, we thought we had to hurry because of Jewish law . . ." Bella whimpers.

"Well, Harriet said since she had the car and she wasn't busy . . ." Sophie adds.

"Quick," I say, going over to Evvie and shaking her, "give me O'Brien's number."

Evvie fumbles though all the papers in her purse, then she looks at me, stricken. "I don't have it. Feinstein made the call."

I look through Greta's kitchen drawers until I find her phone book. "Maybe Jews have to hurry, but what was O'Brien's rush? Why would O'Brien need to cremate her so fast? Don't they go through their own kind of funeral service, like a viewing of the body or a wake or whatever Catholics do?"

Evvie's voice was practically whimpering. "Since there were no relatives . . . And . . . the crematorium had a cancellation. . . ."

With my back deliberately turned away from them, I find the number and dial. I get voice mail which I hate the most of all these so-called modern improvements. I wade through all the instructions to press all the right numbers and after an endless wait on hold I finally get an operator who has to find someone who knows the phone number of the crematorium. The crematorium also puts me on hold, and an electronic voice tells me someone will answer in (pause) four minutes, and then I have to listen to an advertisement about the Neptune Society and be reminded to stop in their gift shop to see their large assortment of attractive urns. Finally I get a receptionist who makes me wait some more until she can find someone with an update on the disposition of the deceased. After too long, I hear what I prayed not to hear. The cremation is over. But if I'd like to come over and light a candle . . . and don't forget to stop at the gift shop. . . .

Through it all, the girls haven't moved. They sit rigidly, practically holding their breath. When I hang up they can tell by my face that the news is not good.

I walk stiffly to the door, turn, and face them.

I know I'm being melodramatic, but I can't help myself. "On behalf of the murderer of Selma, Francie, and Greta, I thank you." With that I walk out on them.

The way I feel right now, I may never speak to any of them again.

30

Nobody's Talking

Even though the weather continues its monotonous daily routine — heat and more heat — the song lyric running through my head is from "Stormy Weather." "Gloom and misery everywhere . . ." It might as well be raining. The grapevine, true to form, is spreading the word: The sisters aren't talking. And Gladdy's not talking to the rest of the girls, either. Buzz, buzz, buzz, but no one knows the reason. The girls, probably out of guilt, are keeping mum, and no one dares ask me. The condo board held a memorial service yesterday for Greta in the clubhouse. The girls attended when they were sure I wouldn't. I suppose everybody said kind words for the deceased and nobody mentioned insulting poems and garbage left smeared on doors.

It is too quiet these days, as if everyone is tiptoeing around us. Waiting for it to blow over or get worse. People still gossip about the murders, but there is much heated dissension as to whether they really were murders or just figments of my imagination. There are no more morning walks, and none of us go to the pool. From my window, I see the girls pile into a cab on Publix day.

I spend much of my time doing heavy thinking. Or else I am at the library commiserating with Conchetta and Barney. They share my consternation about the cremation of Greta. I do take them up to Greta's apartment at a time I knew the girls have gone somewhere, again by taxi. They are bowled over by Greta's artifacts, as I knew they would be. Dear friends — they try to get me out of my depression by saying I mustn't give up my detecting. But what is there to detect? No clues. No body. I really don't expect the killer to drop in on me and confess.

If you made a bet about it you would have won. Detective Morrie Langford calls me the next day and agrees to set up an autopsy. I briefly explain what happened, and I can tell from his voice he is genuinely sorry.

An afternoon shower hits hard, and the air seems almost cool for a few minutes. I decide to walk through the grounds just because I need to move around a little. I miss our exercise time, such as it is.

I find a bench in a quiet area, and I wipe the rainwater off and sit down. A few minutes later I hear two voices, coming toward me, singing happily, although off-key, in Spanish. Millie is awkwardly trying to stroll in her walker and Yolanda is with her, one arm keeping the walker steady. Millie seems genuinely happy. That sight finally makes me smile.

"Hi, Millie . . . hi, Yolanda."

Like twins they answer, *"Buenos días, Señora Gladdy."*

"And *buenos días* to you, too. Where's Irving?"

Millie answers. *"Mi esposo esta jugando cartes."*

"Cartas," Yolanda gently corrects.

"Yolie is giving me *lecciónes* in *Español.*"

"That's wonderful."

Millie giggles. "And I'm giving her lessons in snooping." Now Yolanda puts her hand over her mouth and giggles, too.

Getting into the spirit of it, I ask, "Why are you snooping?"

"Because the children like it. They like to see the dirties. . . ."

"The what?" I ask, curious.

"Hy Binder watches porno movies when Lola takes her nap." Another round of giggles.

"We *vemos* through *las ventanas.*"
More giggles. "And Señora Feder, she walks when nobody looks."

"I don't understand. Harriet walks?"

"No, *la vieja,* the old one," says Yolanda.

Millie imitates it. "She gets out of that old wheelchair and she just sashays around." Millie lets go of the walker to show how and loses her balance. Yolanda and I both grab for her.

Millie starts singing again, *"La cucaracha . . . la cucaracha . . ."* and Yolanda joins in. Together they continue down the path happily singing about a cockroach.

Is it possible? Esther is faking being crippled? It would explain how she managed to see what Greta wrote on John and Mary's door three floors up. And why? To keep Harriet imprisoned? If she can get around, what else has she been up to? Wait 'til I tell Evvie — I stop myself. And remember there is no telling Evvie . . .

I go back upstairs. I try to read, but can't concentrate. The hours drag by. The phone never rings. I guess I never realized how much of my days were dominated by the girls and their unending activities. I try to watch TV. Everything seems stupid to me. Now I am pacing and wondering what I can do to get out of this rotten mood.

The phone finally rings. I jump, so un-accustomed am I to hearing it. What a sur-prise. It's Langford, Sr. Why do I have the feeling the son called his father and told him I am feeling blue?

"I hope you don't mind my calling?"

"Of course not, Jack." I blush and I'm glad he can't see it. It must be genetic. Both father and son seem to be able to make me turn red. "Sorry. I've been ter-ribly distracted."

"Things not going well?"

As if Morrie hadn't told him. "At the moment, my investigation has come to a full stop."

"Then the timing may work to my ad-vantage. May I take you to dinner this eve-ning?"

Suddenly that seems like a wonderful idea. "Yes, thank you."

"May I pick you up at six?"

"No!" I surprise myself at how fast I say that.

"What time would you prefer?"

"It's not the time, it's the place. I don't think it's such a good idea for you to come here."

"*You* want to pick *me* up?" I can hear laughter in his voice.

I am getting frustrated. "No, that's not

what I mean, either."

"What have you got in mind?"

"Maybe we can meet somewhere else?"

"How's this: We can meet halfway between Phases Three and Four. Or how about that palm tree next to the mailbox. You can hide behind it and jump into my car as I speed by."

"Stop laughing at me," I say, laughing myself. "You know what busybodies we have in this place. People talk about me enough behind my back. Why should I add fuel to the fire? I'll meet you off campus, so to speak."

"Is ten miles far enough away? Or perhaps we can meet in Miami? Key Largo? Cuba?"

He got me at last. We are both laughing hard now. I play along. "Well, we can't go to Chinese. Or Italian. Definitely not a deli. We're bound to run into somebody we know. I've got it. Nobody here eats Greek. Do you like Greek food?"

"Mention moussaka and I'll follow you anywhere."

"You're on. Athenian Kitchen. Sunrise Boulevard, six p.m."

"I'll wear dark glasses and a fez."

"And I a babushka and a veil."

"Code names, Boris and Natasha. Which

one do you want to be — the moose or the squirrel?"

"Wrong country. Try Irena and Nico."

"Whatever."

When I hang up I am grinning like a fifteen-year-old. A little ouzo, a little feta, a lot of laughter — just what the doctor ordered. Or was it the detective?

But first, I have a million decisions to make. What am I going to wear?

31

The Dating Game

Look at me! I'm wearing a bra for the first time since I can't remember when. And a smidgen of makeup. Did a little something to my hair. I keep changing my outfit, unable to make up my mind. What image am I trying to project? Am I dressing up or dressing down? I'm making myself crazy. Finally I end up with the first thing I had on. Which I now hate. But I'm exhausted, so this is it. Glancing at the mirror, I'm startled. I don't look like me, the me that's gotten used to living single in these so-called golden years. The me that does nothing more than run a comb through my hair when we go out, just us girls. None of us bother anymore, in terms of attempting beauty. It's comfort that counts. Except for Sophie, of course, but she doesn't know any better.

It's only a dinner, I keep reassuring myself. It's a date, admit it! And if you're spending so much time getting gorgeous, that means you want to impress him. You want him to think you still look good. That you are interested. It means you're actually contemplating — oh, gasp — the possibility of a relationship!

Shut up, I tell myself, and move it already or you'll be late. How much longer are you going to attempt to turn not much into something more? Go, already.

When I enter the restaurant I see Jack talking to the owner. He waves me over.

"You look lovely," he says, then, "There's a complication. A nice one." He smiles.

"What's the name again?" Mr. Thomopolis asks. I know that's his name because his picture is over the cash register, smiling with a group of Little Leaguers.

"Jack Langford."

"No problem. The very minute you get your call." With that he shows us to a table and hands us gigantic menus.

"What's that all about?"

"Right after I spoke to you, my daughter called to tell me she was on the way to the hospital to give birth. Morrie's sister Lisa."

"That is exciting. But don't you want to be there with her?"

"Not too manageable. She lives in New York. It's their third child. I just want to

249

get the news hot off the griddle, so to speak."

Now that that's taken care of, we are facing each other for the first time since Fuddruckers. And yes, he still looks great to me. And he's smiling, so I guess I pass muster.

We make a big to-do about picking from such a huge menu, but finally the drinks are taken care of, white wine for me, beer for him. Moussaka for him, dolmas and a Greek salad for me. That took up a little time, but here we are again looking at each other.

He seems very content with the silence. And I remember that feeling. Belonging to someone. Feeling you fit and all's right with your world. My Jack used to call it the "aha" factor. Meet the right person and you breathe a sigh of relief and your mind says, *Aha, at last. The search is over. You're home.*

"Well," he says, "I don't have anything to report. My life has been status quo. But you — clearly much has been going on. Want to talk about it, or do you want this evening to be your respite from the real world?"

"The latter. Desperately. My world has become too much for me."

"OK, then," he says, smiling. "Read any good books lately?"

And we talk about the kind of books we like (me, good fiction and, of course, mysteries; he, nonfiction, especially history); movies (me, sophisticated comedies and good drama; he, spy thrillers); music (me, opera and Beethoven and swing; he, Mahler, Britten); theater (both agreeing that the last great musicals were in the era of *West Side Story* and *Fiddler on the Roof* and in drama, Arthur Miller and Tennessee Williams); and both of us, crossword puzzles and travel, which we don't do much anymore, and our children (extreme prejudice on both sides).

We laugh and talk and laugh and talk. It's wonderful.

Mr. Thomopolis comes over, smiling. "The phone, Mr. Langford."

Jack excuses himself and follows Mr. T.

I sit there bathing in the glow of happiness. God, how much I've missed this. Someone to share ideas with. Being a couple.

And suddenly I get anxious. What am I thinking! Too late for this. Haven't I spent my widow years assuming I would never love again? Redefining myself as single. Learning to adjust to that life.

I sip my wine as negative thoughts start tumbling about. At my age, it's too late to start over. Give up the known for the unknown? And think of what's involved. Readjusting to a new, unfamiliar man living with you. What's he going to expect? Here's a woman who has all the trappings of old age, from varicose veins to the dire results of gravity on down. This body is gonna turn a man on? Part of the agreement being never to turn on a light at night again? It's one thing for couples to live together fifty years, when the changes are gradual as opposed to shocking.

What about no longer just planning for myself but having to always consider another? The subtle battles. Who will have control. Having to compromise. No more being comfortable alone with one's own self.

And will the apartment need to be kept neater? Will I have to be the housewife again, with the man's wants more important than mine? Will I not be able to read in bed 'til dawn or eat standing in front of the open fridge at midnight? Remember what you've forgotten, Glad, old girl. Living with a man is work. You've got to please him, dress for him, cook for him. Bother. And sex. How much effort will it take to do what used to come easily and naturally? Will it work at all at this age?

You've got your own baggage, now you'd have to take on his as well. A whole new load of relatives to deal with and have to make room for. How much energy is left for this? And let's not forget the downhill countdown, the body's deterioration and potential illnesses. The possibility of having to care for an invalid. And what if that invalid is you? Would you be able to dump that on a stranger? And dealing with death again. One or the other left bereft again. So much risk. So much easier to do nothing. Live the easier life. Without love.

Best to leave well enough alone.

"It's a girl!" Jack appears at the table, beaming. "Six pounds, eight ounces."

I try to recover quickly from my shambling thoughts. "Congratulations, Grandpa." A weak retort.

He looks at me, eyes seeming to pierce into mine. He sits down, reaches over and takes my hands in his.

"I leave you alone for five minutes and you start to think! Stop it immediately! You imagine I don't know what's going on in that beautiful head of yours? That I haven't had every one of those same thoughts?"

I try sarcasm to cover my feelings. "What are you, a mind reader?"

"No, I'm just a person of the same age having all the same doubts and fears and giving myself all the same rationales to run as fast and as far as I can."

My voice sounds shaky to me. "So why don't you?"

"Because hopefully we're wise enough by now not to make the same mistakes we made when we were young. We no longer need to fight those foolish battles anymore. There are different ways to live with someone at this age. A way to make life easier and simpler for both. A way to cherish whatever is left for as long as it lasts, and to have someone at your side to share it."

"But what if . . . what if . . ." I can't say it.

"What if it's only a few years or a year or a month or even a day? Isn't one perfect day worth it?"

I am speechless. Then I start to cry.

32

Back to Reality

I guess I drove home. My car must have made it back on autopilot. Oh, wonderful world of limitless possibilities. Jack Langford. All these years so near and yet so far. We might never have met again had it not been for — murder. Francie, why aren't you here? You would have enjoyed the irony.

Suddenly, out of the corner of my eye, I am aware of something flickering. It's coming from across the parking lot, a ground-floor apartment. Denny's apartment. There is only the barest sliver of dull light shining through the louvers on the front door, but it seems to be moving. Is it a fire? Oh, please, God, no! I quickly park my car and hurry over. The kitchen blinds are shut tight and I can't see anything. I knock, but he doesn't answer. I keep knocking. Finally he speaks to me through the door.

"Who is it?" A mean, unfriendly voice.

"It's me, Gladdy."

"Go away."

"I thought I saw a fire —"

"There's no fire."

I'm relieved, but to my own surprise, I suddenly say, "Denny, may I come in? I'd like to talk to you."

"No. Not now."

"Promise we'll talk soon. All right?"

"Yeah. Some other time."

"All right then. Good night."

I start back across the parking area again and head for my place, my mind wanting to return to pleasant thoughts of Jack. But the sound of Denny's voice has pulled me into the here and now. His behavior in the garden was odd. Now this. It's obvious he's avoiding everyone. One of these days, I am going to make him talk to me and tell me what's wrong. Though I don't want to admit it to myself, I don't want to know. I'm afraid to know. . . .

33

The Living Dead

Denny peered out the peephole and waited until he was sure Gladdy stepped into the elevator.

Moving lethargically through his cramped apartment, he was no longer aware of the putrid smells around him. Of his own body odor from too few baths. Of the clothing he no longer washed. Of the garbage piled up in the kitchen and the filthy dishes in the sink. All he knew was that he was tired all the time. All he wanted to do was sleep. And he couldn't sleep. Life was only bearable when he was in his garden.

He placed a flickering black candle under his mother's portrait and straightened the black crepe he had wrapped around it. He did that every evening before the phone call. It was a ritual he dared not stop.

It was stifling in the apartment. He knew he should fix the air conditioner, but he didn't care that he could hardly breathe.

He didn't care about anything anymore. He only wanted it to stop.

Everything was wrong in his life now. He'd even lost his keys. He never lost keys before!

He had been so happy. Without her. *He had his garden and his jobs for all the ladies. Everyone was so good to him. They gave him presents and food. Nobody ever made him feel bad. Like* she *always did. Why did she have to come back and ruin everything?*

For seven wonderful years he'd thought he was rid of his mother forever. But then on the night before her birthday, she'd called him. How was it possible? And she sounded so strange. It didn't sound like her. But she knew everything about him and reminded him that it was because of him she'd died on this very date, the night before her birthday. He had killed her. Because he was a bad boy. He deserved to be punished. Then he knew it had to be her.

He didn't understand how she could phone him from heaven. She laughed and said they had all the modern conveniences. But he would never know that because he would never go to heaven. Because he was bad.

But why? What did she want from him? She told him, but he didn't really understand. How? he had cried out in anguish. She said she was lonely in heaven and she wanted her friends to join her. She couldn't wait until God was ready to send them. Oh, no, she had to have it her way, like she always did when she was alive. But it was confusing. It made his head hurt to try to understand. His mother never liked those ladies. She didn't have any friends.

Denny kept looking at the clock, waiting for it to be ten. Afterwards, he wouldn't be able to sleep. No wonder nothing got done around here anymore.

He sat on the couch, hands clenched, staring at the clock, praying for it to be over. He didn't want to do this every night, but he didn't dare disobey her. He had tried once. He left the house, so he wouldn't be there at ten when the phone rang. The next day he found a dead rat in his bed. Strangled. He threw up when he saw it. And that night when she called she warned him: The next time it would be his *neck.*

The second hand was nearing the end of the hour. He suddenly realized he had to pee, but it was too late. He had to answer on time. He didn't dare be late.

259

The old grandfather clock chimed the hours. Six . . . seven . . . eight . . . nine . . . ten. Ten o'clock. And the phone rang. Denny, staring at the phone, felt paralyzed. Pick up, Denny, now!

With sweating, shaking hands he lifted the receiver.

"Mama?"

He listened with the growing awareness that he should have gone to the bathroom first. He jiggled his body up and down, trying to control his bladder.

"But I did pick it right up. I did."

"No, the clock isn't wrong, I swear."

"Oh, no, Mama, not another one. Please."

"But, why? Don't you have enough friends up there?"

"No, I don't want to. Why do you say that? I don't want them dead."

"But I don't remember doing that." He shivered with fear. "I can't sleep, so how can I do that in my sleep?"

"Mama, no, I'm not fighting with you. I'm not . . ."

He couldn't help himself and Denny, mortified, could feel the pee running down the inside of his pant legs. He was sure she could see it. She saw everything he did.

His voice was dead now. Dead as he was feeling. "Who is it this time, Mama?"

"Yes, Mama, whatever you say."

Denny hung up the phone and sank to the floor. It was over. For tonight anyway. He stared at the damp spot on his pants and began to sob.

34

Back in Business Again

What a night! When I finally do fall asleep — nightmares galore. Denny was in my tortured night visions. Crying and standing over a grave, waving white flowers and whispering "Not me, not me." When the grave looked like it was opening up — well, that sure woke me up, covered in sweat and absolutely terrified. I shudder to think what the dream was trying to tell me.

That keeps me up a few more hours, pacing, thinking, attempting to read, until I can finally fall back to sleep again.

Around eight a.m. I'm awake again, feeling like I just drove a ten-ton truck to Tallahassee and back. I drag myself into the kitchen and make my morning coffee.

While carrying my cup and my toast to the dining room table where my crossword puzzles await, my eye catches something white on the floor, half hidden under the front door. I retrieve it after setting the coffee down.

And at the same moment the phone

rings. As I answer it, I'm aware that the note is from Evvie. I feel terrible. We've come to this. To talk to me she has to leave a note under my door. *Mea culpa,* as my pal Conchetta would say.

"Good morning," says Jack Langford cheerfully. "Hope I'm not calling too early."

"No, not at all," I say, still preoccupied by the note.

"I just wanted to tell you how much I enjoyed our evening together."

"Thank you. I did, too."

"You sound distracted."

"I'm sorry. I am. I had a fight with my sister and I'm feeling overwhelmed with guilt."

"Not good. Guilt is something we should not have to suffer at our advanced age."

"Easily said . . ."

"I know. Well you do what you have to do to repair the damage and call me when your mind is clear."

"Thanks for understanding, Jack."

After I hang up I read Evvie's note. *Glad. We're still on the job. We have important news about Leo the Sleaze and his real-estate company. They are up to no good. Evvie.*

This is so stupid! What am I supposed to

do — never forgive them? Live here and never talk to them again? Sneak around so that we don't ever run into one another? So Evvie reached out first, attempting to make up. I can guess how much it cost her. I have to let them off the hook even though I'd still like to wring all their necks.

I put on my sweats and walk outside to begin peace negotiations. This is my way of announcing to them that I am willing to begin our daily walks again, and channels are now open for further communication. Immediately, I can feel eyes peering out at me from behind louvered windows.

Sure enough, Evvie is out her door in a flash. Playing it cool, she does her warm-ups without facing me. She calls out to me across the parking area. "So, how did you sleep last night, Glad?"

If she only knew. This isn't the time or place to tell her about my nightmares. I call back. "Pretty good. Only got up twice."

And here comes Bella, peeping out her door to make sure it's safe to make an appearance. Evvie must be nodding at her, because she, too, is now out and moving at her usual snail pace.

"Hi, Gladdy," she calls tentatively at me.

"Hi, Bella," I answer. I can see her grin clear across the way.

Here comes Ida, doing her warm-ups. Head up, nose in the air, and definitely not looking at me. She is not going to say hello. Never one to accept blame for anything, in her mind she did nothing wrong; I'm to blame.

Sophie pokes her nose out the kitchen window. "I'm coming. I'm coming!"

"I think we need to have a meeting," I announce.

"When?" Bella asks eagerly.

"As soon as we can."

"I have a full pot of coffee on." This from Evvie.

Ida finally speaks. Grudgingly. "I'm not in a walking mood anyway. Might as well do it now."

Evvie chimes in. "Sounds good to me. Come on over."

With that, Ida walks right past me to the elevator.

Sophie calls out from inside her door. "I'm almost ready!"

I catch up with Ida at the elevator. From the expression on her face, I can tell she was hoping not to ride with me. We descend without speaking.

Finally, I sigh. "Truce?" I ask her.

"You hurt my feelings. We were only trying to help."

"I know," I say. "Let's get past it."

A pause. Ida isn't about to give me any easy satisfaction. "Well. We'll see how it goes."

But she is still not looking at me as we cross over to Evvie and Bella's building.

As usual it takes a while to get the coffee, cut the bagels, spread the cream cheese, exchange some quick gossip, get settled around the dining room table. The only difference is that everyone is uncomfortable. Ida's body is still turned away from me. Bella is looking nervously from one of us to the other and Evvie can't quite look me in the eye.

Finally everyone runs out of unimportant things to do or say. Evvie, seeing silence as dangerous, taps on the table with her teaspoon. "The meeting of the Gladiators will now come to order." She looks around, "Where's —"

The door bursts open and there's Sophie, half-dressed, looking frazzled, breathless and hyperventilating. She stares at us, just sitting there, puts her hands on her hips, and fires away. "Well, this is a fine kettle of fish and chips! I see you all out on the walkway, so I hurry into my sweats. I come out and you're all gone. So, I figure you went downstairs, but I can't find you on the path, so I figure it was time to go swimming, so I run back in and put on my suit, then I don't see you near the pool —"

Ida puts her hand over Sophie's mouth. "Shah, still! Close your mouth or you'll catch flies."

Sophie jerks her hand away. "Nobody ever thinks about me! You know I'm not good at rushing, and what am I, a mind reader, to know you're all up here at Evvie's? I knocked on everybody's doors!! Is this a way to treat a person?"

Bella jumps up and gets her a cup of coffee as Ida pushes an onion bagel at her. "It's all right. It's over. Sit. Eat. Listen."

"As I was saying," Evvie continues as Sophie noisily accepts the bribes, "the meeting has come to order. We all know all the old business, so we better go straight to what's new. . . ."

Bella gets excited. "Tell Glad what we found out about Leo."

"I was just getting to it."

Ida jumps in. "I was there, too. I'm a witness."

"Anyway, we were heading to the pool when we ran into Tessie. Tessie had news. Selma's apartment finally sold. She heard this from Selma's kids."

"Well, that's good," I say.

"No, it's bad."

Ida can't stand being left out. "So we naturally asked, who did they sell to? And when are they moving in?"

Evvie fairly pushes her. "Will you let me tell it already? Tessie says no one is moving in. A company bought the place. And they got it dirt cheap because it was on the market so long."

"Uh-oh, that's bad," I say. "When that news gets out, the property values will drop and they're plenty low now."

Evvie says, "You know, other people can be a detective, too. I go into the office and look through the condo records and I call up the families of all the people who died in the last six months in all the phases. And guess what?"

Ida bursts in again. "All bought by different companies. With no people moving in anywhere!"

"With one family after another taking cheaper prices after these companies told them what the one before sold for."

Sophie is sitting on the edge of her chair. "So what does it mean? Are they waiting 'til real estate prices go up and they'll sell at higher prices?"

"Hah!" says Evvie. "We bought our units

over twenty years ago, and our dumb luck — everywhere around us condos are worth a hundred thousand and up and we got the only price that never budged! This place always stayed cheap —" She stops suddenly, getting it, eyes wide. "But the real estate it's sitting on must be worth a fortune. . . ."

"So," I say, nodding at her, coming to the same conclusion. "They intend to buy us all out and tear this place down and build something much more valuable."

"Like a fancy high-rise," says Bella.

"Or, God forbid, a shopping mall!" says Ida.

"What's so bad about a shopping mall?" Sophie muses.

Ida swats her with a napkin. "Dummy, so where would you live?"

"Bad, very bad." Now I'm worried, too. "You said 'companies.' More than one?"

"Yes, about a half dozen different companies, but our accountant, Lou, is smart. He starts looking up the companies for me and surprise, surprise, there is one mother company who owns them all, by the name of Sunrise-Sunset, and that takes us squarely back to Leo Slezak."

"That gonif," says Sophie indignantly. "They're out to get all our apartments, one way or the other."

Bella picks up her coffee cup and her hand is shaking so hard the cup rattles. "But would they kill us to get them?"

I say, "Sleaze and his gang may be crooks, but cold-blooded murderers?!"

Ida says, "Makes sense to me. It would explain why they were trying to make us believe they were heart attacks."

"Counting all the phases, he'd have to kill off approximately a hundred and fifty of us," I say.

Ida still likes her theory. "Instead of serial killers we have mass murderers."

"Oh, well, another theory shot," Evvie says, ignoring Ida. She folds her arms, looking determined. "We'll get to the bottom of this mess, don't you worry."

"I have something else to report, though it might not mean anything." With that, I tell them of my funny little conversation with Millie and Yolanda.

Bella is truly shocked. "Esther Feder is not a cripple?!"

Sophie is grinning from ear to ear. "I knew it. I knew something was phony with that old broad!"

"She could be sneaking around when she knows no one is looking, like at night, when Harriet is also sleeping." Bella looks worriedly from one to the other. Then she brightens. "Maybe she and the Kronk hung out by the Dumpsters together?"

"But what could it mean?" Evvie asks, ignoring Bella. "It couldn't mean . . . it couldn't . . ."

"I doubt that," I say, "and besides, look at who told me. Millie? Yolanda? Maybe they made it up."

"I can believe it," Ida says. "She's plenty strong enough. Think of the muscles she has from wheeling that chair around."

"Should we say something to Harriet?" Evvie says.

"I personally am amazed. Someone as smart as Harriet wouldn't catch on?" Sophie is not convinced.

Bella says, "I don't think we should say anything. Not 'til we're sure."

"We could let a mouse run loose in the house and watch her get up and run," Sophie offers.

"Where would we get a mouse?" Bella asks, already contemplating this as a plan.

"Oh, my God," says Evvie excitedly. She quickly looks through her purse-size calendar of events. "That reminds me. I've been keeping track of everybody's birthday in our phase. Esther's birthday is in three days!"

Bella ponders that aloud. "Well, if Esther was the killer, she wouldn't kill herself on the night before her birthday. That would be suicide."

Sophie jumps in, liking this scenario. "So, if she is killed then it would mean she isn't the killer. And she's cleared herself of the crime. Then she wouldn't have to go to jail."

Evvie is excited. "I think we better have a meeting with Harriet, and fast."

35

Warning the Victim-to-Be

The girls and I crowd in to the Feder apartment, a place we hardly ever visit. For a number of reasons. We are rarely invited. And if we are, we are intensely uncomfortable. So much furniture. Very large, ugly, heavy — totally wrong for Florida. The pieces were undoubtedly expensive in their day, but who would want them? There is only one narrow aisle for Esther's wheelchair to traverse from room to room, and it must be difficult for her to manage. No wonder she usually parks it at the front screen door and stays there most of the time. I can't imagine living in a place so claustrophobic. I don't know how Harriet stands it.

As the girls try to get comfortable, I start to work my way up to why we are here. "I'm glad we caught you before you went to work," I say to Harriet.

"You would have caught me all day. I've been switched to the night shift."

Bella groans at that and Harriet eyes her curiously.

Ida looks at Harriet sadly. "Talk about bad timing."

"It's about your birthday," I say to Esther.

"What about it? You gonna make me a party?" She cackles.

Harriet gets it. "You're worried," she says quietly, trying to downplay it.

I nod, as do the girls.

"What about?" Esther demands to know. She wheels her chair deftly about to face us. Bella stares down at her legs. Evvie pokes her for staring. Ida fingers her sharp Hadassah lapel pin meaningfully. Bella sees it and giggles.

"Can't you change your shift back to day?" Evvie asks Harriet, at the same time glaring warningly at the girls.

"No chance," she says. "I made a lot of people switch schedules so I could take my vacation last week. I don't dare ask for another favor."

"What are you talking about?" Esther says, her voice strident now. She looks from one to another of us. Then she gets it. "The night before my birthday. You think —" and with that she makes a cutting gesture across her throat. "Eh, what a crock!"

"We don't want to take any chances,"

Evvie says. "Selma and Francie were killed —"

But Esther interrupts. "Who says they were killed? Only you girls, spreading rumors. I don't see any cops around investigating."

"Mom, be nice. The girls are only trying to help you."

"Who needs their help? I don't. And besides, Greta didn't die just before her birthday."

"Mom," Harriet intercedes. "We all think Greta was killed because she knew the killer."

"We? *We* all think? Suddenly these crackpots are your new best friends? Ha!"

Harriet looks at us, extending her hands, helplessly. I can see Ida getting red hot under the collar, just itching to say something. I shake my head at her.

Esther keeps jabbering. "Then what about Eileen O'Connor? Her birthday passed and she's still around. Too bad. She's such a big mouth, getting rid of her would be a blessing."

"Can't you behave!" Harriet exclaims, embarrassed.

"Frankly, I think her leaving and going to stay with her sister in Boca probably saved her life," I say quietly, trying to ignore Esther's rotten remarks.

Esther folds her arms. "OK by me. Send me to Miami Beach. I wouldn't mind a nice cabana for a week. You could also throw in a Cuban beach boy while you're at it."

Harriet smiles wryly. "That's a great idea. If only we could afford it."

"You would say that," Esther says sarcastically. "You don't let me spend a dime on anything."

Bella is again staring at Esther's feet, but they stay perfectly still under her blanket. Evvie pokes Bella. Sophie snickers.

"At least ask if you can have that one night off?" Evvie is determined to ignore Esther's rudeness.

"I'll try, but you don't know my supervisor."

"Then we have to set up some kind of plan," I say.

"I agree," Evvie says. "We can all sit here with Esther until you get home."

Ida wants to know what time her shift is over.

Harriet tells her it's four a.m.

Sophie groans at that.

"Hello? Don't I have any say in this matter? I don't need you. I don't want you," Esther says. "Don't do me any favors."

"Mom. This is no time to get stubborn."

"The whole thing's stupid anyway. Who'd want to kill me?"

From the looks on the girls' faces, I'd say, right now, four people.

Harriet is exasperated. "Foolish old lady. Why would anybody want to kill Selma or Francie? But they did!"

"Even if I believed all their *chozzerai,* you think I'd be afraid? Just let that guy come. I'll be ready." Esther makes boxing jabs with her hands as if to show what she would do.

Sophie laughs out loud.

"You think I couldn't?" Esther says, annoyed that they are laughing at her show of bravado.

"Mom, please. Don't be ridiculous," Harriet says.

Bella tries appeasement. "What have you got to lose? We could keep you company, play a little cards."

"Big shots! Nosy old biddies. Mind your own business."

Ida is up in a shot. "That does it. Let's go."

Sophie and Bella jump up with her.

Esther smirks and steers herself out of the cluttered living room and heads down the hall to her bedroom, muttering to herself. "As if I'd eat any food from some stranger! You have to be a moron!" Now she is shouting. "Like the TV show, that's my final answer!"

Harriet shrugs. What else can we say? As we start out the door, she whispers to us. "We'll talk later."

From the bedroom, Esther calls out again, "Don't forget to send me a present. Just don't send food!"

We can still hear her cackling when we step outside.

Back to square one. What's that funny saying? No good deed goes unpunished? We're going to have to find a way to save her in spite of herself. From the looks on the faces of my angry cohorts, I'd say I'll have a hard time convincing them.

Under her breath I hear Sophie mutter, "We shoulda let Ida jab her."

36

Double Feature

How can I describe this day? Everyone is on *shpilkes. Shpilkes* — an untranslatable word. It's like going crazy without going crazy. A high state of nervous anxiety. Or — as Ida calls it — ants in your pants.

Today is the day before Esther's birthday and our hands are tied. She won't let us help her. I thought about calling Detective Langford, but what would he say? What the police always say: We can't do anything unless something happens. So, it's up to us without Esther's permission.

The girls are driving me nuts. They are calling every hour on the hour. Do you see anything? Do you hear anything?

At three o'clock, there are multiple knocks on my door. I can see four anxious faces through my kitchen window. Reluctantly, I let them in.

Evvie takes the floor. "We've made a decision. We're going to the movies."

"But first dinner," says Bella.

"There's a great double feature at the

Reprise Theater. Harriet read about it in the papers and called me," says Evvie.

"You'll really love it," says Sophie. "Two murder miseries."

"That's 'mysteries,' " Ida corrects her.

"Whatever."

I look at them in horror. "Are you trying to say we shouldn't stay home and guard Esther? Have you all lost your minds? Who's going to be able to concentrate on a movie!"

"Me!" A unanimous chorus.

"I can't do that!"

"Yes, you can," says Ida.

Sophie throws it to first. "We picked a deli right in the same minimall as the theater."

Bella takes it to second. "We do the early bird at four-fifteen."

Ida makes it to third. "The double feature is from four-thirty to seven-thirty. We'll be home before Harriet has to leave for the night shift."

And Evvie brings it to the plate. "We'll be home before dark. Well, anyway, it won't be too dark."

"Is that the movie?" I ask. "*Wait Until Dark*?"

"No, that's the plan," she informs me.

"So, tell me already." I can't believe I'm

even asking. "What's playing?"

"*Sorry, Wrong Number*," Evvie says. "With Barbara Stanwyck."

"I love Barbara *Sandwich*," Sophie coos. "Is she dead?"

Bella says, "I think so."

"Such a pity, so young," says Sophie.

"And *No Way to Treat a Lady* with Rod Steiger," Evvie adds. "Perfect for this week's movie review on golden oldies. Waddaya think? What with all the murders getting in the way, I haven't had time to write one single review. My fans miss me!"

I am fairly salivating. Two great classics. What am I thinking? This is crazy!

Evvie pokes me playfully. "Admit it, you want to go."

I am pacing now. Torn, and ashamed of myself. "We have a responsibility here!"

"To Miss Ungrateful?" Ida says. "Why should we care?"

"And how will you live with yourselves tomorrow if she's dead?"

That stops them for about a minute.

"The killer won't do anything until it gets really dark," says Evvie.

"You know that for a fact?" I say icily. "He killed Selma around five in the afternoon and Greta early in the morning."

Evvie smiles knowingly. "With all the

noise we've been making, he knows we're watching. He'll have to wait 'til he thinks we're all asleep."

"Some watching. He'll watch us take off for the movies."

"Exactly. That'll fool him. But then he'll think we're trying to trick him. See?"

See? That's about as clear as mud.

Bella and Sophie jump up and down, grabbing my arms, pulling at me, like a couple of spoiled five-year-olds. "Please! Pretty please! Let's go."

"All right," I say reluctantly.

They are all out the door. Ida has to have the last word. "Downstairs in ten minutes, not a second later!"

I can't believe I am sitting in this theater. Those lunatics I live with dragged me so fast, my head is spinning. Rushed to the theater, rushed around looking for a parking spot, fairly dragged me out of the car and raced us all to the deli, so we'd have a whole ten minutes to choke down a dry pastrami on rye. I'm amazed I don't have indigestion.

Why did I go? Because Harriet reassures me she won't have to leave for work until we get home. Because I'm so edgy and the girls so crazed, the movies will relax us.

Believe me, I hedged my bet. I called Langford's office and left him a message. What a world. Even cops have voice mail. Whatever happened to some gum-chewing tough guy saying, "Yeah, waddaya want him for?" My message was to the point. "This is the night before Esther Feder's birthday. If I'm right, she'll die tonight. I hope I'm wrong."

I also intend to phone in between features.

Stanwyck is as wonderful as I remember, as the bedridden invalid who overhears two men plot a murder, and I relax into supreme enjoyment. Then that delicious chilling moment when she realizes she is the target!

Now I find myself staring at the screen. Barbara dials everyone she can think of to get help and I stare, hypnotized, at her hand as it keeps reaching for the phone. What does it remind me of? I think of Selma and Francie and someone else so long ago . . . but who?? It's been nagging at me since all of this started.

I lean over to Evvie. "Who was it who died in Lanai Gardens years ago holding a phone?"

"Wait a minute, this is the good part. Barbara hears someone breaking into the house."

"Evvie, this is important."

"What?"

"Someone died a long time ago —"

"In this movie?"

"No. Pay attention. In our phase."

"Someone we know?"

"Yes, of course. She died trying to get help."

"Shhhhh!" I hear from behind us.

"Sorry," I whisper. I talk lower. "Think!"

"I'm thinking," she hisses at me.

"Be quiet!" someone yells at us.

"Mind your own business," Evvie yells back. "There's a film critic sitting here, you know!"

Someone throws popcorn at us. Ida jumps up, hands on hips. "Who did that!" she shrieks. In a moment, the manager is running down the aisle.

"If you wanna talk, go home and watch TV!" someone heckles.

But it all calms down quickly. This isn't our usual neighborhood theater where everyone talks incessantly throughout every movie. We must be in a theater with real movie buffs.

I call Harriet at intermission. All quiet, she tells me. Have fun, she says.

My mind is not on the opening credits for the next feature. I am suddenly starting to remember what I cannot believe I'd forgotten.

And as if someone on the screen is helping direct my thoughts even further, there's Rod Steiger, a serial killer, standing in front of the portrait of the mother he hates, the reason he kills older women one after another. Putting on disguises to fool old ladies into letting him in. Leaving his trademark, lips painted on the forehead of the dead women with their own lipstick.

We are three quarters of the way through the picture when it finally hits me. Maureen Ryan! Denny's mother. Ohmygod!!!

The pieces are falling into place.

I hit Evvie on her shoulder. "Tell the girls we're leaving!"

"But we're at the thrilling part. Steiger is going after George Segal's girlfriend, Lee Remick!"

"Now! Meet me in the lobby."

I race out to the lobby bank of phones and I dial Harriet's number as fast as I can. The line is busy. Come on, Harriet, get off the line! Or is the phone off the hook because Esther knocked it down as she tried calling for help? I try to calm my hysteria.

The girls tumble out into the lobby, grumbling. This is unheard of. They never leave a movie in the middle. I ignore their complaining. I'm out the door, so they follow.

"We've got to get back now. We've got to stop him."

"Who?" Evvie asks.

"Denny," I say, choking on my traitorous words. There's no more denying what's been staring me in the face all along. Denny's gone bad. "He's going to kill Esther!"

They stop dead in their tracks, but I'm still moving.

"Come on," I yell. "We haven't a minute to waste!"

Quickly, panting with exertion, they run to catch up with me. They are incredulous and frightened now.

We reach my car as I am groping in my purse for my keys. I can't find them. I always put them in the outer pocket. Otherwise I'd go nuts digging for them every time. They have to be in there!

Evvie shoves me nervously. "Open the door already!"

I hiss at her. "I can't open the door because I can't find my damn keys!"

They are not where they should be, and now I grope anxiously all through my purse. Nowhere! And then I see them.

Dangling from the ignition. In all that hurry I locked my keys in! The girls look where I am looking, then back at me, sheepishly.

God keep me from committing murder, as well.

37

Stuck in the Minimall

By now we have quite a crowd of kibitzers around us. Testimony to boring lives, that everyone in the Hollywood minimall has stopped whatever they were doing to witness these little old ladies' embarrassment at being locked out of their car. I am not embarrassed, I am livid. With passersby either jeering catcalls or giving us bad advice, the scene is only adding to my aggravation.

Advice like get a piece of gum and stick it on a stick and drop it down the window. Gum, hard to come by in a group heavily into dentures. A stick, equally hard to find in a concrete shopping area. And the so-called window opening? Merely a sliver of air space.

A reedy voice calls out to us, "How come you don't carry an extra key? I do."

"Gimme permission to smack her," Ida says under her breath.

The girls hover close to me, waving their hands helplessly.

"But how do you know it's Denny?"

Bella whispers behind my head. The girls can't get over the bombshell I threw at them. I can't get over that we are trapped here in this stupid minimall.

"Remember how Maureen died?" I answer, unable to hide my irritation at them.

"Maureen?" Sophie asks, befuddled. "She's been dead, what — six, seven years? What's she got to do with this?"

"Maybe everything."

I have sent Evvie back to the theater to call the auto club. I'm waiting anxiously for her to report back.

Everyone's favorite suggestion is to get a hanger, bend it and push it through. So where do we get a hanger at this time of night? I gaze longingly at Betty's Better Dresses, which is five feet from where I'm standing, and count all the hangers through the locked store windows.

I am desperately trying to control my temper, impatience, and anxiety, but I'm not doing too well.

"I knew we shoulda listened to Hy. He told us to get a car phone," Sophie says, hitting me on my back. "Single women need a car phone to be safe."

"And where would the car phone be right now?" I say icily. "In the *locked car,* that's where!"

"Then we shoulda got a cell phone," Bella whines. "But no, you have to hate progress. And besides, my feet are hurting."

Evvie returns, looking dejected. "Auto Club said forty-five minutes, give or take."

"Then maybe we should call a policeman," says Bella.

"Yeah," Ida says bitterly, "I can just hear us on the nine-one-one. Emergency. Send a cop quick. Tell him to bring a hanger."

Bella continues worriedly, "Maureen died of a heart attack, didn't she?"

"But don't you remember," I say, "she was eating a piece of steak and they thought maybe she choked on it?"

"So?"

"God. I can't believe we didn't remember this before. Food. Isn't this all about food?"

And another, "So?" This from Ida.

But Sophie is finally starting to get it. "Wait a minute . . . she was holding the phone when they found her. *Oy vay!*"

"Do you remember the date?"

"Who can remember that far back?" Bella says.

"I don't mean the actual date. I mean the event."

Evvie makes the connection. "Oh, my

God, it was the night before her birthday!"

"Yes! I'm so stupid! Why didn't I remember?"

"Cause your memory is shot, that's why," adds Evvie helpfully.

Every minute that passes frightens me. I need to know what's happening back at Lanai Gardens!

38

No Way to Treat a Mother

Denny stands in the middle of the living room, unable to catch his breath.

No matter how hard he tries not to look at it, he can't help himself. Slowly, he turns to face his mother's portrait. He feels her eyes following him everywhere. He wants to get out of there, but he can't get his feet to move. It's like those dreams he has when his mother is chasing him with the clothesline that she used to use to tie him to his bed. His feet would go numb and she would always catch him and do all those terrible things to him.

The phone rings. Denny jumps, terrified. Sweating freely now, he stares at the phone hypnotically. Stop ringing, he begs. Make it stop ringing. He puts his hands over his ears but he can still hear the ringing. Save me, he mutters under his breath. Someone save me. Finally, unable to stand it anymore, he answers.

"Hello . . ." He is shaking so hard he can barely stand. "But it's not ten o'clock. . . ."

"I know I'm a bad boy. . . . I know. . . ."

"In the kitchen? When did you put them there?"

"Please, no, don't make me . . ."

"I can't. . . . I can't. . . ."

"Yes, Mama. Right now."

Denny hangs the phone up and walks into the kitchen where a small basket, prettily decorated with a lace cloth, sits there just where she said it would be. And right next to it are his keys, the ones he lost.

Slowly, sickly, he moves back into the living room. He can feel his anger and his impotence rising up in him like bile in his throat. His hand reaches for his toolbox nearby. He opens it and grabs for a screwdriver. In rage he leaps for the portrait and gouges out his mother's face. "No more . . . no more . . ." he sobs.

39

Death by Poppy Seed

I keep looking at my watch as if that will make any difference. The cab we called still hasn't arrived. Neither has the auto club. By now we've lost our audience, and the minimall is nearly deserted. The girls are huddled in a doorway, shivering in the cool night air.

I am beside myself. There is still no answer at the Feders, only the same busy signal. Why can't I reach Harriet? Something is very wrong.

I've called Irving. No answer. He is already asleep, early as usual. With the phone locked away from Millie. I tried Tessie. Not home. I better call Hy . . .

A trio of teenagers walk by. They clank from all the metallic piercings they have hanging from various body parts. Their boom box is booming some ugly-sounding rap.

"Hey, old ladies," one of them calls sarcastically, "waitin' for some action?"

They are very big and scary, but I am at

my wit's end. "Yes," I say, ignoring the innuendo. "Do you know how to break into a car?"

"Are you crazy?" Ida shrieks.

"No, desperate," I tell her.

The boys stop, amused. You can see it in their faces. This ought to be fun. "It'll cost ya," says a huge lump of lard with black and white zebra stripes painted across his bald head.

"How much?" I ask, trying to keep cool while my legs are shaking.

Ida hides behind me. "Don't talk to them. Maybe they'll go away."

"Twenty large," the purple-haired one says, sneering.

I attempt a sneer myself. "How about five small?"

The girls are gasping, all of them now crowding behind me.

Zebra Stripes erupts into laughter.

What few people are still around quickly move as far away as they can.

Bella tugs at me, terrified. "Tell them we don't need them," she whimpers.

I shrug her off. "But we do."

The third one, with dreadlocks and a lime green crocheted skullcap, walks over and surveys the car with a most professional air. I think he's the leader. "Give the ladies a senior discount, Horse," he says, and that starts another outburst of hilarity.

"Fifteen," says Purple Hair, aka Horse.

"Shame on you," says Dreadlocks. "Ain't you got no old grandma?"

With that, he whips out a very thin strip of metal and instantly snakes it through the narrow window opening. Within two seconds I hear the door locks unlatch. And just as fast, the metal is back in his pocket and his hand is outstretched. Even though my own hands are shaking, I get a ten and a five out of my wallet and hand it to him.

They walk off, laughing. "You are one hella hip granny," Dreadlocks calls back.

"Thanks for your help," I answer as I notice both the taxi and the auto club driving into the minimall.

Bella waves her little fingers at the boys and gaily calls out, "Thanks for not killing us."

As he walks out the door and starts to cross the parking area, Denny can smell the sweetness of the poppy-seed rolls he carries.

At Esther's door, he stops. He opens it with his master key and walks inside.

The nighttime silence at Lanai Gardens is abruptly shattered by agonizing

296

screams. Doors and windows are flung open or, in most cases, cautiously cracked, and faces peer out. The braver ones come out and lean over the balconies to see what's happening.

Esther Feder is running, falling, then crawling down the middle of the street. Esther can walk!? is the first shocked response. But what's wrong with her? She is gagging, clutching her stomach and grabbing onto cars for support.

"Help me," she cries.

Half walking, half running behind her is Denny, crying. And oddly, he seems to be carrying a basket of rolls.

She falls down as her legs no longer support her.

"Poison," she screams as Denny reaches her. "Denny . . . you . . . ? Why, why?"

He stands over her helplessly, sobbing now. "She made me do it," he says as he drops to his knees beside her.

"I am a dead woman," Esther Feder cries and then falls silent as paralysis sets in and she can no longer move. Only her eyes stare in horror at Denny as her life slowly drains from her body.

And it is just at that moment that the girls and I arrive home.

40

The Cop and the Private Eye

I walk downstairs, exhausted and depressed from lack of sleep, to where Detective Langford is waiting for me in front of the Feder apartment. He called half an hour ago to tell me he was on his way over, saying he wanted to "touch base" with me.

It is chilling to see the yellow crime scene tape across their door. Poor Harriet. She's gone to work because she can't stand being in the house. I can still see her agonized face when she was called home from the hospital three nights ago. I can still hear her shriek as she threw herself down over her mother's dead body lying on the concrete.

"My fault," she kept sobbing.

My fault. I think bitterly. *My fault. God help me.* Had I stayed home, Esther would still be alive. I would have stopped Denny in time. *Woulda, coulda, shoulda,* as Sophie would say.

The girls are hovering on the second-floor balcony of my building. They are itching to come down and talk to Langford, but too shy to do it on their own. When they see me, the scampering downstairs begins.

Pretending not to see them, I greet Morrie Langford.

"How's Denny?" I need to ask.

"He's still being evaluated at the hospital."

The girls all titter their hellos and Langford politely acknowledges them. I wave them away. They ignore me. Evvie moves in closer. "He must be so frightened," she says.

"I'm sure they have him on meds to keep him calm."

Ida is appalled. "Why is everyone so worried about him? He's a killer."

Morrie starts to walk toward the pool area. "I want to show you something," he says.

We follow him down the path, past the duck pond, and over the bridge that takes us to Denny's garden. The girls follow behind us, keeping their distance.

"With their families' permission we've exhumed the bodies of your friends Selma and Francie. And you were right. Poisoned, both of them." The news hits me hard in the pit of my stomach. Even though

I've always suspected it, finally knowing the truth is a jolt. I hear the girls gasp.

We reach Denny's garden.

"And here's where he got his poison." Langford leans over and plucks one of those beautiful white flowers I'd noticed only recently. "Right in front of everyone's eyes."

Evvie can't stand being left out anymore. She moves in right next to us. "A pretty flower? How is that possible?"

"A deadly poisonous one, Mrs. Markowitz."

Sophie now closes the gap and is breathing down Langford's neck. "You mean, he made them eat a flower?" She is incredulous. "Francie wouldn't eat a flower."

Bella, scampering over, is in tears. "How could he do it? He loved Francie!" Sophie puts her arms around Bella to comfort her.

"How could a flower turn into poison?" Ida closing in fast, so as not to be left out, demands to know.

"I won't go into details," Langford answers, "but it isn't too difficult to crush the leaves and boil them down into a substance he could put in their food."

Sophie stares at the blossoms that have overwhelmed the garden and caused such tragedy. "Who even knows what they are.

I've never seen such things before."

Langford answers her. "They're called oleander."

"I just don't get it," Evvie says. "Denny was a happy man. He had a good life here. He was kind to everyone and everyone liked him. What set him off?"

"Hopefully the doctors will figure it out." Langford starts walking back. "There's something else I want to show you. Maybe it will help you see how disturbed Denny was."

We walk back to our buildings and, with our backs to the Feder apartment, now stand in front of Denny's place, where the other crime scene tape is draped.

Langford moves the tape and unlocks the door. "I have to warn you —" he starts to say, but we've already hurried inside.

At first we can't see anything because all the blinds are drawn, but we can smell something, and the smell is awful. We quickly cover our mouths and noses with our hands.

"Gott im Himmel!" Ida is gagging. "What died in here?"

Langford turns on the lights and we look around, horrified. At the garbage, the filthy dishes, the overwhelming clutter, the candles and the black crepe around Maureen's portrait. And in the center of the portrait, Maureen's face, mutilated beyond recognition.

If I were Catholic, I would cross myself. Instead I utter a silent prayer for poor, sick Denny. Sophie and Bella are crying and holding onto each other. Evvie and Ida are trying hard to be brave.

Langford faces us. "You all knew him, and I assume you've been in his apartment. Was it always like this?"

Everyone is shaking their heads. "Never!" Evvie says vehemently. "He was always proud of how well he kept it up and how neat he was. Even his garden tools and his repair kits were always in good order."

Ida continues, "But we haven't been in here in a very long time."

After a lengthy silence, I ask if we can get a cleaning crew in. That is, if they're through searching.

"We'll be finished after tomorrow," he says. "The doctors will be here to see this, and it will be part of Denny's evaluation."

"He went crazy, that poor boy," Bella whispers. "And nobody knew."

I feel defeated. I look at this abomination. I don't want to believe Denny is a killer. How can I deny his guilt now?

41

M Is for Mothers and Murder

It's a fairly nice memorial service and a very large turnout at the clubhouse considering that Esther Feder did not have any friends. Oh, everyone manages to find some kind words to say for Harriet's sake, but you can sense the strain.

Residents of all six phases of Lanai Gardens show up and no wonder, considering all the excitement. They are still reeling from the information that is slowly trickling out day by day. They really were murders! And Denny Ryan, the killer! That such a thing could happen here . . .

All of us from Phase Two are attending the service. Enya is seated by herself as always. I can see her lips moving, saying Kaddish for the dead. Irving brought Millie with Yolanda's help. Millie is going though a bad stage and Yolanda is becoming indispensable to Irving. He adores her now, and she truly has become a member of his family.

Tessie is greatly subdued now that she

realizes her beloved friend Selma had indeed been murdered. And everyone loved Francie, so that realization is a bombshell. It was bad enough thinking of losing her to a heart attack, but cold-blooded murder . . .

All in all, it's a solemn ceremony and it's not just Esther being mourned here today.

I am ashamed to say I am sitting in the back row, not wanting Harriet to see me. How can I face her feeling all this guilt?

The service is over, and as we all leave the clubhouse, I hear my name being called. Twice.

I hadn't even realized he was there, but it's Jack Langford calling as he walks toward me.

At the same time Harriet speaks my name as well. Alas, she reaches me before Jack does. Jack backs away. I shrug, indicating to him that I am trapped. He pantomimes phoning me. I nod and he leaves.

I look around for the girls, needing a buffer, but they are here and there chatting with neighbors, busily filling in the blanks for those who came in late to our tragedy.

"Can we talk, Gladdy?" Harriet asks in a plaintive tone. I'd rather not, but how can I say no?

"Of course," I say.

We stroll along the path leading back toward our building. We pass Denny's garden, and I quickly avert my eyes from the sight of those beautiful, deadly flowers. Harriet stiffens, so I assume Detective Langford has told her the results of the autopsy.

We find a bench under a palm and sit down. We are silent for a few moments.

Finally she says, "I desperately need to talk to somebody, and you are the one I thought of."

"I'm here and I'm listening."

"I am so angry at myself," Harriet says. "God help me, it's all my fault Mom is dead. And I'm going to have to live with that the rest of my life."

I stare at her in amazement. Here I'm bracing myself for her condemnation of me and she says *she's* at fault? "*You?* It's me. I failed you terribly. It's *my* fault your mother died," I blurt out. "If only I'd been there . . ."

She takes my hand in hers. "Oh, no, don't blame yourself. You tried to warn us. It was one thing to talk about the others getting killed just before their birthdays, but I never believed it would happen to Mom. Never. How could I have been so blind?"

"No one wants to believe the worst. It's only human."

"But I sat in meetings with you, and we even talked about the coincidences with Denny. Then I just denied it all. I'll never forgive myself."

Poor Harriet. She was saying all the things I'd been saying to myself. We both made so many mistakes.

"I hope in time we can forgive ourselves," I say.

"Dear God. I hope so." She turns to me and I can see the anguish in her eyes. "You know what's the saddest part of all? That she pretended to be crippled so I'd stay with her. And I had to find out this way — the way she died — running down the street. Oh, my poor mama, didn't she know? I would never have abandoned her!"

"I'm so sorry, Harriet."

Again we sit silently, then Harriet speaks once more. "I've made a decision, Gladdy. I'm putting the apartment up for sale. Ring up another victory for Mr. Sleaze." Harriet chokes on a laugh at her sorrowful attempt at a joke.

"I'm sorry to hear that."

"I can't live here anymore. Everywhere I turn I see Mom's face. I feel haunted."

"Listen. You don't need to convince me.

Of course you should move. And to some-place cheerful, where there are younger people and especially younger men . . ." I attempt a smile at that. "You've given up all these good years for your mother; now it's time to live your own life."

I hear these tired old clichés coming out of my mouth, but that's what clichés are — truths retold.

Harriet reaches over and kisses my cheek. "I knew you'd understand. I just didn't want to hurt everyone's feelings. You've all been so good to me. And oh, how I'll miss all of you."

We shed a few tears and we both feel better.

We continue our walk, hearts lightened, and Harriet asks my advice about condos and where to live and is open to my sug-gestions, and I am more than happy to try to help her.

Harriet has forgiven me, but I'm not sure I can forgive myself.

42

Feeling the Blues

The girls are cranky. I won't take them anywhere. Sophie insists her cupboard is empty. Ida must get to the bank. Evvie needs to get to the newspaper office. I just want everyone to leave me alone.

Sophie humphs at that with, "Who do you think you are, Garbo?"

Ida snaps, "Just because you're a big shot, you're too good for us now?"

And Evvie adds her bit. "What's eating you?"

I don't know. Yesterday I felt fine. Today I feel terrible and I don't know why. I have no patience for the girls. I take my phone off the hook. The designated driver, wallowing deep in depression, is not available.

I need to think. I sneak out and go to my sanctuary, the library.

No easy getaway. The celebrity must be waved at and yoo-hooed at and smiled at by one and all, in homage paid to the smart person who realized there was a killer in our midst. Just what I need when I am feeling so confused. I try to avoid everyone, but good old Hy grabs me by the arm as I reach my car. Needless to say Lola is her usual five steps behind.

"My fedora's off to you, Glad. You got some kind of balls. Who knows how many more of you old broads he would have iced."

"Gee, thanks, Hy. I'm glad I lived long enough for such a glowing compliment."

"Lola and me, we knew there was something hinky about old Denny. We would have said something but we didn't want to get the kid in trouble."

"I commend your sensitivity." I sidle past him and get into my car.

"Didja hear the latest dumb blonde joke?"

"Some other time." I rev up the engine, hard, and Hy nervously moves out of the way. Taking my opportunity, I quickly drive off.

At the library, my two buddies greet me warmly. I almost relax in their comforting demeanor. They, of course, have heard the news — the grapevine is working overtime. They want to know what they can do to help. But there is nothing. I confess my agony over avoiding dealing with Denny when I knew he was emotionally in trouble.

"All the symptoms of a breakdown were there right in front of me. Why didn't I act? I have no excuse."

Conchetta pours me the inevitable coffee. "Hey, maybe it's because you're only human. Or maybe you can't take care of the whole world all by yourself. The girls are enough of a handful for one person, don't you think?"

"Or maybe it's because I'm getting old and careless. The damn synapses work slower now. It takes forever to react in time."

Barney hands me a doughnut. "Don't go there. It's not true. You made an error in judgment."

"Esther is dead. Harriet's lost her only relative. And Denny's life is over. I don't call that an error. I call that a tragedy."

"I don't mean to belittle your pain," Conchetta says, "but can't you take this to the next level and maybe you'll feel better? It's over. The killings are stopped."

"I've tried to tell myself the same thing, but it doesn't work. Something still feels out of whack."

I pace agitatedly up and down along the shelves of books as Conchetta and Barney watch me with concern. Books, my old friends, are of no comfort to me now.

"What's bothering you?" Conchetta asks.

"Something. But I don't know what."

"Quick! What pops into your head?" Barney asks. "Don't think, just say it!"

I wheel around and face the both of them.

"It's too damn pat!"

I surprise myself at my intensity and at the words that jump out of my mouth so totally unexpectedly.

My friends watch me, waiting, as in my mind I feel a settling.

"It's not over," I say quietly, and I feel the tight muscles in my back begin to loosen.

43

To Sleep, Perchance to Dream

What a nightmare! It jolts me up from a deep sleep. It's so strong that I find myself sitting bolt upright in bed, heart pounding, body sweating.

I was dreaming about two people dressed as ninja assassins, standing in the middle of Oakland Park Boulevard. Having a tug-of-war. And what a tug-of-war it was! I recognized Denny holding the rope at one end, but his opponent's face was fuzzy and unrecognizable. The rope was made of a daisy chain of white oleander flowers. I remember thinking *How pretty,* until I realized that they were entwined around dead bodies! Selma was there. And Francie and Greta and Esther. But then there was Maureen, and Enya's husband and children who were killed in the Holocaust. And there was Enya on her knees, praying. I could hear her whisper. Injustice, she was crying. Injustice.

It is when the dead bodies all turn to me and open their eyes accusingly that I catapult into wakefulness, and fast. Wow!

Someone once told me that if I had a problem I wanted solved, all I had to do was state it before I fell asleep. And by next morning I'd have my answer. Well, last night I went to bed and framed my question, and asked my subconscious to tell me the answer.

I got my answer; now all I have to do is interpret it.

Forget about falling back to sleep. I am wide awake and my mind is going a hundred miles an hour. I make a pot of coffee, but it takes two pots to keep me going. Another night of hardly any sleep. I'll be a wreck tomorrow, but who cares.

So I pace and think and pace and think and talk to myself out loud. I can feel the pieces falling into place. Click. Click. Click. And then I make notes and I'm still at it when it gets light.

I remember my grandchildren, when they were small, loving Bugs Bunny and that funny thing he always said when he made a huge mistake. Well, Bugs, so did I. Boy, did I make a left turn at Albuquerque.

I go over and over my conclusions, and now all I have to do is prove them. Not easy, that. But I know I'm right. Everything fits. I have to tip an imaginary hat to my opponent, tugging at the other end of Denny's oleander rope. I have to give the devil its due.

Plain and simple, *I've been had!* All of us have.

First things first. I have to be patient until Detective Langford gets to his office. I need to ask him one question.

Then I need to get permission to visit Denny. He has all the answers. Only he doesn't know it.

Look out, world. Here comes Gladdy Gold, Private Eye. On track at last!

44

Poor Denny

I'll bet Detective Morgan Langford hadn't had time for his first bitter cup of police department coffee before my call came in. I guessed right and he tells me so.

"How come you're calling and how come this early?"

I'm still rattling around in my bathrobe. I'm too wired to bother getting dressed. "I couldn't sleep. There's an important question I have to ask."

"Not to worry. Everything's moving along smoothly. I told you I'd call and keep you in touch."

I can tell from his voice he is giving me only half his attention. He's probably looking through his day's workload. "That's not the question. Did Denny actually confess to killing Esther and the others?"

"Sort of."

"What kind of answer is that?"

"He admitted his dead mother made him do it, but he doesn't remember doing it."

"Doesn't that answer bother you?"

"Not really. Many psychotics admit to hearing voices."

"Yes, but don't they usually remember doing the killing as well?"

"Maybe it's too traumatic to remember. So he shuts that part out."

"Believe me, if you had known Maureen Ryan, *she's* what he'd want to shut out."

"Why is this suddenly so important?"

"I need a favor, Morrie. Excuse me — Detective. I need to see Denny. As soon as possible."

Now I have his full attention. "That's not a good idea. He isn't in very good shape."

"Why? Didn't the marks from the rubber hoses fade away yet?"

"Very funny, Mrs. Gold."

"*I* thought so." I feel like I'm losing him again. He's covering the phone and talking to someone who's come in and I can hear him rattling through papers. "As your possible future stepmother, I'm asking you to do this for me."

"What did you say?"

I knew that would grab him. "This may change everything. I can't tell you any more right now."

"No, not that. Go back to what you said before that."

I play dumb. "What did I say? I forgot."

Langford sighs, and I know I nagged him into giving in. Besides, he owes me. And he knows it. "Maybe you could help. All we got out of him was gibberish. Maybe he'll tell *you* the truth."

"He's already told you the truth, Morrie. At least the truth as he understands it. Denny Ryan has never uttered a lie in his life."

"All right. All right. I'm a busy man here. I'll arrange it and let you know when."

The sight of Denny makes me want to cry. This big man, in such a small, narrow hospital room with bars. He looks like a big bear with all the stuffing knocked out of him, frightened and confused.

"Did you come to take me home, Mrs. Gold?" he asks plaintively.

"I can't do that right now, Denny, but I do want to help you." Carefully I put my hand in my purse and turn on my tape recorder. I have a feeling I'm going to need it later. Forgive me, Denny.

"I don't like it here."

I look around at the plainness and the coldness. "I don't blame you."

"There's no window. How can I see the sunshine? I need the sunshine."

"I know you do."

"Why am I here?"

"Don't you know?"

"Because of Mama, isn't it?"

Denny is seated on his narrow cot, his legs spread wide, his hands splayed across his knees. How does this poor man sleep at night in that tiny bed? I sit down opposite him on the edge of the one small chair in the room. Our knees are almost touching.

"Is that why you've been so upset lately? Because of your mother?"

He hangs his head, ashamed. "Yes. I'm sorry I've been so mean to you."

"It's all right. I know you didn't mean it. Tell me about your mother."

"That's what those policemen kept asking me, and I told them but they wouldn't believe me. They got me all mixed up. Why did she have to come back? Everything was so good."

"I believe you, Denny. When did she come back?"

"The night before her birthday."

Bingo! I'm excited but I don't show it. I make a quick calculation in my head. Two weeks before Selma died. "How did she come back?"

"She called me on the phone. Ten o'clock in the night."

"The phone? Just like that?" I keep my chatter nonthreatening and interested.

"Yeah. I just finished watching the wrestling show. I like that show and they really don't hurt each other, it's just for pretend." He smiles, then remembers where he is. "And the phone rang and I answered thinking maybe one of the ladies had a problem. Like last week Mrs. Fox thought she had a cricket in the bedroom but it was only the smoke alarm. She was so funny. When I came in she was standing on a chair and hitting the alarm box on the ceiling with a broom and trying to kill the cricket." He laughs hard at that and I join him.

His face turns ashen. "But it wasn't one of my ladies. It was *her!*" He reaches for a cup of water and his hand is shaking. "At first I didn't believe it, she sounded so funny. I could hardly understand her. I thought somebody was playing a joke, like Mr. Hy Binder likes to fool me. But she said it was her and what did I expect, she was calling from a billion miles away. I said yeah, yeah, like they got phones in heaven. Then she got mad and yelled at me and called me Dennis like she used to when she was mad, and said I better pay attention because she came back for a reason."

My God, I think to myself. This is not of

heaven, but of hell.

"And she tells me the names of the CDs on my shelf over my bed and the plants I got in my garden. I didn't have CDs or a garden seven years ago. How does she know all this stuff I ask her? She tells me she can see me plain from up there. She sees everything I do and hears everything I say." He lowers his head in misery. "She always could. Know everything I did."

"Why did she come back, Denny?"

"Because I killed her, that's why."

Oh, no, I think. Not that. "Why do you say you killed her?"

"Because I had this fight with her. I got mad because she wouldn't let me go to the movies, so I ran out. Then Mama ate that steak and choked on it. It was all my fault, because I wasn't there."

"But you didn't kill her. It was an accident." Such guilt this boy suffered all these years.

"She said I had to pay."

"How?"

"By killing all the nice ladies. Every night she called me. Every single night 'til it made me sick and she just kept calling me and she wouldn't let me alone. And then she left that rat in my bed. I didn't want to do those bad things, but she made me. I loved Miss Francie." Denny starts to cry.

"Did you kill them, Denny?" I can hardly breathe waiting for his answer.

"She said I did it when I was sleeping, but I don't remember. But I must have, 'cause they're dead, aren't they?"

"The night Mrs. Feder died, tell me about it."

"Mama called and told me I had to go over there right now and carry some rolls she left in the kitchen. I didn't even know there were rolls in the kitchen, but there they were in a little basket."

Denny puts his head in his hands, shaking hard, as if to rid himself of the demon mother inside.

I take his hands in mine and hold them. "It's all right, Denny. Tell me what you did then."

He looks at me with tormented eyes. "I didn't do nothing. I just stood there in the kitchen. I didn't want to hurt Mrs. Feder. But if I didn't . . ." His eyes tear.

"How long did you stay there?"

"Maybe an hour. But I had to do what Mama said. So I went outside. I looked careful each way — she said make sure nobody saw me — so I went across the street and went inside, and just then Mrs. Feder started screaming she was dying and she ran in the street and I ran out after her."

"Did she eat any of the rolls you brought?"

"No. Like I told you, I just got there."

"The garden, Denny. I need you to tell me something."

Denny frowns, worried. "Everything's gonna die if nobody waters."

"I promise your garden will be taken care of. The white flowers, Denny, where did you buy them?"

He smiles. "Aren't they pretty, those whachamacallits? I always like to read the little tag that comes on them, but those flowers never got a tag."

"They're called oleander."

I watch his face for a reaction and there is none. He doesn't have a clue. "They didn't have a tag when you bought them? That's unusual."

When he answers me, my heart skips a beat.

"I didn't buy them. They were a present."

"From whom, Denny?" I know the answer, but I need to hear him say it. When he does, I send a silent prayer to God to thank Him.

I promise Denny he'll be home soon, and that's a promise I intend to keep.

45

Scavenger Hunt

I call an emergency meeting of the Gladiators and they march promptly up to my apartment where the coffee and bagels are already waiting. Why is it nothing can be done without food as part of the proceedings? The girls are all atwitter. Anything out of the ordinary is met with eagerness.

I tell them we are going on a scavenger hunt.

"You mean like when we were kids?" Evvie asks me.

"Something like that." I don't dare tell them about my visit to Denny and its result. It would blow them away, and within five minutes, since they are incapable of keeping a secret, everyone in the building would hear about it. That mustn't happen. What we accomplish today is crucial.

I'm encouraging their nosiness. As Sherlock would say, the game is afoot. I dramatically announce that by the end of today they will be amazed and dumbfounded. It will be a day they will never forget. I can sense them fairly drooling with anticipation. You want to know the secret of staying alive? Stay curious.

Well, that sure got their juices going and they started a barrage of questions, like what are we doing and why and where and when, which I immediately nip in the bud.

"Listen, dear friends and sister. Later for questions and answers. Now we have work to do."

I hand them each a sheet of paper and they read what's written with puzzled looks.

"But what does it mean? . . ." starts Bella, and I shush her.

"Just do everything it says to do, and over dinner tonight you'll find out. I know it doesn't make sense right now. It will later."

"But —" says Sophie.

"No buts."

"I really, really need to ask this question," Sophie says pleadingly. "Where are we eating?"

"No place you've ever eaten before."

They are all so excited they can hardly contain themselves. "At least give us a name," says Bella.

I smile. I am on such a high today that I feel silly. So, I improvise. *"Dinner at the Homesick Restaurant."*

"Huh," says Ida. "I never heard of it."

"Or you can join me at *My Dinner With André*."

"Who's he? You're bringing a stranger?" asks Sophie.

"You might like the *Fried Green Tomatoes at the Whistle Stop Cafe*."

"That sounds awful," says Ida.

"Or how about *Dinner at Eight*?"

"But you said five," Bella wails in confusion.

I stop. This is cruel, since they haven't a clue to what I'm talking about. Except for Evvie, who's beginning to catch on and is watching me as if I've got a screw loose. "I'm only teasing. You'll learn the name of where we're eating when we get there. Come on, get in the spirit of the game."

The girls study their sheets of paper.

"I need the applesauce crumb cake in an hour," I say to Ida. It's her finest creation. "Can you do it?"

"Of course," she says proudly.

"But we already talked to Meals on Wheels," Evvie reminds me.

"Go in person. That might jog their memories," I say.

"How are we supposed to get around? Are you driving us?" Ida demands to know.

"No, I have my own errands to run. Take taxis."

"Taxis?" Sophie, the cheapskate, asks in horror. "Spend our own money?"

"All right," I say wearily. "I'll pay you back."

"I see a lot of walking on this one," Ida points at her paper.

"A little real exercise won't kill you."

"Every phone booth?"

"Every single one."

"So, what's the prize?" Sophie asks. "For winning the scavenger hunt."

Evvie shakes her head. "We're all doing this together, Soph. There's no winner."

"Oh."

"Believe me," I tell them, "you'll all be winners. Now the most important thing of all: Tell nobody anything! Talk to no one. And I mean *no one*. Not one person! Can you do that?"

I get a chorus of yeah, sures.

"This is a matter of life and death. No mistakes this time." This is my only reference to the Kronk cremation catastrophe and they hear me loud and clear. Now I get steady nods of assent.

"Promise. Swear to me on your children's heads."

This is the most serious of all promises, and one by one they swear.

And we are off and running.

46

Book Soup

The girls haven't stopped talking about food the whole drive over here. Visions of pot roasts and chicken livers dance in their heads, so naturally when I stop the car at the Lauderdale Lakes public library they are puzzled. Especially since the library is closed.

I give no explanations. I walk to the back entrance, I knock three times for dramatic effect, and it is unlocked for us by Conchetta. With Barney right alongside. I do the introductions. Conchetta Aguilar and Barney Schwartz meet my girls. They all shake hands, most bewildered. And even more so when Barney identifies them by the books they read that I take out for them.

"Bella," he says. "The lady of the romance novels. Large print. And Evvie and her Hollywood biographies and Ida who likes best-sellers and Sophie who likes *Reader's Digest*."

Evvie beams. She's getting into the spirit of this. "So that's what you meant when you called off the names of restaurants. They were book titles. And a few movies, too."

I wink at her, but Ida is not pleased. "OK," Ida says, hands on hips. "Just what is going on here?"

"Yeah," says Sophie, whose mind is never far from the subject of food, glaring at me, "I thought we were going out for dinner."

"We are out. And we are going to have dinner. What we have to do tonight is very private, and this is as private as we can get."

"I brought in food that I cooked at home," Conchetta says cheerfully, leading us into the main reading room. There along the checkout counter are hot plates with an assortment of covered dishes. "I hope you'll like Cuban food."

There is much consternation at this.

"What's Cuban food?" Bella asks nervously.

"Hot and spicy," Barney says mischievously.

Conchetta jabs him. "You know I kept the spices down."

The girls peer suspiciously into each pot as Conchetta lifts the lids and identifies them. "*Potaje de frijoles negros, masa de puerco fritas* with mango sauce, fried plantains and rice, with *boniato* and chimichurri." She opens all but the last.

"I never eat beans," says Ida, recognizing only one word. "They give me the gas."

I grab a plate. "Well, I'm excited here. I can hardly wait to try these."

The girls continue to hang back, except for Evvie who also takes a plate. "Hey, I'm game to try anything. What's a plantain, Conchetta?"

"Like bananas."

"And chimi . . . whatever?"

"That's a green sauce with garlic and lime juice you can dip your bread in. I'll finish translating. The *masa de puerco* is a pork dish. *Boniato* is sweet potatoes. *Mojo* is another sauce. And the *potaje* is a wonderful black bean soup."

So Conchetta, Evvie, Barney, and I pile up our plates, but there is no forward movement from the others.

Barney breaks into laughter first. "Let's put the girls out of their misery," he says as he unveils the contents of the last pot. "Stuffed cabbage, for the less adventurous of the Jewish delegation. Compliments of my mom."

Needless to say there is a rush on the stuffed cabbage.

"Save room for the apple strudel afterwards," he adds, grinning.

As we spread out at the library tables, which Conchetta has set prettily for us with tablecloths and linen napkins, I glance over the pages Barney hands me: their research on oleander. I nod vigorously. "I knew it!" I say victoriously.

"You were right on target. From the time the victims ingest, they go through severe abdominal pain and heart palpitations, paralysis, then death."

"But it takes an hour or so before they die, and that's the big issue here," I say.

The girls look at me, befuddled.

"Isn't it about time you filled us in, Glad?" Evvie asks. "Why are we getting phone numbers of telephone booths and visiting Meals on Wheels?"

"In a moment, the big picture." I smile as I see Bella and Sophie, one by one, taking tiny portions of Conchetta's food, liking what they taste and coming back for more. Not so Ida, of course. "Did anyone at Meals remember anything?"

"You were right about going to see them," Evvie says. "One volunteer remembered that on the date that Selma died, someone ordered a meal, then at the last minute came in and insisted they better

330

deliver it themselves to a frightened elderly aunt. He remembered it because it never, ever happens that way."

"Good. Good. Could he identify the person?"

Evvie shakes her head. "He didn't think so. All he remembers was someone in a baseball cap and sunglasses."

"But at least we know it happened. And the phone booths? How many did you find?"

"Five of them, between Lanai Gardens and across the street at the Florida Medical Center," reports Sophie.

"Excellent."

"And what about my applesauce crumb cake?" Ida asks. "What on earth was that for?"

"To bribe a chubby bank teller, who loves to eat, to do the unthinkable — give me confidential information. Which she did."

"So, all right already, I'm about to bust from not knowing," Sophie says. "So, tell us already!"

"Since we're in a library, let me tell you all about it — in a story."

47

The Very Sad Story
of a Very Foolish Mother

Six pairs of eyes are riveted on my face. Six sets of ears are listening to my every word. Dinner is forgotten. Even dessert is forgotten. Not a chair is allowed to squeak. Since the earliest campfire, the storyteller has held his audience enthralled as he spun out tales that made the dark a little lighter and life a little clearer. And so I, a storyteller, begin my tale.

"Once upon a time there lived a very foolish old woman. After her husband died the old woman was afraid of being alone. Since she had no one in the world but her daughter, she was determined to make her daughter live with her and take care of her. The daughter didn't want to, so the old lady pretended to be crippled and tricked the daughter into moving in."

I already hear the whispers starting.

"The old woman happened to be quite rich."

"Shush," Evvie hisses.

"But she wouldn't share any of her money with her daughter. This turned out to be her biggest mistake. So what little money the daughter had was what she earned at her job, or what her mother doled out to her. This made the daughter very angry. She couldn't stand her mother, but she pretended to everyone that she loved her. All the while she kept waiting for her mother to die. Her mother boasted how long people in her family lived, and she just kept on living."

There's more whispering and plenty of speculating.

"Be quiet!" Evvie says.

"The daughter finally got tired of waiting." And here I stop for a very long attention-getting pause. Then softly, "So Harriet Feder decided to kill her mother."

Suddenly all movement comes to an abrupt halt. Dead silence. Then all hell breaks loose.

"What!" Evvie cries out.

"Say that again!" Ida says.

"What are you talking?" Sophie asks.

"Why didn't I bring my hearing aid?" Bella whines. "What did she just say?"

"Harriet wanted to kill her mother!" Evvie exclaims.

Ida is about to explode. "Harriet!? But what about Denny? I thought yesterday he admitted killing Esther!"

Sophie is benign about change. "So, today he didn't."

"Oy, could we start all over again?" Bella whines, leaning her good ear in.

"Then who killed the other girls?" Sophie asks.

"She killed them all."

I promised them they would be amazed. And dumbfounded.

"Glad, are you sure?" Evvie asks.

"All the pieces fit. It's the only thing that makes sense."

The uproar and general carrying-on stops abruptly because I start talking again, and they aren't about to miss one single breath of the rest of *this* story.

"But Harriet knew if she killed Esther, no matter how cleverly she did it, she would still be the prime suspect, especially when it would come out eventually that her mother was worth nearly four hundred thousand dollars."

Another round of sputtering.

"Oy gevalt," Bella cries.

"You found that out at the bank, with my applesauce crumb cake!" Ida shrills triumphantly.

I smile. She's got it.

"That's a lot of money, four thousand dollars," Bella says.

"Not four thousand, forty thousand," says Sophie in amazement.

"Everybody needs hearing aids around here," Ida says impatiently. "That was *four hundred thousand!*"

Sophie reaches nervously for her strudel. "Who could have so much money besides a Donald Trump?"

"I am going to smack the next one who opens her mouth!" says Evvie angrily. "*I am trying to hear this!*"

Everyone quiets down. For the moment. I continue.

"So she came up with this idea. What if there was a serial killer loose who was murdering old women, and poor Esther just happened to be one of them? But Harriet decided a phantom serial killer was too risky. It had to be someone who could be caught so that she'd never be suspected. And she found the perfect patsy: simpleminded Denny."

Bella gets so agitated, she falls off her chair. Barney and Conchetta help her back on.

I'm determined not to let anything sidetrack me, and I just keep talking.

"So she did some snooping and found out exactly how Maureen Ryan died. Maureen died while eating food. Died reaching for the phone. Died on the night before her birthday. So Harriet recreated the pattern. The food our unlucky friends would eat would be poisoned. And where would she get the poison? Why, from the oleander that happens to grow in Denny's garden, a plant Harriet gave Denny as a present."

"I still don't know how Francie would eat a flower," Sophie insists.

"My very clever friends, Conchetta and Barney, did some research. Guess what they learned from Harriet's hospital résumé?"

"She used to work in a lab?" Evvie guesses.

"Right on," Barney says. "Toxicology is one of her specialties."

"So the die was cast as to who would be the victims: the next birthdays to come up in Phase Two before Esther's. If you recall, Harriet managed to point out to us how nice it was that Denny made a birthday calendar of everyone in our Phase. Calling our attention to Denny knowing everyone's birthday."

This time Evvie interrupts. "That was

when we were clearing out Francie's apartment. She just showed up. And said she was too sad about Francie to go to work."

I nod. "She planted the hint so that I would figure out that it was too coincidental that these women would die in order of their birth dates. Three birthdays came up before her mother's. Selma, then Francie. However, lucky Eileen O'Connor became rightfully nervous, and saved her life by going to her sister in Boca Raton."

"And she doesn't even like her sister," Sophie has to add.

"Greta Kronk, who prowled around at night, probably saw Harriet going in and out of Francie's apartment, so she had to die, too. Then everything was set up for the one murder she was waiting for: her mother."

I am aware that it's very quiet now. I think they're all in shock. I take Denny's tape out of my purse and put it on the table.

"Now she had another problem to solve. How to pin it on Denny. Happy-go-lucky Denny. Who would believe he'd kill anyone? She had to make it look like Denny was having a breakdown. She had to drive him crazy. How? She brought back his awful mother from the grave to haunt him."

"*Jesucristo,*" Conchetta says, crossing herself. "The woman is a devil!"

"Maureen is back?" Sophie asks in amazement.

"I never did like that woman," Ida says.

"I went to see Denny yesterday and he told me all about it."

"Wait a minute," Evvie interrupts. "You went to jail without me?" Then she stops, chagrined. "Sorry."

"You can hear it on this tape. Denny, who had been terrified of his mother when she was alive, actually believed she had returned from the dead to frighten him again. Calling him up on the phone every single night and tormenting him."

"Wait a minute," Bella asks. "She could call from heaven?"

Ida snorts. "How do you know it wasn't from hell?"

"Whatever," Bella says, "they're both long-distance. Maybe it was only from the cemetery. That's local. Do you think she used an eight-hundred number?"

"Will you silly twits stop it!" Evvie says. "Maureen is dead. Harriet was making the calls!"

"Oh, so how was I supposed to know that?" Bella says, feeling put upon.

I continue relentlessly. "Harriet called

Denny from different phone booths, either near the apartment when she was home so she could sneak in and out quickly, or near the hospital when she was on night shift. She didn't use her home phone because that could be traced."

"The phone booths you sent us to today," Sophie says, finally getting it.

"And so, pretending to be Maureen, she told Denny he had to kill Selma first, then the others. She really did a job gaslighting him."

"I remember that movie," Evvie says, "with Charles Boyer and Ingrid Bergman. It was named after a light fixture."

"She actually got Denny to believe he did the killings, even though he kept saying he didn't remember. She told him he did it in a trance. Since Esther was going to be the last murder, he had to be caught."

I stop to take a drink. My mouth is dry. The girls are itching to ask questions, but I motion them to wait until I'm finished.

"She had it timed perfectly. She cold-bloodedly fed her mother dinner with poisoned poppy-seed rolls."

Sophie can't stand it. She has to interrupt. "Esther told us she'd never eat food from a stranger!"

"Well, she didn't," says Bella.

"Better she lived with a stranger than that daughter from hell," Ida adds.

"Then later she tells us she had to leave early for the hospital, thus establishing her alibi. She calls Denny, as Maureen, and tells him he must go to Esther's house immediately with the other rolls she left in his kitchen. By that time the poison would have taken effect, Denny would be at the scene of the crime, and we'd be home from the movies in time to catch him."

"But we got home late from the movies —" Evvie starts.

"And let's remember whose idea it was for us to go to that movie," Ida says, arms crossed, brimming with outrage. She mimics Harriet. 'You girls go out and relax. You'll be home just when I'm going to work. We're covered. So have a good time.' That *farbissener!*"

"She needed us to be away from Esther's apartment," Evvie says, feeling awful. "She knew us all too well. I feel so ashamed."

"She conned everybody, Ev. But it turns out this time Denny didn't obey his 'mother.' He stayed home for an hour before he could bring himself to leave. And we were delayed that long getting home. It didn't matter. Denny was caught red-handed leaving her apartment anyway."

Barney pours us all another round of sangria. Bella is fanning herself; the wine is getting to her.

He says, "I'll bet she was in some sweat when the call didn't come in at the hospital at the time she expected, with the sad news about her poor, dear, dead mother."

I continue. "She needed one more element for this vile crime to work. She had to make sure the first deaths were seen as murders and not heart attacks. She certainly couldn't be the one to point that out, and that's where yours truly came in. The next perfect sucker. I began to suspect on my own, but she had to make sure I went down the trail she pointed out, and that explains why Harriet Feder, who never seemed to be able to escape her mother, suddenly was always available. Wherever we were, she turned up. I kept looking for someone whose behavior had changed, and it took me a long time to realize it was Harriet's."

Evvie says, "So that's why she was able to show up in the clubhouse when we had our big meeting."

"And I bet she took her vacation just so she could keep an eye on us." Ida sniffs with righteous indignation.

"That's how she found out everything

we knew," Evvie says.

"She really did have Esther spying on us for her!" says Ida.

"She didn't make any mistakes, did she?" Conchetta asks.

"But she did. She left a piece of the Meals on Wheels package in Selma's apartment," says Evvie.

"No mistake," I say. "That was her way of leading us away from heart attack to someone who came to Selma's apartment to poison her. Someone delivering Meals on Wheels."

"Aha," says Sophie, now seeing it. "She picked up the food, poisoned it, and then delivered it to poor Selma, may she rest in peace."

"I get it," says Ida. "She also left the cake crumbs in Francie's sink. But the cleaning lady cleaned up before you figured that out."

"You can bet she arranged it so that poor Denny would find the bodies, further freaking him out," I add. "Then she points it out to us, the 'coincidence' of Denny having a master key and finding the bodies."

Barney is puzzled. "But why so elaborate a plan? Why not murder the women outright, rather than go to such lengths to make it seem like heart attacks at first?"

Evvie is so excited, she's fairly jumping out of her chair. "Wait a minute. She knew you wanted a body to autopsy, a body that would prove it was murder, yet Harriet's the one who got us to get Greta cremated."

"It was all about timing," I say. "That would have the cops investigating too soon, and that might have gotten in the way of killing her mother. And she couldn't wait until after her mother had died to get us to think about the earlier murders. Suspicion would immediately fall on her. She couldn't take that chance."

Barney is incredulous. "She makes Lizzie Borden seem like an angel."

"Four hundred thousand is a lot of incentive," I say. "Can you imagine her frustration? Year after year knowing she was rich and not being able to get at the money."

We're all exhausted, especially me. We drink our wine and nibble at our dessert, lost in our troubled thoughts.

"What put you on to her, Glad?" Barney wants to know. "I mean I have to hand it to her, it was a perfect plan."

"It was almost perfect. My realizing that Greta Kronk didn't write the last poem, and Denny arriving too late with the rolls, got me thinking. I just could not believe, no how, that Denny could kill anyone. Nor could Denny have written that poem or managed the sophisticated ways she got the poison to each of them. If she hadn't tried to set him up, I might never have figured it out."

"She outsmarted herself. We've got to call Detective Langford," Evvie says, tugging at me. "Right now. Tell him everything."

"Yeah," says Sophie, "put that *kurveh* in jail and let poor Denny out!"

"So why are you waiting?" asks Bella.

Barney says, "I think I know. Everything we've heard tonight — it's all circumstantial."

"What's that mean?" Sophie asks.

"It means even if Langford agrees with us, we can't prove a thing."

"But you said she made a mistake with the poppy-seed rolls," says Evvie.

"Still not proof. It could be argued that Denny made her eat the rolls earlier as well."

"So how is your story going to end?" Bella asks worriedly.

"You aren't going to let her get away with it?" Ida demands.

All eyes look to me for a solution. I've already given this a lot of thought and I share it with all my helpers.

"If we want a happy ending, we're gonna have to do the impossible. We're going to have to make Harriet Feder confess."

My coconspirators look at me as if I'm crazy.

"Why would she do a stupid thing like that?" Evvie wants to know.

"I think I have an idea," I tell them.

48

Now What Do We Do?

Detective Langford and I have been talking for a very long while. He's actually told his switchboard not to interrupt us, although a number of police personnel have looked in the door to get a glimpse of me. Who knows what he's told them, but it can't be too bad, because they're smiling.

He's read my summary of why I know Harriet is the murderer. And listened to Denny's tape. He's questioned me on every single point until I'm hoarse from talking. Finally he stops.

"Gladdy Gold, you are an amazing woman."

"So," I say impatiently, "does that mean you think I'm right or not?"

"I'll tell you what makes me sure you're right. Something you don't even know yet."

"What's that?" I smile. Justified at last.

"Something very odd came up in Esther's autopsy. There were bruises all over her body that were unexplained. The medical examiner wondered if they were self-inflicted, since all the contusions were in places she could get to. Thanks to your very thorough analysis, we know now that Harriet abused her mother."

I gasp, then shake my head and feel such overwhelming sorrow for Esther. "Oh, God, that, too?"

"And for a long time. There were very old bruises as well."

I jump up, agitated. Morrie looks at me, surprised. "Sorry," I say, "you really threw me with that."

I walk around the room to calm myself. There's a wall of black-and-white photos. Morrie at his cop graduation. Morrie posing with a huge marlin that he caught. Morrie and his dad, Jack, and his mom, Faye, circa 1970, arms around one another. Jack with dark curly hair. Yes, I think, I do remember Faye.

"Gladdy, you still with me?"

I turn back to Morrie. "Esther joked to us about being beaten, but of course, we didn't believe her. We thought it was her pathetic attempt to get attention, but it was a cry for help, wasn't it? And Harriet probably beat her even more every time she did that."

"Sad, but probably true."

"Why didn't Esther just give her the damn money?" I cry out, frustrated.

"Probably because she knew Harriet would leave her, and being alone seemed worse to her. We'll never know."

"So what do we do now?"

"You're right. It is circumstantial. We could bring her in for questioning, and what we would get is a poor, grieving daughter, highly insulted and how dare we say such things? She will deny, deny, deny. This kind of woman won't crack because she knows we don't have any proof."

"But what if we do a lineup — the man in Meals on Wheels might identify her."

"But you said that the guy *thinks* he remembers someone in a baseball cap. And he wasn't very sure at that."

"She could have been seen at one of the phone booths."

"We can try asking around, but I'll bet she was very careful. Probably disguised herself there as well."

"What about at the lab? Maybe someone saw her boiling the oleander —" I stop myself. Harriet was never careless. I'm dejected. "We can't let her get away with it."

"Don't give up. Even though the evidence is purely circumstantial, people have been convicted on it. We won't let her walk."

"What can you do?"

"Start a full investigation. We'll follow through on every single piece of information you've given us. Hopefully, we'll get her in time."

"Can you stop the bank from giving her Esther's money?"

"Unfortunately, no. Had it been insurance money, it would have been a different story."

"Unless Esther didn't leave it to her." I know I'm kidding myself. "I'm sure she did."

"We'll find out."

"An investigation could take a long time and she might still get away with it, couldn't she?"

"It's possible."

I shrug. "I may have an idea. I think I could get her to confess."

He takes a long look at me. "And what miracle are you thinking of performing, Gladdy Gold?"

"Think about it. We have a real advantage right now. She has no idea we're on to her. She's happy. She's packing. She's shopping for a new place to live. She's smug. She thinks she fooled us all. Maybe we can catch her off guard."

"How?"

"I may know a way to trap her."

Morrie Langford leans back in his chair, puts his feet up on the desk, and grins at me. "You solved the case and now you're gonna trap the killer. I am very impressed. This I gotta hear."

So I told him.

49

Poor Harriet

"Doesn't it seem like a lot of people are at the pool today?" Harriet asks me as we walk toward the clubhouse.

I answer her in this perky mode I've affected for the occasion. I'm hoping it hides my stark terror. I'm also wearing my brightest orange-peel sundress, hoping color will give me courage. "Just another beautiful day in sunny Florida, and the natives are taking advantage."

I fling a casual wave toward the sunbathers, and a few casually wave back. But most of them ignore us.

"How funny," Harriet says. I glance over to where she's looking, and there are my girls dressed for swimming. Then I realize what she's commenting on. Next to each of their lounge chairs is a peculiar object — a bathroom plunger, a fly swatter, a rolling pin. I groan inwardly. I told them to bring weapons. That's what they brought!

I move along quickly. I don't want her lingering. "You never know when you'll need a fly swatter," I toss back at her.

She catches up to me. "Your friends are so quaint."

Needless to say the usual Muzak is playing over the loudspeaker at full volume.

We pass the pool, make a right at the palm tree, and arrive at the clubhouse.

"Oooh, how sweet," says Harriet, feigning delight, as she sees the huge, garish sign over the door. The girls and their helpers really put their all into it, using lots of Day-Glo colors. It reads, for my taste, low on subtlety:

"Farewell Harriet,
We Hope You Get All You Deserve!"

"We really shouldn't be here 'til everyone arrives for the party; we'll spoil the surprise," I say, all sugary, "but I wanted to give you my gift in private."

"And I can't wait to see it. I really always thought of you as my favorite person."

"Why, thank you. I'm honored."

"It's because you're the only smart one around here."

Or so gullible, Harriet? "No, you're really the smart one."

We go inside, and the girls have done a great job. Multicolored streamers everywhere. Lots of balloons. All kinds of photos. And a great big sign reading, *"Good-bye Harriet, So You'll Never Forget Us,"* and signed by just about everyone in Phase Two.

Harriet puts her hand over her heart. "I am so touched."

She wanders around the room looking at the photos and the pretty little flower baskets made for the tables, while I move around fiddling with this and that.

Finally she turns back to me, eyes wide in anticipation, and I smile with equal brightness.

"So what's this wonderful mysterious gift you're giving me?"

I take a deep breath and plunge in. "Me."

She looks puzzled, and rightly so. "Me, what?"

"Just me. I am giving you the gift of me. Since you've lost that dear, sweet woman, your mother, I am offering to take her place in your heart."

Her voice is getting this teeny-tiny edge. "Gladdy, what are you talking about?"

"Well, you're about to blow this joint and have a wonderful life, and I want to share it with you."

Her eyes are like slits now. "I'm afraid

I'm still not following you."

"No, it's *me* wanting to follow *you.* I see us taking trips around the world. I always did want to see Paris. And maybe after that, buying a gorgeous mansion somewhere. I'd like to suggest the Bahamas. That's always been another dream of mine. With four hundred thousand dollars you can buy anything!"

Her hand grips a chair now, very tightly, I notice. She forces out a phony laugh. "Wherever did you get an idea like that?"

"A little birdy told me." I giggle nervously. "A chubby little bird at the bank."

"How dare anyone discuss my personal finances!" Harriet knows exactly who I mean. "I'll have that fat pig fired!"

Chalk one up for the home team. She isn't denying it. And it's nice to see her temper has a short fuse.

Then she realizes what she's admitted, and pulls up short. "I hope you'll keep my little secret," she says coyly.

"Why on earth would your mother live here if she had all that do-re-mi?" I ask in all innocence.

"My mother was very eccentric. I didn't want anyone to know. It was very embarrassing for me to be here, when we could have gone anywhere. You can see that."

"I certainly can, and now that you are free to do anything you want, I want to share in your fun."

"Will you stop saying that!" She actually stamps her foot.

I smile. She's starting to lose it.

She pulls herself back under control. "You're acting very strangely today, Glad. It's not like you."

"That's 'cause I'm giddy with excitement. I see a chance for me to get out of this dump and live in the manner to which I'd like to get accustomed. After all I did for you, I deserve it."

Harriet is having trouble holding still. She moves erratically around the tables, her fingers beating little tattoos on their surfaces. I can sense she'd like to walk out right now, but she has to find out what I know.

"Just exactly what did you do for me?"

"I helped you get away with murdering your mother." I say it very calmly and I'm proud of myself. Considering my heart is pounding and my stomach is in a knot the size of Chicago. I want out of here myself. It's the memory of Francie, who died for nothing, that keeps me going.

She stops moving and stands very still. I can almost hear the wheels clicking.

"I mean I didn't know I was doing that, but you so cleverly led me down that garden path, and little old me just did everything you wanted me to."

I can't take my eyes off her because I'm scared to death of what she might do. And believe me, she can't take her eyes off me. So I babble on.

"That's just it, you see. You wanted me smart and you wanted me dumb. You can't have it both ways. I needed to be smart enough to pick up all the clues you left for me, so I would come to the conclusion that Selma and Francie had been murdered. It wouldn't do for the medical reports to remain heart attacks. Then you wouldn't be able to kill your mother, who was really the intended victim. You needed a serial killer to take the heat away, because otherwise you'd be the prime suspect."

"You're crazy!" she says, low and ominously.

"No, but speaking about crazy — that was brilliant, the way you brought back good old dead Maureen to drive Denny nuts."

"Denny!" she says, almost snarling. "Who gives a shit about that retard! They should have drowned him when he was born!"

I am shaken by the force of her hatred,

but I know I mustn't show it. "Poor, sweet Denny who couldn't kill a mosquito, let alone someone like Francie whom he worshipped! So that's how I finally figured it out — if he didn't do it, you did it. For the money."

Harriet starts toward the door. "I'm walking out of here, you lunatic."

"So, go. What's holding you?"

She stops as I knew she would. "Why are you making this up? What did I ever do to you?"

Now she moves very close to me. I can feel her breath on my skin. She grabs me by the shoulders and shakes me. I hold very still and don't try to resist, though every instinct in me wants to fight her. Or, at least, scream.

"You silly cow!" she hisses in my ear. "Who would ever believe a story like that!" Then she stares into my eyes to see if I'm telling the truth. "Who did you tell?"

I manage to keep my eyes steady. Please, God, let her believe me. "Nobody, yet," I say. "Nobody *ever* — if you take me with you when you leave."

She relaxes her grip and slowly backs away from me. She actually smiles. "So you want to blackmail me, you greedy old fool."

"Something like that," I say, as casually as I can, considering that my jellied knees are about to give way.

"But what about your dear friends, those ugly, stupid women you spend all your time with? How could you bear to leave them?" The fangs are really out now, and her voice is dripping acid.

"Try me. See how fast I pack."

I can feel her analyzing her options. Can she kill me here and now and get away with it? Or should she promise me anything until she can find another Dumpster?

"I don't think so," she says icily. "It's your word against mine. Nobody would believe a senile old fool like you who has nothing to do but read too many murder mysteries."

"They'd believe my proof." I whip out of my pocket a sheet of paper and read: "Five five five-six two four three, five five five-seven seven six three, five five five-five two two eight — need I go on?"

"What the hell's that supposed to be?"

"The phone numbers in the phone booths you used here and next to the hospital to call poor, pathetic Denny every night at ten o'clock. There will be a record of his number being called when I hand it to the police to check."

"That does it!" she shouts, lunging for me. "I've taken enough of your crap!" She knocks me against the wall. I grab at her hair and pull.

"Stop it!" I scream at the top of my lungs, holding on for dear life. "You might have gotten away with beating your mother up all these years, but you won't get away with hurting me!" Instinctively, my eyes look toward the door.

The twisted expression on Harriet's face is terrifying. "Bitch! You're too smart for your own good! Watch me!" She smashes her hand against my mouth and, although I'm in agony, I instinctively bite as hard as I can. She pulls away, shrieking.

"Murderer! Why did you have to kill them that way? Why!?" I shout at her, now crying bitter tears. "They died in such pain!"

Her voice hisses back at me. "Maybe I liked seeing them suffer! Maybe it was *fun* getting rid of you old miserable pieces of garbage! Maybe I was doing society a big favor! Wasting space, still living when you should have died long ago. Who needs you, you pathetic, brain-dead losers. With your goddamn wheelchairs and walkers. With your shriveled-up, useless bodies. Even your families have deserted you. Even they wish you were dead!"

With what little strength I have left, I butt my head into her stomach and ram as hard as I can. With ease, she lifts me away from her and knocks me down on the floor.

"Damn you! You're dead, old lady, you're finished!" she shouts at the top of her lungs.

If ever I heard an exit line, that was it. Practically crawling, I manage to get out the front door as fast as my arthritic knees let me.

And fall into Evvie's arms.

"Come back here, you bitch," Harriet screams, rushing out the door. "I'm not through with you —"

Harriet stops dead in her tracks as she is aware of two things at once. Everyone who was around the pool is now standing in front of the clubhouse. And her voice is reverberating over the loudspeaker: ". . . through with you . . ."

I manage to smile, though every bone in my body is hurting. Harriet stares, thunderstruck. Hostile faces stare back at her, and then she sees Detective Langford, off to one side, grimly looking at her. And next to him is Denny Ryan.

"Hey, Harriet," I say.

Harriet whips around to glare at me.

"I'm sure glad Hy finally taught me how to use the PA system."

50

The New Old
(Not an Oxymoron)

Picture this. Time seems to be standing still. Nobody is moving.

I am reminded of a game we used to play when I was a child, called Statues. (Do kids still play that?) The leader would yell "Freeze!" and everyone would stop immediately, caught in some dramatic pose or another. The leader would turn around and there we'd be, statues frozen in time. Who would move first?

Today it will be Evvie.

She turns toward Langford, terribly upset. "Why didn't you go in to help my sister! Harriet could have killed her!"

"No," I interject. "He was right not to. You know I had to go all the way."

"You did a hell of a job," Langford says to me, slowly starting to walk forward, his eyes never leaving Harriet.

And Harriet's eyes never leave him.

"It was too dangerous. It was crazy to

try it!" Evvie says.

"But it was the only way, dear Evvie."

"With a lot of help from my acting lessons," she adds, finally relaxing, wanting her due.

"You bet," I say, kissing her cheek.

"Do you need a doctor, Gladdy?" Langford asks me as he continues his move toward Harriet.

"I'm fine, really," say I, the stoic, but boy, will I be black and blue tomorrow morning.

"But did you have to call this place a dump?" Ida whispers.

"Yeah," says Sophie, "and couldn't you put in a nice word for us?"

The crowd parts for Langford as if they are the Red Sea, and he, our Moses. Everyone watches him intently.

"I want a lawyer," Harriet says.

"Why do they always say that?" Bella wants to know.

"Harriet Feder," Langford says, "you are under arrest for the murders of Selma Beller, Francine Charles, Greta Kronk, and Esther Feder . . ."

There is much murmuring and sighing at these names. Sophie is practically jumping up and down from the drama of it all.

Bella says, "Again like in the movies."

Sophie pokes her. "This is better than the movies. Come on, let's move closer."

Ida, queen of grudges, is enjoying the sight of payback at last. She announces, "I knew it was her all along."

The other three give her a dirty look.

As Langford continues to recite the Miranda warning, the three girls, holding hands and weapons, move sideways and forward for a better angle. "I hope he pulls out his gun," Bella says, shivering with anticipation.

"Nazi!"

Everyone looks around.

And there is Enya, eyes wild, rushing toward Harriet, hands fashioned into claws. "Nazi!" she is moaning and sobbing. "My *shayner kindlach,* my Jacov . . . They put my beautiful babies to die. Put them out of their misery, they said, pushing them into the ovens. The world would be better off without them, they said. Oh, *Gott im Himmel!* God, where was God?? Why didn't God stop them! Why didn't God stop *you!*" The clawed hands stretch to Harriet's face as if to scratch and tear at it. "*You* are one of them! *Nazi!*"

But the hands go limp, trembling, impotent. Harriet looks down on her, pitiless.

Enya, finding a last bit of strength somehow, spits in her face.

With that, she runs off sobbing.

Silence. Everyone is transfixed by what has just happened. Then someone calls out. "Yes, Nazi!" And a chorus of people echo the vile word, reaching for one another for comfort.

"My God!" Ida says. "She never cried. Never! Not in fifty years!"

Harriet takes a few steps back, wiping at her face, as the group rage builds.

And suddenly there's Tessie pushing past Langford, through the crowd to Harriet, who cringes at the sight of her. Tessie, all two hundred fifty pounds of her, lifts her arm, opens her hand, and smacks Harriet's face with a sound as loud as a gunshot.

"This is for my Selma!" she cries.

The crowd, now caught up in the hysteria, goes wild, moving erratically, yelling and calling her names. Harriet, forgetting caution, begins to run across the lawn away from them. I suddenly find myself thinking of a famous story of long ago, Shirley Jackson's "The Lottery," about a public stoning. Is it turning into that?

"Stop!" Langford shouts at the crowd. Frustrated, because he can't push through the mass of elderly folks, he is stuck.

Utter chaos. "Somebody do something!" A voice in the crowd yells. "Don't let her get away!"

The crowd is now speeding up in Harriet's direction.

"And they're off!" Sol Spankowitz shouts, elbowing Irving as if they were at the starting gate at their beloved Hialeah.

The three Gladiators go rigid in shock as Harriet heads right for where they are standing.

Ida punches Sophie. "Spread out! Block her! Move!"

"A klog iz mi!" Sophie cries. "And me in my flip-flops!"

Puffing away on short, stubby legs, disregarding osteoporosis and every other ailment, the girls spread out and take blockade positions. With weapons aloft, they prepare to attack. Sophie wields her toilet plunger. Bella, her fly swatter. Ida, her rolling pin. Ida, in her usual choler, shouts, "So we're ugly and stupid, are we, you . . . you ugly, revolting . . ."

But they are no match for Harriet, who lifts hundred-pound weights at the gym. She plows through them, knocking them away as if they were bowling pins. Bella is down, still gripping her swatter. The other "weapons" go flying, but amazingly Sophie and Ida manage to cling to Harriet like a couple of swamp leeches. Harriet keeps running, unable to shake them, dragging them behind her as Sophie hangs on to the tail of her blouse and Ida clutches the belt of her pants suit.

Langford is trying to find an opening, but by this time the Red Sea has closed and he is falling farther behind. "Stop! Everyone stop!" he calls. "Let me through!"

Exhausted, Sophie can no longer hold on, and she falls by the wayside, plopping down like a rag doll. Evvie reaches her and, without breaking stride, gets her to her feet and pulls her along.

The crowd of seniors, giving it their all, is still trying to catch up, but at their ages, and physical conditions, and those old legs — not to mention the metal walkers — they don't stand a chance.

Ida, the bulldog, is still clutching the back of the belt of Harriet's pants suit. Her feet are being dragged along, her body almost scraping the lawn, as Harriet tries to shake her off. But she's gamely hanging on, working like an emergency brake and slowing Harriet down a little.

I look for Langford, but he's now on the ground under Tessie, who accidentally tripped over him, God help him.

Sol, still at the track, announces, "Harriet, carrying a one-hundred-ten-pound handicap, is four lengths ahead. Langford is blocked at the far turn. The rest of the pack is losing ground. What a race for a trifecta!" Sol is jumping up and down in excitement. "Whadda ya know — Harriet's now passing the long shot, Denny, who is the only one not running after her!"

That's not quite accurate. Denny and I are the only ones standing still. Evvie left me long ago to join the fray. My body hurts too much to move. But the muscles of my mouth still work. "Denny!" I shout. "Go get her!"

Denny, who has been watching it all, befuddled, reacts to the sound of my voice.

"It's all up to you now!"

His slow mind is processing what I am telling him.

"After all she did to you, don't let her get away!"

Denny may not be swift of mind, but he sure is swift of foot. Like a greyhound after the rabbit, he takes off after Harriet, who is now right in front of him, still lumbered with the stubborn Ida.

And just in time. Ida has finally lost her grip and has tumbled down next to the duck pond. "Shit!" she cries out in disgust, as she realizes what she's landed in. Poor Ida. The ducks quack at her, having had the last laugh.

Denny is breathing down Harriet's neck. She sees him coming and panics. She turns quickly trying to avoid him, but in her confusion she's now running back toward the crowd. Seeing her mistake, she tries to turn again, but Denny is on her. He grabs her by the arm and with the other hand hammerlocks her around the neck, holding fast. The two of them stand there, panting.

Sol catches up to them and starts gesturing with his fists. Now Hy is there, joining Sol, dancing up and down, jabbing along with him. "Hit her. Knock the broad out!"

"Don't lose her!" Irving yells, and he puffs up to them, his hands punching air.

Denny studies the three excited, jabbing men. Harriet is about to break loose.

"You're not my mama!" he yells, and with a neat left uppercut, he knocks Harriet out cold.

Sol grabs Denny's arm and pulls it up high. "The winner and new 'champeen,' Denny Ryan!"

The crowd cheers.

The running stops.

The kvetching begins. "I lost my

glasses." "I need my nitroglycerin." "My bathing suit is ruined." "Does somebody have a seltzer? I have such a thirst."

My girls and Evvie come back to where I'm leaning. They are panting and disheveled. Sophie's lost both of her pool sandals. Ida's French twist has come undone. I won't even describe her clothes. Bella is hyperventilating. I hug them all. "I told you to bring weapons. That's all you could come up with?"

Bella holds up her fly swatter proudly. "There's a lot of flies who wouldn't agree with you."

"You were brave and wonderful and I love you all." We all hug and kiss again.

I'm surrounded by all the well-wishers congratulating me. I thank them profusely for their gallantry. And boy, am I glad no one dropped dead of a heart attack from all that exertion!

"Best entertainment we ever had at the clubhouse," says Mrs. Nettie Fein from Phase Three, tugging at her support hose that came flopping down in the chase.

Yolanda leads Millie to me. They are both giggling. With a terrible Spanish accent Millie says, *"Basura, malo, hasta la vista, bueno."*

"What, in the name of heaven," Evvie

asks, "does that mean?"

Yolanda answers in equally bad English. "I teach Millie, she teach me. Means good riddance, bad rubbish."

Leo, the Sleaze, is smiling. "Gotta hand it to ya, Glad. You took a fixer-upper and turned it into a fast seller!"

"Good show!" chorus the Canadians.

My heart swells with pride that word of mouth brought out nearly fifty "extras" from the other five phases, who turned up to give me moral support and bear witness.

As the accolades keep coming, I glance toward the lawn and watch someone familiar reach down to help Langford up. Morrie balefully looks up into his father's eyes. "You look like hell, boy," I hear Jack Langford saying as he grins. "Wait 'til the guys at the station hear about this. Done in by a bunch of old fogies!"

"Dad!" Morrie says, horrified. "You wouldn't!"

Jack sees me looking. He waves at me and I wave back.

We all watch Detective Morgan Langford (who is not only disheveled, but limping) take the handcuffed, and still groggy, Harriet away.

"I hope she gets the chair," Hy says cheerfully.

"God forbid," Ida retorts. "Life in prison without parole. I wanna see how she likes it when *she* gets old!"

"Like you're gonna be around to find out?" Evvie asks, sarcastically.

I put my arms around Hy and hug him. "No, but Hy will be here. He can tell us."

We all have a great big laugh at that. And it feels wonderful to laugh again.

Do I feel good. Considering how bad I hurt. At last the forgotten ones have had their day. We senior citizens fought back. We reserve our right to live.

We are the new old.

51

All's Well . . .

What a celebration we had last night! All six phases attended. The Manischevitz Malaga kept flowing, the klezmer band kept playing, the deli platters never ran out. I even sneaked in a dance with Jack and the girls never saw us. Which made me face the fact that I haven't gotten around to telling them about him. And wait until Evvie hears. . . . Well, they're going to find out today, heaven help me.

It's ten a.m. and no sign of the troops yet. Probably hungover like everyone else and slept late. Oops, I spoke too soon. Four bleary-eyed faces peer in at me through the open louvers.

"Coffee," a desperate Evvie begs.

"Bagels, or I'll perish," adds Sophie.

"With a schmear," continues Bella.

Ida, as usual, has to be different. "I could go for some scrambled with a little lox. And maybe a slice of Bermuda onion."

"Come on in, the kitchen is open. The cook is up."

In they march. "I'm so tired I could sleep for a month," Sophie announces cheerfully.

"But wasn't it wonderful?" Bella says, sighing. "A day and a night to remember."

Ida says, "My favorite moment was when Denny floored Harriet."

"Mine was seeing you on the grass with the ducks." Sophie chuckles at the memory.

Ida scowls. "You would. My best pool lounging outfit is ruined!"

"Did you see that Enya came to the party?" I comment. "She was actually talking to people."

"And even smiling," comments Sophie.

"So out of killing came a mitzvah. Enya joined the living again." Evvie's eyes tear up.

"And Denny," I say, and this time it's my eyes tearing. "Just sitting there shyly as everyone came up and said how glad they were that he came out all right."

"Wasn't it nice of the Haddassah women in Phase Four to clean up Denny's apartment for him?" Bella says happily.

Ida comments, "I hope they got rid of that battle-ax's portrait. Right smack into the Dumpster!"

"You know what Tessie told me?" Sophie

says. "She's thinking of moving. After knowing what really happened to Selma, she says she can't bear living here next door to her apartment anymore."

"And speaking of moving," Evvie says proudly, "I cornered the Sleaze and told him we're on to him. Don't be surprised if there's a 'for sale' sign on *his* place soon."

"Yeah, that was some party," Sophie says contentedly. "Even the Canadians had fun after a few belts of the Manischevitz."

"But," says Ida, "what I really want to know is who gets Esther's four hundred thousand dollars?"

"Good question." Evvie turns to me. "Glad, maybe you can ask Langford."

"Poor Morrie," I say, laughing. "We totally demoralized him."

"Do we get a reward for catching Harriet?" Bella asks cagerly. "Maybe they'll give *us* the money."

Ida sniffs. "In your dreams."

Bella keeps shaking her head. "I just can't get over it. How could it be?"

"How could what be?" asks Ida.

"Harriet, a killer." Bella reaches for an onion bagel for comfort. "And she was such a nice Jewish girl."

As they pile around the kitchen table, digging into the basket of bagels, they plan the day. Ida must go to the bank, Bella to the cleaners. Sophie looks at me, with my head full of curlers. "Looking at you reminds me. I could use a trip to the beauty parlor. I'm thinking, maybe, of dyeing again. I'm fed up with Champagne Pink. What do you think about Strawberry Blonde?"

"Now that you mention it," says Evvie, eyeing me suspiciously, "what's with the curlers?"

"I'm setting my hair. What does it look like?" It's starting, I think to myself. I am reminded of Bette Davis's famous line in *All About Eve*: "Fasten your seatbelts, it's gonna be a bumpy night."

"Since when?"

"Since today."

Now everybody stops to study me. Ida picks up my hand as if I had leprosy. "Is that nail polish?"

"Curlers? Nail polish? What's going on?" Evvie wants to know.

"I'm giving myself a makeover."

"Since when are you a fashionable plate?" Sophie asks.

"Hey," I throw at them, "you're all big-shot detectives now, so detect."

With time only to grab a macaroon or two for dessert, they have at it.

"You're maybe going somewhere to-night?" Sophie ventures.

"Yes. Out," I answer.

"To the library?" Bella adds.

"Who wears pink polish to a library?" Ida argues.

Sophie is now sniffing about the apartment for clues. Evvie is standing with her arms folded. I can tell she doesn't like this one bit. It feels like it won't be good news for her. And she's right.

Sophie shrieks from the bathroom. "There's a bottle of Chanel Number Five on the sink!"

Evvie glares at me. "You haven't worn perfume since your daughter's wedding eighteen years ago!"

By now Ida and Bella have dashed into the bedroom in time to hear Sophie say, "And take a gander at this!"

Ida calls out. "It's her best silk shantung."

Evvie's voice is ominous now. "Ditto worn at the same wedding."

"Not really," I correct her. "That was blue. This one's green. It's only seven years old."

"And her good fake pearls," Bella now calls. "With the matching teardrop earrings."

The girls all converge back in the dining area. Now everyone is staring at me.

"I detect," says Ida officiously, "since you're getting so gussied up, you are going someplace nice."

"I also detect," says Bella, "since you didn't tell us about it, you're going by yourself."

"Where would you go alone?" Evvie demands to know. "You take me everywhere."

I take a deep breath and plunge in. "Who said I was going alone?"

Silence. Finally, "So . . . who are you taking?" Ida demands.

"Actually, I'm going on a date."

Shock. Surprise. Consternation.

"Waddaya talking?" Sophie says, irritated. "You haven't had a date in a hundred years!"

I smile. "Not quite. It only seems like it."

"A date?" Evvie asks, genuinely startled.

"Really? A date?" Bella asks, grinning.

"Don't I speak English? A. Date. With. A. Man!"

"Impossible," Evvie says. "What man?!"

"A man I met a short while ago." I'm really not trying to torture them. I'm just afraid to tell them.

"Oy," Sophie says. "Say it already. This

is like having a mammogram from a nurse with icy fingers."

Evvie is flabbergasted. "How can you meet anybody? You're never out of my sight for a minute."

I grin impishly. "Well, obviously I was out of your sight for more than a minute. I met him the day Greta soaped my car and flattened my tire. When I went to that bookstore party near the garage."

"That was weeks ago. How come you didn't tell me?" Evvie is now indignant.

"I was going to, but then Greta got killed and it went right out of my mind."

"Oh. So it's a first date," says interrogator Evvie.

"Actually, a second."

Evvie is speechless. Ida picks up the grilling. "That slipped your mind, too?"

"Actually, I was mad at you guys then. You just had Greta cremated."

"That's no excuse!" Evvie says sharply.

"Excuses, excuses," singsongs Sophie.

"Yeah, you just didn't want to tell us," Ida says. "Why? Is he ugly?"

"Actually, he's very handsome and actually, he lives in Lanai Gardens and actually, you all know him."

"Enough with the actuallys already," says Ida. "So actually, what's his name already?"

I take a deep breath. "Jack Langford."

Click. Click. Click. Click. Four minds are data-processing.

"Phase Six," says Ida.

"His wife, Faye, passed a few years ago," remembers Sophie.

Evvie is stunned. "Langford? You said Langford?"

Bella claps her hands gleefully. "Morrie's father!"

"I can't believe you didn't tell me," Evvie says, unable to let it go.

"I guessed," Bella says proudly. "I saw them dancing last night. Making goo-goo eyes at each other." She giggles.

They turn to her, amazed.

"And you didn't say a word?" says Evvie, wanting to choke her.

Bella shrugs. "I forgot."

Ida glares at her.

"So, kill me," Bella says in a huff.

Sophie moves in closer to me, conspiratorially. "So, are you having an affair?"

"Sex?!" Ida spits out the loathsome word. "That's disgusting! You're too old!"

I can't take anymore. This is torture. "Well, girls, I'm removing the curlers. Five minutes and we go on our errands." With that I start to leave them in the dining room to stew.

As I pass them, I try to ignore their expressions. Bella grinning. Ida horrified. Sophie intrigued. And my beloved sister, just plain flummoxed.

Whew. I'm glad that's over.

This evening, as we drive away from the building in Jack's Cadillac, I look back to see the girls leaning over the third-floor balcony watching us. Boy, do I feel guilty.

"Don't look back," Jack says, smiling. "You'll turn into a pillar of salt."

"I knew we should have met at the Greek restaurant."

"No more Greek odysseys. We're out in the open now. Let the chips fall where they may. You only live once."

I poke him in the shoulder. "Any more clichés you want to throw at me?"

"Just testing to make sure you're paying attention."

"So now what do we do?" I move closer. His aftershave smells so good. He actually dressed in a suit and tie for me. Oh, my, it's been such a long time. He puts his arm around my shoulder.

"We negotiate."

"I'm not giving up my apartment."

"Who asked you to?"

"Maybe we'll only get together on week-ends."

"If that's what you really want."

"Don't ask me to give up my new profession. The phone is ringing off the hook with people needing private eyes."

"I have no problem with you supporting me."

"I'm not cooking."

"Fine. I'll cook."

"Ha-ha. You're English. No, thanks."

"I am a good cook. Ask Morrie."

"Right. And for breakfast you'll serve bangers and bacon and fried eggs and fried tomatoes and blood sausage. With enough cholesterol to kill a horse."

"Who needs breakfast? We're gonna live on love."

We are both laughing by now. He pulls over, turns off the ignition, takes me in his arms, and kisses me.

And inside my head I hear aha, aha, aha.

Acknowledgments

MY EVERLASTING THANKS
To the women of Hawaiian Gardens, who shared their laughter and their tears: Helen, Arlene, Eva & Snookie

IN MEMORIAM
Family at Hawaiian Gardens

My beloved dad, David, Aunt Rose and Uncle Hy, Aunt Bronia

THESE TWO I OWE REALLY BIG
Caitlin Alexander
Lynn Vannucci

THIS GANG I ALSO OWE
My sons, Howard and Gavin, and daughter-in-law, Leslie. Always on my side.

My wonderful grandchilden, Alison, Megan, James & Amara. For just being themselves.

Sister Judy and adopted sister Rose. Who

tried hard (and failed) to make a bingo player of me.

Margaret Sampson & the Women Who Walk On Water Book Club of Green Bay & Dykesville, Wisconsin. My first readers and supporters.

MY SPECIAL READERS —
FAMILY & FRIENDS
Ginger Leibovitz, Harriet Rochlin, Dick Katz, Doug Unger, Dolores Raimist, Jack & Ruth Kay, Guiamar Sandler, Adrienne Goldberg, Sandy Carp, Joan Cohen.

All characters, though inspired by knowing the women at Hawaiian Gardens, are fictitious. Fort Lauderdale is, of course, real, but I have changed many of the locations for the sake of plot. Continental Restaurant, everybody's all-time early-bird favorite, is closed, but it remains alive forever here.